FATHER'S DAY 1982

D0152620

THE
PHYSICIAN
IN
LITERATURE

THE PHYSICIAN IN LITERATURE

Edited,
with an Introduction by
NORMAN COUSINS

THE SAUNDERS PRESS
W. B. Saunders Company
Philadelphia • London • Toronto

The Saunders Press
W. B. Saunders Company
West Washington Square
Philadelphia, PA 19105

IN THE UNITED STATES
DISTRIBUTED TO THE TRADE BY
HOLT, RINEHART AND WINSTON
383 Madison Avenue
New York, New York 10017

IN CANADA
DISTRIBUTED BY
HOLT, RINEHART AND WINSTON
55 Horner Avenue
Toronto, Ontario
M8Z 4X6
Canada

THE PHYSICIAN IN LITERATURE

© 1982 by W. B. Saunders Company. Copyright under the Uniform Copyright Convention. Simultaneously published in Canada. All rights reserved. This book is protected by copyright. No part of it may be reproduced, stored in a retrieval system, or transmitted in any form or by any means, electronic, mechanical, photocopying, recording, or otherwise, without written permission from the publisher. Made in the United States of America.

Library of Congress Cataloging in Publication Data

Main entry under title:
   The Physician in Literature

   1. Medicine—Literary collections.
I. Cousins, Norman.   [DNLM: 1. Medicine in literature—Collected works.   WZ 330 P578]
PN6071.M38P5   808.8'35261   81-50841
                                     (WBS)   AACR2

W. B. Saunders Company ISBN: 0-7216-2739-0
Holt, Rinehart and Winston ISBN: 0-03-059653-X

Print Number 9 8 7 6 5 4 3 2 1

First Edition

The Editor and his publishers gratefully acknowledge permission to reprint the following:

An excerpt from MR. SAMMLER'S PLANET by Saul Bellow. Copyright © 1969, 1970 by Saul Bellow. Reprinted by permission of Viking Penguin Inc.

From ARROWSMITH by Sinclair Lewis. Copyright 1925 by Harcourt Brace Jovanovich, Inc.; renewed 1953 by Michael Lewis. Reprinted by permission of the publisher.

From SHOOTING AN ELEPHANT AND OTHER ESSAYS by George Orwell. Copyright 1950 by Sonia Brownell Orwell; renewed 1978 by Sonia Pitt-Rivers. Reprinted by permission of Harcourt Brace Jovanovich, Inc.

From MRS. DALLOWAY by Virginia Woolf. Copyright 1925 by Harcourt Brace Jovanovich, Inc.; renewed by Leonard Woolf. Reprinted by permission of the publishers.

From Dylan Thomas, THE DOCTOR AND THE DEVILS. Copyright © 1953 by Hedgerley Films, Ltd., 1966 by New Directions Publishing Corporation. Reprinted by permission of New Directions.

From Louis-Ferdinand Celine, JOURNEY TO THE END OF THE NIGHT, translated by John H. P. Marks. Copyright 1934 by Louis-Ferdinand Celine. Reprinted by permission of New Directions.

"The Use of Force" From William Carlos Williams, THE FARMERS' DAUGH-TERS. Copyright 1938 by William Carlos Williams. Reprinted by permission of New Directions.

"The Injury" From William Carlos Williams, COLLECTED LATER POEMS. Copyright 1948 by William Carlos Williams. Reprinted by permission of New Directions.

From MY YOUTH IN VIENNA by Arthur Schnitzler. Translated by Catherine Hutter. Copyright © 1968 by Verlag Fritz Molden, Vienna-Munich-Zurich. Copyright © 1970 by Holt, Rinehart and Winston. Reprinted by permission of Holt, Rinehart and Winston, Publishers.

From OUT OF MY LIFE AND THOUGHT by Albert Schweitzer. Translated by C. T. Campion. Copyright 1933, 1949, © 1961, 1977 by Holt, Rinehart and Winston. Reprinted by permission of Holt, Rinehart and Winston, Publishers.

Excerpt from MYSTERY, MAGIC AND MEDICINE by Howard W. Haggard, M.D. Copyright 1933 by Howard W. Haggard, M.D. Reprinted by permission of Doubleday & Company, Inc.

"Diabetes" From THE EYE-BEATERS, BLOOD, VICTORY, MADNESS, BUCKHEAD AND MERCY by James Dickey. Copyright © 1968, 1969, 1970 by James Dickey. Reprinted by permission of Doubleday & Company, Inc.

Excerpt From BACK TO METHUSELAH by George Bernard Shaw. Reprinted by permission of The Society of Authors on behalf of the Bernard Shaw Estate.

From F. Scott Fitzgerald, *Tender is the Night*. Copyright 1933, 1934 by Charles Scribner's Sons; copyright renewed 1961, 1962 by Frances Scott Fitzgerald Lanaham. Reprinted with the permission of Charles Scribner's Sons. From Ernest Hemingway, "Indian Camp" (Copyright 1925 by Charles Scribner's Sons; copyright renewed) From *The Short Stories of Ernest Hemingway*. Copyright 1938 by Ernest Hemingway; copyright renewed. Reprinted with the permission of Charles Scribner's Sons.

From OPIUM—THE DIARY OF A CURE by Jean Cocteau. Reprinted by permission of Grove Press, Inc., Copyright © 1958 by Grove Press, Inc.

Specified excerpts From MARK TWAIN'S AUTOBIOGRAPHY, Volume I by Mark Twain, edited by Albert Bigelow Paine. Copyright, 1924, by Clara Clemens Samossoud. Reprinted by permission of Harper & Row, Publishers, Inc.

From THE MAGIC MOUNTAIN, by Thomas Mann, translated by H. T. Lowe-Porter. Copyright 1927 and renewed 1955 by Alfred A. Knopf, Inc. Reprinted by permission of Alfred A. Knopf, Inc.

From THE PLAGUE, by Albert Camus, translated by Stuart Gilbert. Copyright 1948 by Stuart Gilbert. Reprinted by permission of Alfred A. Knopf, Inc.

"The Art of Healing" Copyright © 1969 by W. H. Auden. Reprinted from EPISTLE TO A GODSON, by W. H. Auden, by permission of Random House, Inc.

Excerpt from "The Interior Castle" from THE COLLECTED STORIES OF JEAN STAFFORD. Reprinted by permission of Farrar, Straus and Giroux, Inc. Copyright © 1946, 1969 by Jean Stafford. Copyright renewed © 1973 by Jean Stafford.

Dedication

To all the people who helped me with this book, beginning with my colleagues at the UCLA School of Medicine who went far out of their way to make me feel at home in a new setting—in particular, Dean Sherman Mellinkoff, L. Jolyon West, Carmine Clemente, Bernard Towers, William Winslade, and Milton Greenblatt. I am especially indebted to Dean Mellinkoff, who provided me with the opportunity to emphasize the place of literature and philosophy in the education of medical students.

Caroline Blattner and Eric Nath were my prime collaborators. Mrs. Blattner worked on the basic architecture of the book, helped in the preparation of the notes, did the proofreading, and presided over the multiple retypings. Mr. Nath helped to screen and assemble the basic materials. Shannon Jacobs assisted me in my early days at UCLA. Susan Schiefelbein, then Senior Editor of Saturday Review, *was involved in the early planning for the book and in bringing together the initial materials. John L. Dusseau, of the Saunders Publishing Company, drew upon his vast store of literary knowledge in drawing up the outline for the book. Howard E. Sandum, also of Saunders, is owed special thanks for his encouragement.*

This dedication would be incomplete without mention of Dr. Omar John Fareed, whose idea it was that my proper place in life was at a medical school, and Dr. Franklin D. Murphy, who initiated steps to bring it about.

CONTENTS

CLINICAL DESCRIPTIONS IN LITERATURE *183*

DOCTORS AND STUDENTS *207*

THE PRACTICE *271*

THE PATIENT

AN ENDURING TRADITION

INTRODUCTION

It should be no surprise that almost every novelist or dramatist of any consequence—from Aeschylus to Walker Percy—has had something to say about doctors. The writer deals with the universals of human experience—and the struggle not just to stay alive but to get the most out of life is at the epicenter of those universals.

To the writer, the physician is not just a prescriber of medicaments but a symbol of all that is transferable from one human to another short of immortality. We may not be able to live forever, but we persist in the notion that the physician possesses the science and the artistry that will provide us with endless deferrals. We cannot be persuaded, apparently, that the physician does not command all those fastnesses where the secrets of life are stored. To be able to listen to the human heart and draw meaning from its slightest vibrations or whispers, to be able to take a tiny droplet of blood and perceive its vital balances, to convert electric markings into precise knowledge of the body's chemical complexities—all these may represent science to the doctor, but to the patient they are powers that come from the gods.

Writers have not had to imagine the patient's condition. They know at first hand all the frailties and uncertainties and loneliness that the physician is expected to banish. For writers, all too often, have been deeply troubled patients themselves. They have a direct acquaintance with the doctor's little black bag and know the value of the physician's touch and the healing power of his presence.

Imagination and the art of writing go together. And, since imagination is the basic ingredient of hypochondria, writers have had little difficulty in suffering from all sorts of symptoms. Consider Proust, his windows shut and his blinds tightly drawn, seldom emerging from his flat, living in a habitat certain to intensify his ailments, only a few of which were organic, but all of which kindled his imagination. The greater the writer's uncertainty about his/her health, the greater the dependence on the physician. It is here that we observe an element of reverence in the attitude of many writers towards physicians—if not of their persons, then of their roles. For when the writer becomes a patient, his dependence on the physician is no less epic than it is with anyone else. Naturally, this leads to unreasonable expectations of the powers of the physician. Consider as evidence the way many writers describe the arrival of physicians at a critical time. The family is huddled in dreadful uncertainty around the bedside; but the presence of the physician produces a miraculous change of spirits. It is not always possible, of course, for the physician to bring about the looked-for miracles. This collision of hope and reality provides a good test of the writer's ability to deal with heightened emotions.

It is natural that writers, in dealing with ultimate confrontations, should find the doctor such a convenient literary resource. The physicians may vary widely in their personal and philosophical behavior, but they all offer rich material to the novelist. Voltaire writes dispassionately in *Candide* of the helplessness of physicians when confronted by venereal disease—a penalty attached to the deepest of pleasures. Alexander Pope takes such paradoxes in stride but also takes the view that the physician should not be expected to be kinder than God. Boris Pasternak, true to the Russian literary tradition, sees the physician as the embodiment of all the mixed emotions that the human tragi-comedy can produce. There is no standardization of attitudes or responses—nor can there be—but the physician never lets the writer down. The entire field of medicine offers infinite materials to the novelist.

Of all the Russian writers, perhaps none has exhibited greater fascination with the doctor than Tolstoy. He brings all his gifts of descriptive irony to the account of the physician who treats Ivan Ilych. The doctor is supreme, invulnerable, and possesses a confident claim on the future. The patient is dependent, tentative, and a sure loser. A somewhat similar perception of the physician emerges in Dostoevski's *Crime and Punishment*. The sufferings of the ill are far more memorably described than are manifestations of compassion by the physician. Even when the physician is in love with his patient, as in Turgenev's "The District Doctor," there is a perceptible distance in the relationship between the doctor and the object of his affections. Is this a reflection of the traditional reserve doctors are supposed to maintain in their relationship with patients? (Medical students will think of *Aequanimitas*, by Sir William Osler.) Or is it a manifestation of the eternal loneliness in the Russian soul, portrayed so powerfully by Gogol in "The Diary of a Madman"? What the Russian writers are trying to tell us, perhaps, is that human beings are never really able to shatter their loneliness and that physicians, whatever their magic, are capable only of limited rescues. This generality is not as morbid as it seems, for there is always the relieving and redeeming virtue of the interim triumph, the discovery that improvement and prolongation of life are the attainable prizes, and therefore can also be a sustaining reality.

In the English novel, the physician tends to be treated more as an institution than as a person. One thinks of Emily Brontë's description in *Wuthering Heights* of the physician whose professional detachment keeps him from becoming a vitally needed emotional resource for the patient. Not that the physician is callous; he is acting in the institutionalized way that doctors are supposed to act. The physician whose towering sense of authority leads him to make arbitrary decisions is seldom better described than in Wilkie Collins's *Moonstone*. Thomas Hardy's Dr. Fitzpiers in *The Woodlanders* seems to feel his special station entitles him to exploit the affections of the heroine. Samuel Butler's observations about the institution of the doctor may be no more satirical than those of his contemporaries, but there is no mistaking the underlying resentments that are sometimes part of the physician's quixotic attitudes towards his patients.

What about the physician's vaunted heroic role? In all cultures, this role is as real as it is substantial. If the demigod concept is resisted by a minority of novelists, it is not because writers are unmindful of the exalted station of the doctor, but because novelists are merchants of paradox and searchers after warts. Even when they are unabashedly idealistic, writers reveal in their work their conviction that reality is best portrayed through contradictions. And the physician's calling enables him to preside over lives in a way that is the envy of politicians and, indeed, of all those who by calling or temperament try to steer people. It is inevitable that physicians, who are supposed to possess life-and-death powers, should be so often idealized by most people and ascribed with virtues equal to their authority. But the novelist is careful not to ignore the juxtapositions and complexities of character that make the physician credible.

In any case, the writer's fascination with the physician has been a continuing characteristic of world literature—and the contemporary American novel is no exception. For example, Hemingway, both in his short stories and novels, makes use of his special knowledge as a doctor's son. The loneliness and despair of the ill people in his books are in stark contrast to the lofty estate of the physician. For the physician comes and goes at will, in contrast to the desperation and immobility of the patient. William Faulkner's doctors are perhaps more philosophical than are Hemingway's: they look not just at illness but at life. In the same vein, John Steinbeck's Dr. Burton, from *In Dubious Battle*, manifests a curiosity not just about the workings of the human body but about society; he is thereby justified in addressing himself to the interaction between the two. Even when Steinbeck's doctors are erratic and deeply flawed, as in *Cannery Row,* they remain the rallying points for a surrounding humanity. Walker Percy, himself a doctor, sees the tragic human weaknesses in doctors, especially in his *Love in the Ruins,* but he also sees a vital human spark inherent in the physician that touches off lifegiving energies and prospects. Ring Lardner, chronicler of picturesque character and speech, portrays the physician not just as a mediator with death but as a protector of those who are easily gulled or made to look ridiculous in the eyes of their fellows.

In the contemporary world novel, it is doubtful if any writer has imparted a more epic quality to the physician than Boris Pasternak. Dr. Zhivago learns and grows from the suffering he has seen—both at the home bedside or in the hospital room and on the battlefield. His experiences, far from making him indifferent to suffering, enlarge his sensitivity and his view of life even as they help connect him to the great events of his time.

From *Dr. Zhivago* we learn that the responsible physician is more than just a scientist able to make a difficult diagnosis; he is a human being whose skill depends as much on his knowledge of life as it does on his knowledge of disease. Proper treatment calls for an awareness of human uniqueness and for sensitivity to all the elements of human potentiality. Poetry cannot replace prescriptions but it can widen perceptions. What we learn from the world's great literature is that the best education for the physician is a blend of science and the liberal arts, which is to say, a knowledge of the elusive aspects of human uniqueness that are no less important than the medical and technical aids used by the physician in combatting disease.

For many years, the liberal arts have been downplayed in medical education. The assumption is made that undergraduate education will meet the rounded needs of a student and that, therefore, the graduate school can afford to concentrate on the particularized requirements that go with a professional career. But the assumption is unjustified. Undergraduate students who intend to go on to medical school tend to steer away from the liberal arts. They do so in the belief that their chances for admission to medical school are strengthened in direct proportion to their demonstrated excellence in the sciences. The result is that they put most of their scholastic energies into studies that deal with quantifiable matters. Hence they arrive at medical school in a state of educational disequilibrium. And, since medical schools are under increasing curriculum pressure to incorporate all advances in medical knowledge, they have little or no room for remedial education in the liberal arts.

The result is that many graduates are deprived of their rightful cultural heritage. This is not a minor deprivation. It affects the total ability of the physician to deal with the complex equation that is represented by an individual patient's illness. That illness is often the result not just of an encounter with a pathological organism but of a way of life. The physician must, therefore, construct a context for his scrutiny of the patient. He must be able to assess the possible role of the patient's full environment in contributing to the illness. In short, the wise physician understands the ease with which modern society transfers its malaises to the individual. He comprehends the variations of stress in modern family life and in relationships in general. He understands disappointment, rejection, blocked exits. He has an appreciation of what is required to make an individual whole again.

Literature helps the medical student to analogize the patient, to make connections between the experiences of the race and the condition of the individual, and to fit the individual into a world that is not as congenial as it ought to be for people who are more fragile than they ought to be.

Finally, what the world's great literature tells us about medicine is that few things are more important than the psychological management of the patient. Hippocrates and Galen and the other early greats of medicine may not have known about endorphins, encephalins, gamma gobulin, epine-phrine, interferon and the entire range of neuro-transmitters. But they knew a great deal about the totality of the human organism and the interaction of all its parts. Galen made the observation that, not infrequently, breast malignancies occurred in women who were suffering from melancholia. A person's outlook on life, especially one's attitude toward illness, can be a vital factor in the onset and course of a disease. The wise physician, when making a prognosis, does not confine himself or herself to the virulence of the particular micro-organism involved or the nature of an abnormal growth; the wise physician makes a careful estimate of the patient's will to live and the ability to put to work all the resources of spirit that can be translated into beneficial biochemical changes.

Few things are more encouraging about recent medical research than the information being developed about the wide array of secretions produced by the brain—secretions that have a role in maintaining health and overcoming illness. Richard Bergland, of the Harvard University School of Medicine, has resurrected the French view from a century or more ago that the human brain is not just the seat of consciousness but a gland; indeed, the most prolific gland in the human body. This fact is strengthened by the findings of Carmine Clemente, head of the Brain Research Institute of the

School of Medicine at the University of California, Los Angeles. Dr. Clemente has estimated that the number of secretions in the brain may exceed 1000. Not all these secretions are locked into the autonomic nervous system. A substantial number of them are activated by thought processes and by the emotions. It is not necessary, for example, to run a race in order to stimulate the production of epinephrine. Merely the contemplation of a challenge or a danger can cause the mind to trigger the production of chemical changes.

Writers such as Dickens, Hardy, Tolstoy, and Dostoevski subjected their various characters to recurrent strain. They would serialize their stories prior to publication in book form; each installment would end with an impending crisis in order to arouse interest in subsequent chapters. The extraordinary trials to which the fictional characters were subjected would have produced any number of cases of adrenal exhaustion in real life. Obviously, we don't need great novels to tell us that the ability of human beings to tolerate stress is incontestably finite. But those same novels help us to recognize that attitudes are vital factors in enabling people to meet serious problems, whether they take the form of illness or crises of circumstance.

A related value of fictional illnesses is that they tend to rescue us from exaggerated feelings of resentment towards medical anecdotes. Few trends in modern medicine are more conspicuous than the almost automatic rejection of anything that smacks of an anecdote. Almost automatically, anyone who has a medical incident to relate can expect someone in his audience to dismiss or downplay it because it is an "anecdote." Yet hostility to anecdotes can be badly overplayed. Distinctions need to be made. An account of what appears to be a remarkable cure in a single case has little standing. Any recommended new therapy must rest on a wide base of testing and experience. But even a single account of a patient-physician episode can be significant. Anything bearing on that relationship may have supreme educational value. It is translatable and transferable to general experience. When we read that a patient has gone into shock because of the physician's lack of artistry in conveying information, we cannot dismiss the account as "only an anecdote." It is all too easily replicated. We need no more than a single case as an example of what to avoid.

Writers are natural producers of anecdotes. This is what they are supposed to be. The anecdote is their stock in trade. We absorb these anecdotes and we learn from them. I now give a course in a medical school on the physician as perceived by the writer. Nothing is more interesting to me in that course than the willingness of students to take fictional anecdotes more seriously than they do examples from real life. Fortunately, by the end of the course, many of them come to recognize that even isolated incidents in human experiences can be repeated and are therefore significant. The novelist, by dealing with individual occurrences, helps to protect medical students from the overworked tendency to think statistically.

Oliver Wendell Holmes, one of America's most distinguished physicians and philosophers of medicine, once proposed some perennial questions for doctors:

How does your knowledge stand today?
What must you expect to forget?
What remains for you to learn?

Winds of change now blow throughout American medicine, and one of the most promising zephyrs is the growing recognition that a good medical education involves more than science. The questions Dr. Holmes proposed are essentially philosophical, for they cannot be answered without reference to the history of man's intellectual and scientific development, without relating one's learning and occupation to the needs of the society, without retrospective and prospective compass points. In short, they cannot be adequately answered without some exposure to the cluster of intellectual disciplines that come under the heading of the humanities, by which is meant not just the general range of human experience but the creative arts and the way people come to terms with life.

Science puts its emphasis on research and verifiable fact; art and philosophy put the emphasis on creativity and values—values that come out of the memory of the race and that have something to do with the importance of being human, values that are conscious respecters of the unknown factors in the human equation. Among the recent discoveries in the practice of medicine is the fact that human beings come equipped with resources for healing that are best mobilized not by detached scientific efficiency, but by communication and supportive human outreach.

BASIC to any education is one unchanging fact—that is, that facts do not stand still. A great deal of what medical students are now learning in their formal scientific education will become outdated within a decade or two after graduation. It is obviously and remorselessly true that the factual base of medicine has steadily changed in response to new findings about the nature of disease and the treatment of disease.

What endures, too, is the system for teaching scientific knowledge even if the knowledge itself tends to be fragile. I refer to the scientific method. The *way* new facts are discovered and developed; the *way* these facts are scrutinized and put to the test; in short, the *way* theory is translated into practice—this is what endures and what gives science its essential character. Respect for the scientific method is a vital ingredient in any medical education.

There is no conflict between the scientific method and the need in the medical curriculum for subjects that deal with human values. Values constitute a moral system that transcends change. When values are strong enough and good enough, changes in science can be fitted into the lives of people, making it unnecessary to fit people into change. The way people are dealt with as patients can be as important as all the other treatments they receive in the attempt to ease or cure their ills. That is, the effectiveness of the doctor as scientist is tied to his or her qualifications as artist and philosopher—to those intangible credentials that have to do with character and personal dimensions.

The separate paths that the sciences and humanities have taken in search of truth are now converging in the wake of new findings. Human survival may depend upon man's ability to work within nature rather than in opposition to it—as well as upon the ability to control the proliferation of knowledge that threatens to overwhelm us. The convergence is bringing about a new unity that cuts across disciplines. We are seeing a new breed of scientific humanists and humanistic scientists. The separation of the two intellectual worlds is giving way to a realization that they are both dependent on the conditions of creativity and on the need to accept responsibility for their work. The trend has been moving away from scientists who make public proclamations about the morally antiseptic nature of their calling and who detach themselves from the effects of their theories and discoveries. By contrast, more and more scientists insist that they are in a better position to understand the significance and implications for society of their discoveries than are the official decision-makers who may be paying their salaries or subsidizing their work. And, just as scientists are divided, so humanists are split on issues of human values. The point is that the real division is no longer between the two cultures described by C. P. Snow but between those who attach primary importance to human life and those who view their own discipline as sovereign.

The explosive proliferation of scientific knowledge in the past few decades has left knowledgeable members of the human species feeling unsettled, uncertain, even out of control. Young people have good reason to question the adequacy of an education that has separated them from the questions that bear upon their own future, the future of mankind, and the quality of life—which, incidentally, has a bearing on health.

Common to the sciences and the humanities is the human urge to understand the universe and man's connection to it. The failures that have pockmarked history have come at times of philosophical poverty. Man may enlarge his objective techniques and even his knowledge, but he cannot change the basic fact that his position in contemplating the great questions is inherently subjective.

The science and art of medicine converge at the point where physicians become basically concerned—as traditionally poets have been—with the whole of the human condition. "I feel convinced," wrote Claude Bernard, "that there will come a day when physiologists, poets, and philosophers will all speak the same language."

The editor hopes that this book, by providing a wide cross-section of the physician in literature, may also illuminate the expectations of the patient—expectations that may seem unreasonably large at times but that are inevitable in any situation that calls for healing.

The editor is fully aware that dozens of compelling pieces from the world's literature are not included in this book. In acknowledging this fact of conspicuous omissions, I plead personal preference and the hope that, if this volume serves a useful purpose, another work of similar nature may be possible.

NORMAN COUSINS

THE
PHYSICIAN
IN
LITERATURE

RESEARCH AND SERENDIPITY

The best research laboratory is a serendipitous arena—a place where unplanned but significant things can happen. Most people have yet to understand that research cannot be expected to go forward in a straight line from theory to materialization. Creative research is full of detours, and those who have their eyes fixed only on a clearly defined objective may miss important signs along the way. Edward Jenner, with his findings on smallpox; Sir Alexander Fleming, with his observations on penicillin moulds; and Ignaz Philipp Semmelweiss, with his astute observations of the causes of puerperal fever, have demonstrated, each in his own way, the fact that the powers of observation may represent the most important ingredient in "luck." The imaginative researcher must be prepared to spot and pounce upon happy surprises. The ideas in this chapter speak to those surprises.

SIR FRANCIS BACON
Advancement of Learning

SIR FRANCIS BACON (1561-1626) in his *Novum Organum* replaced the logic and philosophy of the Greeks with inductive reasoning, establishing the modern scientific method. Bacon was a scientist, philosopher, politician, and historian who was as interested in the phenomenon of the total human being as he was in the possibilities of thought. He felt that learning should always be dynamic and opposed the tendency of scholars to convert respect for Aristotle into a form of worship. If scholars are lucky, he believed, their work will be critically examined and eventually replaced by other theories.

And Celsus acknowledgeth it gravely, speaking of the empirical and dogmatical sects of physicians, *That medicines and cures were first found out, and then after the reasons and causes were discoursed; and not the causes first found out, and by light from them the medicines and cures discovered.* And Plato in his Theætetus noteth well, That particulars are infinite, and the higher generalities give no sufficient direction; and that the pith of all sciences, which maketh the arts-man differ from the inexpert, is in the middle propositions, which in every particular knowledge are taken from tradition and experience. And therefore we see that they which discourse of the inventions and originals of things, refer them rather to chance than to art, and rather to beasts, birds, fishes, serpents, than to men.

WALTER B. CANNON
The Way of an Investigator

———◄◇►———

WALTER B. CANNON (1871-1945), professor at Harvard Medical School, is one of the great names in twentieth century American medicine. He was as much a man of letters as he was a man of medicine. He pioneered in the concept of homeostasis and in the study of the effects of emotions on the body's chemistry. Medical students who read *The Way of an Investigator* in full may wish to read his *Wisdom of the Body,* which reflected Cannon's characteristic respect for the wonder and mystery of human life.

In 1754 Horace Walpole, in a chatty letter to his friend Horace Mann, proposed adding a new word to our vocabulary, "serendipity." The word looks as if it might be of Latin origin. It is rarely used. It is not found in the abridged dictionaries. When I mentioned serendipity to one of my acquaintances and asked him if he could guess the meaning, he suggested that it probably designated a mental state combining serenity and stupidity—an ingenious guess, but erroneous.

Walpole's proposal was based upon his reading of a fairy tale entitled *The Three Princes of Serendip.* Serendip, I may interject, was the ancient name of Ceylon. "As their highnesses traveled," so Walpole wrote, "they were always making discoveries, by *accident* or *sagacity,* of things which they were not in quest of." When the word is mentioned in dictionaries, therefore, it is said to designate the happy faculty, or luck, of finding unforeseen evidence of one's ideas or, with surprise, coming upon new objects or relations which were not being sought.

Readers who remember Bible stories will recall that Saul, the son of Kish, was set forth to find his father's asses, which were lost. In the discouragement of his failures to find them he consulted one, Samuel, a seer. And Samuel told him not to set his mind on them for they had been found, but to know that he was chosen to rule over all the tribes of Israel. So it was announced, and the people shouted their approval. Thus modest Saul, who went out to seek lost asses, was rewarded by a kingdom. That is the earliest record of serendipity I am aware of.

Probably the most astounding instance of accidental discovery in either

4

ancient or modern history was the finding of the western hemisphere by Columbus. He sailed away from Spain firm in the faith that by going west he would learn a shorter route to the East Indies; quite unexpectedly he encountered a whole new world. It is noteworthy that he was not aware of the significance of what he had found. Indeed, it has been said that he did not know where, in fact, he was going nor where he was when he arrived nor where he had been after his return, but nevertheless he had had the most unique adventure of all time. He realized that he had had a remarkable experience and, by extending the knowledge of what he had done, he laid a course which others might follow. Such consequences have been common when accident has been favorable to one engaged in a search and the enterprise has proved fruitful.

In the records of scientific investigation this sort of happy use of good fortune has been conspicuous. A good example is afforded by the origin and development of our acquaintance with electrical phenomena. It is reported that some frogs' legs were hanging by a copper wire from an iron balustrade in the *Galvani* home in Bologna; they were seen to twitch when they were swung by the wind and happened to touch the iron. Whether the twitching was first noted by Luigi Galvani, the anatomist and physiologist, or by Lucia Galvani, his talented wife, is not clear. Certainly that fortuitous occurrence late in the eighteenth century was not neglected, for it started many researches which have preserved the Galvani name in the terms "galvanize" and "galvanism." And it also led to experiments by his contemporary, Volta, on the production of electric currents by contact of two dissimilar metals—and thus to the invention of the electric battery—experiments so fundamentally important that Volta's name is retained in the daily use of the words "volt" and "voltage."

Such were the accidental beginnings of the telegraph and indirectly of the telephone, radiobroadcasting, and the promise of practical television. And such also were the beginnings of our knowledge of animal electricity. We now use it, for example, to indicate the disordered state of the heart, because every cardiac contraction sends forth through our bodies an electrical wave, a wave that has a different shape according to the damage in the heart muscle. Only recently have we begun to employ animal electricity to give us information about conditions in the brain. That marvelous organ composed of many billions of nerve cells can display rhythmic electrical pulsations and, when extremely delicate instruments are applied to the scalp, they can reveal the different types of pulsations in rest and activity and the modification in some states of disease.

Even in the growth of electrical science, serendipity has played important roles. It was by pure chance that the mysterious relation between electricity and magnetism was discovered. At the end of a lecture the Danish physicist, Oersted, happened to bring a wire, which was conducting a strong current, to a position above and parallel to a poised magnetic needle. Previously, and by intent, he had held the wire perpendicularly above the needle but nothing happened; now, however, when the wire was held horizontally over and along the needle's length, he was astonished to note that without any visible connection the needle swung around until it was almost at right angles to its former position. With quick insight he reversed the current in the wire and found that the needle then deviated in just the opposite way. Later, Faraday not only confirmed the report that an electric current in a wire can move a magnet but also demonstrated that a moving magnet can cause a current to appear in a wire. From these trifling and casual happenings has gradually evolved our vast modern electrical industry with its immense generators and its ingenious arrangements for distributing extensively over great areas the power which provides us with many highly prized conveniences—light in dark places, a cool breeze on a summer day, heat for our morning toast, refrigeration for perishable food, sparks in motor cylinders, the automatic management of complex machines, safety at sea, and multitudes of devices helpful in our daily lives. When we consider the prodigious and intricate involvement of electricity in the affairs of mankind throughout the world, Galvani's frogs' legs may be regarded as almost equal in historical importance to the caravels of Columbus.

In the biological sciences serendipity has been quite as consequential as in the physical sciences. Claude Bernard, for example, had the idea that the impulses which pass along nerve fibers set up chemical changes producing heat. In an experiment performed about the middle of the last century he measured the temperature of a rabbit's ear and then severed a nerve which delivers impulses to that structure expecting, in accordance with his theory, that the ear deprived of nerve impulses would be cooler than its mate on the other side. To his great surprise it was considerably warmer! Without at first knowing the import of what he had done, he had disconnected the blood vessels of the ear from the nervous influences that normally hold them moderately contracted; thereupon the warm blood from internal organs was flushed through the expanded vessels in a faster flow and the ear temperature rose. Thus by accident appeared the first intimation that the passage of blood into different parts of the body is under the government of nerves—one of the most significant advances in our knowledge of the circulation since Harvey's proof, early in the seventeenth century, that the blood does indeed circulate in the vessels.

Another striking instance of accidental discovery has been described by the French physiologist, Charles Richet, a Nobel laureate. It was concerned with a peculiar sensitiveness toward certain substances—such as white of egg, strawberries, ragweed pollen and numerous others—that we now speak of as *anaphylaxis* or *allergy*. This may result from an initial exposure to the substance which later becomes poisonous to the victim. The phenomenon had been noticed incidentally before Richet's studies, but because it did not receive attention its characteristics were virtually unknown. In his charming little book *Le Savant*, he has told the story of how quite unexpectedly he happened upon the curious fact. He was testing an extract of the tentacles of a sea anemone on laboratory animals in order to learn the toxic dose. When animals which had readily survived that dose were given after a lapse of some time a much smaller dose (as little as one-tenth), he was astounded to find that it was promptly fatal. Richet declares that at first he had great difficulty in believing the result could be due to anything *he* had done. Indeed, he testified that it was in spite of himself that he discovered induced sensitization. He would never have dreamt that it was possible.

Pasteur was led by chance to his method of immunization. One day an old and forgotten bacterial culture was being used for inoculating fowls. The fowls became ill but did not die. This happening was illuminative. Possibly by first using cultures that had little virulence and then repeating the injections with cultures of greater virulence, the animals could be made to develop resistance to infection gradually. His surmise proved correct. By this procedure, as readers of his dramatic biography will remember, he was able to immunize sheep against anthrax and human beings against rabies.

It was an accidental observation which ultimately resulted in the discovery of insulin and the restoration of effective living of tens of thousands of sufferers from diabetes. In the late eighties of the last century, von Mering and Minkowski were studying the functions of the pancreas in digestion. While attempting to secure more evidence they removed that organ from a number of dogs. By good luck a laboratory assistant noticed that swarms of flies gathered round the urine of these animals, a fact which he mentioned to the investigators. When the urine was analyzed, it was found to be loaded with sugar. Thus for the first time experimental diabetes was produced, and the earliest glimpse was given into a possible cause of that disease. We now know that small islands of cells in the pancreas produce an internal secretion which exerts control over the use of sugar in the organism. And we know that when these islands are removed or damaged, sugar metabolism is deranged. An extract from the island cells provides the diabetic sufferer with the insulin he needs.

An unforeseen contingency may occasion scientific advances because of the serious problem it presents. A striking instance is afforded in the use of polished rice. There was no reason to anticipate that the polishing of rice would be harmful to those who depended upon it as a food. Yet removal of the covering from the kernels produced in myriads of victims the disease, beriberi, resulting in immeasurable sorrow and distress. As has been pointed out, however, the study of beriberi, thus unwittingly induced, disclosed not only the cause of that disorder but also started explorations in the whole realm of deficiency diseases and thus led to the discovery of some of the most intimate secrets of cellular processes.

A recent instance of serendipity was the finding of vitamin K, lack of which deprives the blood of an essential element for its coagulation. The Danish investigator, Dam, and his collaborators were working on chemical changes in a certain fatty substance in chicks. They noted that the animals on a special restricted diet often suffered from extensive internal hemorrhages. When the diet was changed to seeds and salts, the bleeding failed to occur. By critical tests the abnormal condition was proved to be due not to lack of any previously known vitamin but to lack of a specific agent contained in the liver fat of swine as well as in certain vegetables and in many cereals. This agent, vitamin K, has proved to be important in surgery. For example, patients afflicted with jaundice, owing to an obstruction in the bile duct, can be relieved by operation; unfortunately in jaundice, however, blood clots very slowly; an operation, therefore, may be attended by disastrous bleeding. This danger can now be readily obviated by feeding vitamin K (with bile salts), for it restores to an effective concentration the deficient element of the clotting process, a benefaction which has come to human beings from a chance observation on chicks.

In the life of an investigator whose researches range extensively, advantages from happy chance are almost certain to be encountered. During nearly five decades of scientific experimenting instances of serendipity have several times been my good fortune. Two experiences I mention elsewhere, but not in relation to serendipity. One was stoppage of the movements of the stomach and intestines in times of anxiety. The other was the strange faster beating of the heart, after all its governing nerves were severed, if the animal became excited or if sympathetic fibers were stimulated in some remote region of the body. This effect, due to an agent carried to the heart by the circulating blood, led to the discovery of *sympathin*. Both phenomena were quite unexpected. Proof that the stoppage of digestive movements was due to emotion was the beginning of many years of research on the influence of fear and rage on bodily functions. And the unraveling of the mystery of sympathin led ultimately to prolonged studies on the chemical mediator that serves to transmit influences from nerve endings to the organs they control.

There are many other examples of serendipity which I might detail; among them Nobel's invention of dynamite, Perkins's stumbling upon the coal-tar dyes, and Pasteur's finding that a vegetable mold causes the watery solution in which it is nurtured to change the direction of the light rays as they pass through. Dynamite placed gigantic powers in the hands of man; the coal-tar dyes have fundamentally affected such varied activities as warfare, textile industries, and medical diagnosis; and Pasteur's casual observation has developed into an immense range of chemical theory and research.

Three legends of accidental leads to fresh insight serve to introduce the next point, which is quite as important as serendipity itself. I refer to the presence of a prepared mind. It is said that the idea of specific gravity came to Archimedes as he noted by chance the buoyancy of his body in water. We have all heard the tale, illustrative even if not authentic, that the concept of a universal law of gravitational force occurred to Isaac Newton when he saw an apple fall from a tree while he lay musing on the grass in an orchard. Of similar import is the story that the possibility of the steam engine suddenly occurred to James Watt when he beheld the periodic lifting of the lid of a tea kettle by the steam pressure within it. Many a man floated in water before Archimedes; apples fell from trees as long ago as the Garden of Eden (exact date uncertain!); and the outrush of steam against resistance could have been noted at any time since the discovery of fire and its use under a covered pot of water. In all three cases it was eons before the significance of these events was perceived. Obviously a chance discovery involves both the phenomenon to be observed and the appreciative, intelligent observer.

I may now add to these legends and their illustrative significance the history of that marvelously powerful enemy of infection, penicillin. In 1929 the English bacteriologist, Alexander Fleming, reported noticing that a culture of pus-producing bacteria underwent dissolution in the neighborhood of a mold which accidentally contaminated it. This was the pregnant hint. A careless worker might have thrown the culture away because of the contamination. Instead, Fleming let the mold grow in broth and thus learned that there passed into the broth from the mold a substance which was highly efficacious in stopping the growth of a wide range of disease-producing germs and destroying them. Furthermore he learned that, when injected, this substance was not itself harmful to animals. The mold, a variety of Penicillium, suggested the name "penicillin." The long struggle of Howard Florey and his associates at Oxford in purifying and standardizing this highly potent agent and in proving its value in human cases cannot be recounted here. The record, however, reports one of the most striking instances of immense value that can result from a combination of chance and an alert intelligence; and shows how a brilliant discovery is made practical by hard labor.

Long ago Pasteur recognized that when accident favors an investigator it must be met by sharp insight, for he uttered the wise and discerning dictum, "*Dans les champs de l'observation, le hasard ne favorise que les espirits preparés.*" Even before Pasteur, Joseph Henry, the American physicist, enunciated the same truth when he said, "The seeds of great discoveries are constantly floating around us, but they only take root in minds well prepared to receive them."

In the course of human living no one can tell what new circumstances may arise, nor can one predict the moment of their arrival. Tomorrow opportunities may appear the seizure of which or the neglect of which may have long-lasting and fateful consequences. There is a tide in the affairs of all of us, whether investigators or not, which "taken at its flood leads on to fortune," and not taken, may lead on to failure or misfortune. In other words, the unexpected is frequently happening in our ordinary lives, much as it happens in the realm of exploration and scientific research. Chance throws peculiar conditions in our way and, if we have intelligent and acute vision, we see their importance and use the opportunity chance provides.

If we are to benefit by opportunities for securing fresh insight and for enlarging our experiences in untried directions we must be well equipped with knowledge of the past. Only when we know what has been done by earlier contributors can we judge the present scene. We can then bring to bear, in unanticipated circumstances, the memories of bygone events. A historical reference in a speech or in literature or a name in a poem is enriched with a wider fringe of meaning if we embellish it with associations from our own store of knowledge. "In Xanadu did Kubla Khan a stately pleasure-dome decree" are words which do not demand information in order to appreciate their musical beauty, but if we know the story of Kubla Khan as the poet knew it and are acquainted with Oriental magnificence, the words have an extensive and peculiar significance. Furthermore, when the mind has been abundantly prepared, there is always the favorable possibility of continuing enrichment as we grow older. We bring to the reading of literature or history, to the unpredictable incidents of travel, to the illuminating moments of conversation, and to the varied adventures of the passing years, a substantial basis on which can be gradually developed manifold interests and pleasurable relations with our fellows and our surroundings.

Another implication in Pasteur's dictum that chance favors the prepared mind is the importance of avoiding rigid adherence to fixed ideas. It is quite natural for the unenterprising intelligence to find a comfortable security and serenity in a set of conventional opinions which have been satisfactorily prearranged. The unusual is promptly dismissed because it does not fit into the established plan. To persons who live according to pattern, adventures in ideas are impossible. Actually we dwell in a world which is not settled, not stationary, not finally immobilized. It presents all manner of possibilities of novel and unprecedented combinations and readjustments. Consequently, wisdom counsels keeping our minds open and recipient, hospitable to new views and fresh advances. We err if we dismiss the extraordinary aspects of experience as unworthy of attention; they may be the little beginnings of trails leading to unexplored heights of human progress. In a world organization which is in flux, in an anxious society groping its way possibly to new forms should we close our eyes and refuse attention? The solutions may arrive quite unheralded. Unless we are willing to weigh novel ideas and methods on their merits and to judge them justly, we may not be participants in momentous decisions, but instead may be worried and unhappy bystanders.

Most of my illustrations of serendipity have been drawn from the physical and biological sciences. In political, economic, and social affairs, likewise, important and pressing questions are calling for responses. A better world for all of us will be ours when these questions are answered. Many new discoveries are needed in order that these questions may be answered. How can we find ways to achieve more perfect justice among men? How can there be a fairer distribution of the abundance agriculture and industry can produce? What conditions can be devised that will promote good health and effective medical care? How can we be freed from the distress caused by great oscillations between financial booms and depressions? What can be done to reduce crime and the number of criminals, to stabilize family life, and to avoid or rectify numerous other maladjustments? Discoveries that will yield deeper insight into modes of resolving these urgent, difficult and apparently baffling social problems are likely to be made by minds characterized by learning and by liberality, ready to take prompt advantage of fortunate events which, amid extremely complex situations, are sure to appear. Quite unforeseen possibilities will unexpectedly spring forth, chances of serendipity which the sagacious can utilize.

HOWARD W. HAGGARD
Mystery, Magic and Medicine

————◦❀◦————

HOWARD W. HAGGARD (1891-1959) was the Director of the Laboratory of Applied Physiology at Yale and editor of the *Quarterly Journal of Studies on Alcoholism*. In *Mystery, Magic and Medicine* he laments the digression from scientific medicine after Hippocrates.

Scientific Medicine Is Born–and Dies

It was among the ancient Greeks that the earliest principles of scientific medicine were formulated. And it was among the ancient Greeks that the first complete separation of religion and medicine took place. It was they who first removed mystery from medicine and made it a practice, not of magic, not of religion, but of common sense and observation and logical deduction. This step was perhaps the most important one that has ever occurred in the whole long history of medicine. But it was a step forward in medical progress that was not maintained, for, as we shall see, altho for a brief period the Greeks gave medicine the dignity of a science, it was not held at this level. After the decline of Greece it again sank into the depths of mystery and magic, from which only after the lapse of centuries was it rescued, revived as a science, and finally nurtured into the medicine of today—a medicine which is giving the people of the world the healthiest period that man has ever known.

It is sometimes difficult for us who live in this period to comprehend the extreme hazards of life that existed in bygone days. The medicine of savage peoples did little to prolong life or alleviate suffering other than thru its influence upon the mind. This same statement applies in great measure to the medicine of Grecian days and to that of medieval times. At as late a period as four hundred years ago the average length of life was only eight years; today it is fifty-eight years. Behind those bare figures for the short length of life in bygone days is a tragic story of suffering, sorrow, and untimely death. They were the hazards of life borne in resignation by mankind, from which medical science, particularly in the last seventy-five years, has spared us. One can well give credence to the statement, then, that medical science is the strongest force acting in modern civilization toward human betterment. Modern civilization, as we shall see, is built upon, only made possible by, modern medical science.

And the germ of this science which after centuries was to develop into such a beneficent growth was formed in the days of Grecian civilization—twenty-three hundred years ago. The man who gave us the beginning of science in medicine was a Greek named Hippocrates. Probably no character in all history has thru a single principle exerted so great an influence upon civilization, upon the conditions of humans, as did he whom we revere as the father of modern medicine. Hippocrates separated medicine from mystery and from religion. From his day onward mystery, magic, and medicine cease to be the entire theme of these pages, for he gave us science and medicine.

In the days prior to the work of Hippocrates Grecian medicine was in the hands of a religious organization, the priests of Aesculapius, the deified Grecian hero of medicine. The marble temples dedicated to this God were on the country hillsides, overlooking the blue Aegean. Olive groves and columned porticoes made them beautiful sanatoria. Beyond the entry of each was a statue of Aesculapius, represented as a bearded man of kindly mien holding a staff about which twined a snake—the caduceus, the emblem of the physician even to this day. Beside him were representations of his daughters, Hygieia and Panacea.

The ill applied for admission to these temples. They slept before the statue of the God. In their dreams he and his daughters were supposed to minister with divine healing to the worshippers. The following day the priests would administer such simple medicaments as their knowledge provided, perform crude surgical operations, and prescribe baths and diet. Good and rational medical attention you would say? Seemingly so, but here was its great drawback. These healing priests assumed no responsibility. The Gods, so they said, brought disease; the Gods and only the Gods could relieve it. The priests could intercede for divine aid, but they had no incentive to seek the cause of disease or to search for means for cure and prevention. Under such a system of medicine no progress could be made; for all its dignified and beautiful surroundings the ancient Grecian medicine was, in principle at least, no better than that of early savage men. The will of deified heroes had come in to replace the malign influences of spirits; but the change indicated progress of religion, not of medicine.

It was Hippocrates who brought about a drastic reform in this temple cult of healing, and his great accomplishment was to relieve the gods of their responsibility for the prevention and the treatment of disease and to place that responsibility where it belonged—squarely upon the shoulders of man.

Hippocrates separated medicine from religion. And then for this now for-the-first-time independent field he supplied a philosophy and an ethics that were destined to be the great guiding influences of future medicine. Hippocrates did not create the medical knowledge of his time; the Egyptians long before the Greeks had observed symptoms and had found some practical remedies. The medical knowledge of isolated facts recorded upon their stone tablets often seems fully as great as that which Hippocrates possessed. No doubt it was. But here is the great difference. Hippocrates took these isolated facts, this empirical knowledge, and coördinated it; he made it into a flexible science. Other men had observed the symptoms of disease, but it was Hippocrates who first sat beside his patients and painstakingly sought out symptoms and recorded them; and these symptoms were to him not an end in themselves but indications of an underlying condition, a struggle between the patient and the disease which affected him. He took clinical case histories. He founded the bedside method which was to become the distinctive attribute of all great physicians. Having recorded the symptoms of his patients, Hippocrates after wide experience was able to define and classify diseases. Thus he founded the art of diagnosis and prognosis. But throughout all his work his attention was centered upon the patient, not merely upon his symptoms; he dealt with the man as well as with the disease. He kept in his practice the balanced relation between science and art which was to be the distinguishing quality of all great clinicians in all ages.

The descriptions of diseases left by Hippocrates were based on keen and careful observation; they stand today as models of their kind. After his time such accurate observations were not again made in medicine for over eighteen hundred years.

Hippocrates attempted to turn medical thought away from mere speculation toward accurate observation and common sense. He said, ''To know is one thing; merely to believe one knows is another. To know is science, but merely to believe one knows is ignorance.'' It was a difficult path that he pointed out for medicine to follow, one that involved intellectual honesty. Only the highest types of men have the intelligence, the independence, the integrity, and the courage to admit their errors and seek without bias after the truth. Such are they who have given us modern medicine.

But in the years between the days of Hippocrates—the very peak of ancient Grecian culture—and the rise of the modern period, civilization was to decline and with it medicine. Within a century after Hippocrates the decline was already in evidence. Speculation, dogmatization entered the field of medicine to displace observation and clear reasoning. Rival schools sprang into existence; and the men of these schools were more interested in making converts to their dogmas than they were in carrying on unsullied the great principles that Hippocrates had defined.

Three hundred years after Hippocrates, Corinth, the "light of Greece," was destroyed by Roman armies, and Grecian medicine was taken into Rome. At that time the Roman medicine was like that of the Greeks prior to Hippocrates, a matter of the will of the Gods. Grecian medicine displaced the Roman religious medicine, but it was already a deteriorated practice, rapidly losing the impetus given to it by the Father of Medicine.

Once only among the Romans was medicine raised to nearly the dignity that Hippocrates had given it. In the period covered by the century before and the century after the beginning of the Christian Era, medicine made progress in the hands of such men as Celsus, Dioscorides, Aretaeus, and Galen. It is probable that Celsus was not a physician but instead a wealthy patron of science and literature. He compiled in an encyclopedic manner the medical knowledge of his time. And centuries later in the period of the Renaissance his works were among the first medical books to be printed; they were selected largely because of his elegant literary style.

Dioscorides, a Greek army surgeon in the service of the Emperor Nero, owes his fame to the fact that he originated the *Materia Medica*. During his travels with the army he studied the medicinal herbs of the countries thru which he passed; he described more than 600 plants and plant substances, some 90 of which are still in use today. He recorded as an anesthetic for surgical operations the mandragora wine, which was to become famous in medieval medicine. The *Materia Medica* of Dioscorides was to remain the authoritative work on this subject up to the 17th century.

The next great physician of the Roman period was Aretaeus. Like Hippocrates he was essentially a clinical observer, and it is to him that we owe classical accounts of pneumonia, tetanus, emphysema, the aura of epilepsy, and the earliest accurate accounts of insanity.

It was Galen, the last of the great physicians of the Roman period, who was destined for centuries to influence medicine more than any other man. Indeed the period from his time until the 17th century is essentially one of Galenic domination in medicine; the period from the 17th century onward is the revival of Hippocratic medicine.

Galen was unquestionably the most skilled physician of his time, but his lasting fame rests on the fact that he performed experiments to demonstrate the facts of physiology. He essentially formulated the experimental method, which after his time was to lie dormant until the 17th century, when it was revived in the momentous work of Harvey in the demonstration of the circulation of the blood.

Galen was a great physician, but he lacked the intellectual honesty and breadth of vision that Hippocrates had possessed. Hippocrates opened the wide road of medical advancement; Galen closed it, and it remained so closed for nearly 14 centuries. Galen was a theorist; he had an answer for every question, an explanation for every phenomenon. Although his logic was good, his premises were often bad. But it was his logic, his dogmatism, that appealed so strongly to the men of subsequent centuries. His works, rather than those of Hippocrates, were to become the guiding influence, the final authority in all medical matters, until, in fact, it was to become almost a heresy to doubt Galen.

Galen in his therapy inclined strongly to medicaments made up of many vegetable ingredients. His poly-pharmacy in herb doctoring became the much fought over "Galenical system" of the Middle Ages and the Renaissance.

We have mentioned the outstanding men of Roman medicine but not the outstanding contribution of the period: that was sanitation. The Grecian cities were small and remained small because no provision was made for sanitation. In Rome the streets were paved; sewers and aqueducts were built. Clean streets, pure water, and sewage disposal, three of the main assets of public health, had their first practical application. And this practice, which was destined to be revived centuries later and to influence profoundly the 19th and 20th centuries, fell into disuse after the Roman days. Even in Galen's time the empire was declining. Many causes have been given for this decline—social, political, economic—but there was also a medical one, for in these centuries the enervating and deadly malaria had gained a foothold in Italy. Under its influence the people deteriorated. Plagues and pestilences increased in prevalence. Rome fell to the barbarians. But before it fell, medicine had deteriorated; vendors of quack remedies had their shops on the streets; the calling of the physician passed into the hands of professional poisoners, and courtesans who peddled drugs. Medicine ceased to be a science. It again became mystery and magic.

The Contribution of the Orient

After Rome's fall such medical practice as prevailed was essentially in the hands of priests; it was the period of Monastic medicine. For us, in a day when literacy is the common heritage of all civilized men, it is difficult to visualize the social situation that prevailed, to visualize Western Europe with a population in which only the priests could read and write, in which the common man was little better than a slave. It was not that these people had become a degenerated stock; from their progeny centuries later the great medical leaders were to develop and the great scientists who were literally to revolutionize the world in which we live. What was lacking in the Middle Ages was inspiration, the free spirit of aggressive advancement that had given Greece its great intellectual leaders and Rome its martial triumphs.

The Middle Ages represent probably the greatest experimental demonstration of the influence of environment in shaping the characters of men. And this environment was one of submission to recognized authority— unquestioning submission to Church and Feudal Lord preached and exemplified before the child from birth. Potential genius was suppressed or directed into channels barren of practical results.

Now in these years, while the people of Western Europe are living in their walled cities, filthy, undrained, pestilential, while they are suffering from frightful epidemics of disease, while infant mortality rises and length of life declines, let us turn from them to a people of the East who have the liberal aggressive spirit so lacking in the West, a people who are destined to preserve the medical science of the Greeks and Romans.

At the end of the 7th century the Arabs had swept from Arabia thru the Eastern Roman Empire and over Egypt, North Africa, and Spain. The very fate of Western Europe had hung in the balance until the Arabs were defeated in the Battle of Tours in 732. Once settled in their new lands, the Arabs built up their civilization; they turned to cultural pursuits; they were interested in science. They translated the Greek and Roman manuscripts into Arabic, and within two centuries Arabic civilization had developed to a high level.

During the reign of such liberal rulers as Harun al-Rashid of *Arabian Nights* fame, the sciences were patronized extensively. But there were peculiar attributes of the Oriental mind and the Oriental religion which permeated Arabic medicine. And these peculiarities were destined to leave their mark strongly upon the medicine of Europe in subsequent centuries.

The Arabic tendency was toward disputation, hair-splitting disputation. They admired and applauded clever, subtle logic rather than sound and rugged principles. Their way of thinking was as different from that of the Greeks as were the architectures of the two countries—the Grecian columns clear and simple against the sky, the Arabic filigree detailed and intricate.

The theorizing of Galen, his subtle, showy explanations, appealed to the Arabs; the rugged principles of Hippocrates did not. They adapted Galen's theories, his dogmas, and his poly-pharmacy to an Arabic form. Soon at their hands Galen's theories became dogmas; his beliefs took on the forms of axioms as irrefutable as the basic axioms of geometry.

The Arabic knowledge of medicine was to be transplanted into Europe and along with it the peculiar tendencies of Arabic medical thought. And the Europe into which this medicine was to come was one in which, as we have said, authority was accepted without question. Thus the Europeans were to venerate Galen rather than Hippocrates and to accept the works of Galen with an almost religious veneration.

This medicine that is to reach Europe, filtered as it is thru Arabic culture, is a version of Galen flavored strongly by its Arabic contact. A vast amount of stone lore is added; a sturdier fund of pharmacy than Galen's is supplied, an advantage more than counter-balanced by a diminished knowledge of anatomy, for the Arabs made no dissections of the body; some astrology, some mystery, some magic find their places in it; and above and beyond all is an unhealthy tendency to displace the search for truth by the sterile process of disputation.

The Arabic precursors of European medicine were more aggressive clinicians than were their European successors. Great figures stand out among their physicians. There is Rhazes of the 9th and 10th centuries, who described diseases with a fidelity worthy of Hippocrates. He was the first physician to give a clear description of smallpox and measles. And there also a century later was the great Avicenna, whose influence upon European medicine was paramount. His lasting fame rests perhaps upon his production of alcohol and sulphuric acid, the two substances from which, many centuries later, ether was made, one of the great blessings to humanity, as a safe and trustworthy anesthetic. But his immediate fame rested on his books, destined to become the most popular medical literature of Medieval Europe. In spite of his excellent clinical observations his influence was bad. He confirmed in the minds of Europeans, already inclined in that direction, the belief that mental gymnastics, refined argumentation, was more desirable than the drudgery of original investigation. And, perhaps worst of all, he preached the belief that surgery was inferior to medical practice and indeed an entirely separate branch of medicine. When, as late as the time of Frederick the Great, the Prussian Army surgeons as part of their duty shaved the officers of the army, they owed this mark of their degradation to the day when Avicenna cast surgery into disrepute.

It was this great Arab who advanced the doctrine that cautery should be used instead of the knife and thus added cruelty to a practice already horribly cruel—surgery without anesthesia. In justice it must be admitted, though, that the use of the cautery and of boiling oil in treating wounds had one advantage: it helped to control infection in an age when antiseptics were unknown. When some five centuries later the great French surgeon, Ambroise Paré, discarded these practices of Avicenna, there can be little question that infection increased in prevalence. Three hundred years more were to pass before Joseph Lister made his announcement of the antiseptic principle.

We have dwelt to greater length on Arabic medicine than it of itself deserves here—save for one fact. Unlike the practices of China or India or Japan this Arabic medicine is to have a profound influence upon the medicine from which our own of today has developed. So we shall turn now from Arabic medicine already in its zenith, soon to be stationary and then decadent, to Europe of the 11th and 12th centuries. These are the years when Arabic influence is first felt, radiating from Europe's one medical school, that of Salerno, a small seashore town near Naples. Here under Arabic influence medicine is taught for the first time in the medieval period as a separate branch of science, in distinction to the Monastic medicine prevalent elsewhere.

But the Salernian School was not to be the guiding influence of European medicine; it was a feeble, very feeble, light in a great wilderness. It is best remembered by its famous medical poem said to have been prepared for Robert Duke of Normandy, son of William the Conqueror, the *Regimen Salernitanum*, essentially a compendium of practical advice replete with jingling lines such as "Joy, temperance, and repose slam the door on the doctor's nose." After the invention of printing it went thru some 240 editions, and portions of it were translated into English at the time of Queen Elizabeth under the title *The Englishman's Doctor*. The translator was the famous Sir John Harington, inventor of the water-closet.

The outstanding medical contribution of the School of Salerno was the writings of Roger of Palermo. He prescribed burnt sponge for goiter, used mercury salves for skin diseases, and sutured the intestine over a tube, but he preached the healing of wounds by second intention in the Galenic belief that pus formation was a necessary and desirable part of the reparative process. This problem of wound healing is to occupy much attention during the period extending from these years to the 19th century and the time of Lister. In all these years only three men before Lister upheld the doctrine that wounds should be so treated that pus did not form. Two of them came in this Medieval period—Theodoric, Bishop of Cervia, and Henri de Mondeville. The third was the great Swiss of the early Renaissance—Paracelsus.

We now come to the thirteenth and fourteenth centuries—a period characterized for our story by the Crusades to the Orient, the rise of universities, and epidemics of the Black Death. These epidemics, which wiped out nearly half of the sparse population of Europe, were followed by that amazing hysterical outburst, the dancing mania. At that time the population of Western Europe was less than that of the British Isles alone today.

The rise of medical schools, especially at Naples, Palermo, and Montpellier, impinged upon Salerno so that it was destined to lead but a feeble existence until 1811, when it was abolished by Napoleon.

The Crusades were avenues thru which Arabic medicine was brought in its full force into Europe. And as we have said, it was a Europe peculiarly receptive to this dogmatized version of Galen. The Arabic medicine was accepted and venerated; it furnished endless material for sterile argument but no inspiration for progress. If we seek thru these years for men who advanced medicine, our search is nearly fruitless. Two only, and they surgeons, stand out. One is the Henri de Mondeville of the 13th century whom we have mentioned as a supporter of the Hippocratic belief that wounds should be kept clean and allowed to heal free from pus if possible. His influence was not great. The other was Guy de Chauliac, a man of rare talents and noble character, who by his example helped to elevate surgery to a more dignified position, who believed—a revolutionary concept in those days—that a knowledge of anatomy was essential to surgery. But Guy de Chauliac, in direct opposition to Theodoric and Mondeville, advocated the meddlesome treatment of wounds and the application of salves and plasters. His influence was so strong that his beliefs retarded the progress of surgery for some six centuries.

Of medical progress in Europe there is little to record until the 16th century. The intervening years were years of sterile disputations. Galenic—Arabic Galenic—medicine had taken its hold upon the medical profession and the clergy with nearly the strength of the precepts of the Bible and in an age when it was heresy to doubt the Bible.

To find any notable progress arising from medicine in these years we must turn to one branch of it—pharmacy—and to a progress that is essentially social rather than medical—one of enormous benefit to mankind. For the pharmaceutical beliefs of the times led to exploration; and the exploration resulted in great geographical discoveries—including that of America.

Here again we find the Arabic influence. The pharmacy of the East employed the herbs and plant products native to the Orient—aloes, benzoin, camphor, cinnamon, cloves, cubebs, ginger, musk, opium, pepper, and rhubarb. In adopting Arabic medicine the physicians of Europe likewise adopted the products of Arabic pharmacy. A brisk trade resulted in what today we should call mainly spices, but which in those days were highly desirable medicaments. The caravan routes of trade were slow and expensive, and so explorers set out in ships to find a shorter route for the spice trade. Vasco da Gama sailed round Cape Horn; Columbus sailed to America, believing he had reached India. And for centuries afterwards the seaboard countries of Europe strove for the supremacy of the spice traffic, the lightest and most lucrative cargo a ship could carry, for in those days products common to our kitchens as well as the shelves of our pharmacists commanded enormous prices.

The struggle for the spice trade was a struggle for naval supremacy. In turn Venice, then Portugal, then Holland, and finally England became mistress of the seas, and each in turn so rose as a by-product of pharmacy. But since their naval achievements were only by-products, we must leave their story to the general historian and return to our original subject: mystery, magic, and medicine.

HANS ZINSSER
As I Remember Him

<hr/>

HANS ZINSSER (1878-1940) served as a bridge between the medical profession and the intelligent lay public. He personified the quintessence of the cultivated physician, like Holmes, who thought deeply about life and its meaning—and not just about the repair of the organism. His autobiography, *As I Remember Him*, like *The Education of Henry Adams*, was written in the third person. It is an example of his ability to think objectively about his experiences in medicine and also to express subjectively his discovery of the wellspring of his own being.

America had before this time many medical schools. But with few exceptions they were "proprietary" ones—that is, privately founded corporations of groups of physicians and surgeons who organized courses without a well-conceived educational plan, often without hospital facilities. In a few places, this was being corrected by intelligent faculties who voluntarily placed themselves under university control, or allied themselves with well-run hospitals. But taken as a whole the situation was a deplorable one, lacking any uniformity in educational standards, care in the choice of teachers, laboratory or clinical facilities. In a few places, owing largely to financial support, university influence was gaining power, and in Philadelphia, Boston, Ann Arbor, and New York, schools of increasing strength developed. An especially strong pressure for improvement was exerted by President Eliot, at the Harvard school. The situation was distinctly improving before 1880 and probably was on its way to better things, largely under the influence of the young men returning from Europe. But, at best, this would have been slow and might have taken many wrong turnings had it not been for the opening, in 1893, of the Johns Hopkins Medical School. Whether we attribute it to good fortune or to extraordinary wisdom, the group eventually assembled at Hopkins—Osler, Welch, Halsted, Mall, Howell, and Abel—became the model for American schools, and it was not long before men trained by them became the leaven that raised the general level of all other progressive institutions.

But Johns Hopkins had an endowment and a hospital of its own. It was equipped with laboratories and backed by a university. Few other places could, even with the best will, meet the new requirements. By 1900, great improvement had taken place. But the country was still full of second-rate proprietary schools and university schools that were limping along in penury. Then came Abraham Flexner's report to the Carnegie Foundation.

Oh, Abraham Flexner! We have fought with you on minor points, have alternately admired and disliked you, have applauded you for wisdom and detested you for opinionatedness. But in just retrospect—layman as you are—we hail you as the father—or, better, the uncle—of modern medical education in America. You did, on occasion, hit below the belt, yet in the spirit in which the Christian knights slashed off the infidels' heads while shouting "Kyrie Eleison!" it was your report—uncompromising, cruelly objective, courageous and incisive—which opened the eyes of the medical profession to the state of their training schools, aroused public opinion to the need of better education of the guardians of health, and set the floodgates of the golden streams of philanthropy in medical directions.

For a decade, Abraham Flexner—backed by the huge resources of the Rockefeller Foundation and, indirectly, by similar funds; and advised by such wise men as Welch, Mall, Edsall, Pierce, and less wise ones who, like R.S., gave unsolicited advice which he did not follow—dominated the educational situation in medicine. Meanwhile, laboratories were founded in the schools; young men of spirit, training, and ambition enlisted; professorships were bestowed for promise and accomplishments; and research institutes began to step up the pace of creative production.

One reads the increasing mass of literature on the origins of the great American fortunes of the nineteenth century, and one takes bicarbonate of soda. But however one feels about that, one must acknowledge that the preëminent position of American medicine to-day would have been impossible without a certain amount of rich malefaction in the eighties and nineties.

Thus, modern American medicine is, in a way, a phoenix arising from the ill-smelling ashes of a big business that is forever gone.

THE ROLE OF
THE PHYSICIAN

Should the physician be, primarily, a crusader against illness, a research scientist, a personal counselor, a philosopher, a moral force in society—or a combination of all these and more? The authors in this section emphasize different roles of the doctor. All of them are compelling. The poignant question arising out of all these varying concepts and roles is whether it is humanly possible for any person to fulfill so many expectations.

Physicians mend or end us,
Secundum artem; but although we sneer
In health—when ill we call them to attend us,
Without the least propensity to jeer.

Byron.

Happy the doctor who is called in at the end of the disease.

French Proverb.

A good surgeon operates with his hand, not with his heart.

Dumas.

No one tries desperate remedies at first.

Latin Proverb.

Medicine, the only profession that labors incessantly to destroy the reason for its own existence.

Lord Bryce.

25

W. H. AUDEN
The Art of Healing

———⧯———

W. H. AUDEN (1907-1973), one of the leading names in British and American poetry for more than a quarter-century, was the son of a distinguished physician. During the Spanish Civil War he served as an ambulance driver for the Loyalists. His poetry draws upon this special knowledge, in this instance, a memorial to his own doctor who died of diabetes.

(IN MEMORIAM DAVID PROTETCH, M.D. 1923-1969)

Most patients assume
dying is something they do,
   not their physician,
   that white-coated sage,
never to be imagined
   naked or married.

Begotten by one,
I should know better. "Healing,"
   Papa would tell me,
   "is not a science
but the intuitive art
   of wooing Nature.

Plants, beasts may react
according to the common
   whim of their species,
   but all humans have
prejudices of their own,
   which can't be foreseen.

To some, bad health is
the interest in their lives,
    others are stoics,
    a few fanatics,
who won't feel happy until
    they are cut open.''

Warned by him to shun
the nod-crafty, the sadist,
    and the fee-conscious,
    I knew when we met
I had found a consultant
    who thought as he did,

    yourself a victim
of medical engineers
    and their arrogance,
    when they atom-bombed
your ill pituitary
    and overkilled it.

    "Every sickness
is a musical problem,"
    so said Novalis,
    "and every cure
a musical solution":
    you knew that also.

Not that in my case
you heard any shattering
    discords to resolve:
    to date my organs
still seem pretty sure of their
    self-identities.

For my small ailments
you, who were mortally sick,
    proscribed with success:
    my major vices,
my mad addictions, you left
    to my own conscience.

Was it your very
predicament that made me
    sure I could trust you,
    if I were dying,
to say so, not insult me
    with soothing fictions?

    Must diabetics
all contend with a nisus
    to self-destruction?
    One day you told me:
"It is only bad temper
    that keeps me going."

    But neither anger
nor lust are omnipotent,
    nor should we even
    want our friends to be
superhuman. Dear David,
    dead one, rest in peace,

    having been what all
doctors should be but few are,
    and, even when most
    difficult, condign
of our biassed affection
    and objective praise.

ROBERT BURTON
Anatomy of Melancholy

———◦◦◦◦———

ROBERT BURTON (1577-1640) was vicar of St. Thomas, Oxford, and keeper of the library at Christ's College. He was a scholar of medicine, history, literature, science, and theology. His *Anatomy of Melancholy*, from which this selection is drawn, was at one time considered standard fare in the education of liberal arts students.

With all virtuous and wise men, therefore, I honour the name, and calling, as I am enjoined to honour the Physician for necessity's sake. The knowledge of the Physician lifted up his head, and in the sight of great men he shall be admired. The Lord hath created medicines of the earth, and he that is wise will not abhor them. But of this noble subject how many panegyricks are worthily written! For my part, as Sallust said of Carthage, 'tis better to be silent than to say little. I have said, yet one thing I will add, that this kind of Physick is very moderately and advisedly to be used, upon good occasion, when the former of diet will not take place. And 'tis no other which I say than that which Arnoldus prescribes in his 8th Aphorism: A discreet and godly Physician doth first endeavour to expel a disease by medicinal diet, then by pure medicine; and in his ninth, he that may be cured by diet must not meddle with Physick. So in the 11th Aphorism: A modest and wise Physician will never hasten to use medicines, but upon urgent necessity, and that sparingly too; because (as he adds in his 13th Aphorism): Whosoever takes much Physick in his youth shall soon bewail it in his old age; purgative Physick especially, which doth much debilitate nature. For which causes some Physicians refrain from the use of Purgatives, or else sparingly use them.

ALBERT CAMUS
The Plague

———————⟨∞⟩———————

ALBERT CAMUS (1913-1960), French novelist, journalist, and playwright, has been identified with the Existentialist movement but steadfastly denied any affinity with that philosophy. He had a profound effect not just on French literature but on social philosophy. His observations on bubonic plague were drawn at first hand while he lived in Algiers.

During the first few weeks Rieux was compelled to stay with the patient till the ambulance came. Later, when each doctor was accompanied by a volunteer police officer, Rieux could hurry away to the next patient.

But, to begin with, every evening was like that evening when he was called in for Mme. Loret's daughter. He was shown into a small apartment decorated with fans and artificial flowers. The mother greeted him with a faltering smile.

"Oh, I do hope it's not the fever everyone's talking about."

Lifting the coverlet and chemise, he gazed in silence at the red blotches on the girl's thighs and stomach, the swollen ganglia. After one glance the mother broke into shrill, uncontrollable cries of grief. And every evening mothers wailed thus, with a distraught abstraction, as their eyes fell on those fatal stigmata on limbs and bellies; every evening hands gripped Rieux's arms, there was a rush of useless words, promises, and tears; every evening the nearing tocsin of the ambulance provoked scenes as vain as every form of grief. Rieux had nothing to look forward to but a long sequence of such scenes, renewed again and again.

*   *   *

"What did you think of Paneloux's sermon, Doctor?"

The question was asked in a quite ordinary tone, and Rieux answered in the same tone.

"I've seen too much of hospitals to relish any idea of collective punishment. But, as you know, Christians sometimes say that sort of thing without really thinking it. They're better than they seem."

"However, you think, like Paneloux, that the plague has its good side; it opens men's eyes and forces them to take thought?"

The doctor tossed his head impatiently.

"So does every ill that flesh is heir to. What's true of all the evils in the world is true of plague as well. It helps men to rise above themselves. All the same, when you see the misery it brings, you'd need to be a madman, or a coward, or stone blind, to give in tamely to the plague."

Rieux had hardly raised his voice at all; but Tarrou made a slight gesture as if to calm him. He was smiling.

"Yes." Rieux shrugged his shoulders. "But you haven't answered my question yet. Have you weighed the consequences?"

Tarrou squared his shoulders against the back of the chair, then moved his head forward into the light.

"Do you believe in God, Doctor?"

Again the question was put in an ordinary tone. But this time Rieux took longer to find his answer.

"No—but what does that really mean? I'm fumbling in the dark, struggling to make something out. But I've long ceased finding that original."

"Isn't that it—the gulf between Paneloux and you?"

"I doubt it. Paneloux is a man of learning, a scholar. He hasn't come in contact with death; that's why he can speak with such assurance of the truth—with a capital T. But every country priest who visits his parishoners and has heard a man gasping for breath on his deathbed thinks as I do. He'd try to relieve human suffering before trying to point out its excellence." Rieux stood up; his face was now in shadow. "Let's drop the subject," he said, "as you won't answer."

Tarrou remained seated in his chair; he was smiling again.

"Suppose I answer with a question."

The doctor now smiled, too.

"You like being mysterious, don't you? Yes, fire away."

"My question's this," said Tarrou. "Why do you yourself show such devotion, considering you don't believe in God? I suspect your answer may help me to mine."

His face still in shadow, Rieux said that he'd already answered: that if he believed in an all-powerful God he would cease curing the sick and leave that to Him. But no one in the world believed in a God of that sort; no, not even Paneloux, who believed that he believed in such a God. And this was proved by the fact that no one ever threw himself on Providence completely. Anyhow, in this respect Rieux believed himself to be on the right road—in fighting against creation as he found it.

"Ah," Tarrou remarked. "So that's the idea you have of your profession?"

"More or less." The doctor came back into the light.

Tarrou made a faint whistling noise with his lips, and the doctor gazed at him.

"Yes, you're thinking it calls for pride to feel that way. But I assure you I've no more than the pride that's needed to keep me going. I have no idea what's awaiting me, or what will happen when all this ends. For the moment I know this; there are sick people and they need curing. Later on, perhaps, they'll think things over; and so shall I. But what's wanted now is to make them well. I defend them as best I can, that's all."

"Against whom?"

Rieux turned to the window. A shadow-line on the horizon told of the presence of the sea. He was conscious only of his exhaustion, and at the same time was struggling against a sudden, irrational impulse to unburden himself a little more to his companion; an eccentric, perhaps, but who, he guessed, was one of his own kind.

"I haven't a notion, Tarrou; I assure you I haven't a notion. When I entered this profession, I did it 'abstractedly,' so to speak; because I had a desire for it, because it meant a career like another, one that young men often aspire to. Perhaps, too, because it was particularly difficult for a workman's son, like myself. And then I had to see people die. Do you know that there are some who *refuse* to die? Have you ever heard a woman scream 'Never!' with her last gasp? Well, I have. And then I saw that I could never get hardened to it. I was young then, and I was outraged by the whole scheme of things, or so I thought. Subsequently I grew more modest. Only, I've never managed to get used to seeing people die. That's all I know. Yet after all—"

Rieux fell silent and sat down. He felt his mouth dry.

"After all—?" Tarrou prompted softly.

"After all," the doctor repeated, then hesitated again, fixing his eyes on Tarrou, "it's something that a man of your sort can understand most likely, but, since the order of the world is shaped by death, mightn't it be better for God if we refuse to believe in Him and struggle with all our might against death, without raising our eyes toward the heaven where He sits in silence?"

Tarrou nodded.

"Yes. But your victories will never be lasting; that's all."

Rieux's face darkened.

"Yes, I know that. But it's no reason for giving up the struggle."

"No reason, I agree. Only, I now can picture what this plague must mean for you."

"Yes. A never ending defeat."

Tarrou stared at the doctor for a moment, then turned and tramped heavily toward the door. Rieux followed him and was almost at his side when Tarrou, who was staring at the floor, suddenly said:

"Who taught you all this, Doctor?"

The reply came promptly:

"Suffering."

Rieux opened the door of his surgery and told Tarrou that he, too, was going out; he had a patient to visit in the suburbs. Tarrou suggested they should go together and he agreed. In the hall they encountered Mme. Rieux, and the doctor introduced Tarrou to her.

"A friend of mine," he said.

"Indeed," said Mme. Rieux, "I'm very pleased to make your acquaintance."

When she left them Tarrou turned to gaze after her. On the landing the doctor pressed a switch to turn on the lights along the stairs. But the stairs remained in darkness. Possibly some new light-saving order had come into force. Really, however, there was no knowing; for some time past, in the streets no less than in private houses, everything had been going out of order. It might be only that the concierge, like nearly everyone in the town, was ceasing to bother about his duties. The doctor had no time to follow up his thoughts; Tarrou's voice came from behind him.

"Just one word more, Doctor, even if it sounds to you a bit nonsensical. You are perfectly right."

The doctor merely gave a little shrug, unseen in the darkness.

"To tell the truth, all that's outside my range. But you—what do *you* know about it?"

"Ah," Tarrou replied quite coolly, "I've little left to learn."

Rieux paused and, behind him, Tarrou's foot slipped on a step. He steadied himself by gripping the doctor's shoulder.

"Do you really imagine you know everything about life?"

The answer came through the darkness in the same cool, confident tone.

"Yes."

Once in the street, they realized it must be quite late, eleven perhaps. All was silence in the town, except for some vague rustlings. An ambulance bell clanged faintly in the distance. They stepped into the car and Rieux started the engine.

"You must come to the hospital tomorrow," he said, "for an injection. But, before embarking on this adventure, you'd better know your chances of coming out of it alive; they're one in three."

"That sort of reckoning doesn't hold water; you know it, Doctor, as well as I. A hundred years ago plague wiped out the entire population of a town in Persia, with one exception. And the sole survivor was precisely the man whose job it was to wash the dead bodies, and who carried on throughout the epidemic."

"He pulled off his one-in-three chances, that's all." Rieux had lowered his voice. "But you're right; we know next to nothing on the subject."

They were entering the suburbs. The headlights lit up empty streets. The car stopped. Standing in front of it, Rieux asked Tarrou if he'd like to come in. Tarrou said: "Yes." A glimmer of light from the sky lit up their faces. Suddenly Rieux gave a short laugh, and there was much friendliness in it.

"Out with it, Tarrou! What on earth prompted you to take a hand in this?"

"I don't know. My code of morals, perhaps."

"Your code of morals? What code?"

"Comprehension."

Tarrou turned toward the house and Rieux did not see his face again until they were in the old asthma patient's room.

*   *   *

"Man isn't an idea, Rambert."

Rambert sprang off the bed, his face ablaze with passion.

"Man *is* an idea, and a precious small idea, once he turns his back on love. And that's my point; we—mankind—have lost the capacity for love. We must face that fact, Doctor. Let's wait to acquire that capacity or, if really it's beyond us, wait for the deliverance that will come to each of us anyway, without his playing the hero. Personally, I look no farther."

Rieux rose. He suddenly appeared very tired.

"You're right, Rambert, quite right, and for nothing in the world would I try to dissuade you from what you're going to do; it seems to me absolutely right and proper. However, there's one thing I must tell you: there's no question of heroism in all this. It's a matter of common decency. That's an idea which may make some people smile, but the only means of fighting a plague is—common decency."

"What do you mean by 'common decency'?" Rambert's tone was grave.

"I don't know what it means for other people. But in my case I know that it consists in doing my job."

"Your job! I only wish I were sure what my job is!" There was a mordant edge to Rambert's voice. "Maybe I'm all wrong in putting love first."

Rieux looked him in the eyes.

"No," he said vehemently, "you are *not* wrong."

Rambert gazed thoughtfully at them.

"You two," he said, "I suppose you've nothing to lose in all this. It's easier, that way, to be on the side of the angels."

Rieux drained his glass.

"Come along," he said to Tarrou. "We've work to do."

He went out.

Tarrou followed, but seemed to change his mind when he reached the door. He stopped and looked at the journalist.

"I suppose you don't know that Rieux's wife is in a sanatorium, a hundred miles or so away."

Rambert showed surprise and began to say something; but Tarrou had already left the room.

*   *   *

The difference in his old friend's face shocked him. The smile of benevolent irony that always played on it had seemed to endow it with perpetual youth; now, abruptly left out of control, with a trickle of saliva between the slightly parted lips, it betrayed its age and the wastage of the years. And, seeing this, Rieux felt a lump come to his throat.

It was by such lapses that Rieux could gauge his exhaustion. His sensibility was getting out of hand. Kept under all the time, it had grown hard and brittle and seemed to snap completely now and then, leaving him the prey of his emotions. No resource was left him but to tighten the stranglehold on his feelings and harden his heart protectively. For he knew this was the only way of carrying on. In any case, he had few illusions left, and fatigue was robbing him of even these remaining few. He knew that, over a period whose end he could not glimpse, his task was no longer to cure but to diagnose. To detect, to see, to describe, to register, and then condemn—that was his present function. Sometimes a woman would clutch his sleeve, crying shrilly: "Doctor, you'll save him, won't you?" But he wasn't there for saving life; he was there to order a sick man's evacuation. How futile was the hatred he saw on faces then! "You haven't a heart!'' a woman told him on one occasion. She was wrong; he had one. It saw him through his twenty-hour day, when he hourly watched men dying who were meant to live. It enabled him to start anew each morning. He had just enough heart for that, as things were now. How could that heart have sufficed for saving life?

No, it wasn't medical aid that he dispensed in those crowded days—only information. Obviously that could hardly be reckoned a man's job. Yet, when all was said and done, who, in that terror-stricken, decimated populace, had scope for any activity worthy of his manhood? Indeed, for Rieux his exhaustion was a blessing in disguise. Had he been less tired, his senses more alert, that all-pervading odor of death might have made him sentimental. But when a man has had only four hours' sleep, he isn't sentimental. He sees things as they are; that is to say, he sees them in the garish light of justice—hideous, witless justice. And those others, the men and women under sentence to death, shared his bleak enlightenment. Before the plague he was welcomed as a savior. He was going to make them right with a couple of pills or an injection, and people took him by the arm on his way to the sickroom. Flattering, but dangerous. Now, on the contrary, he came accompanied by soldiers, and they had to hammer on the door with rifle-butts before the family would open it. They would have liked to drag him, drag the whole human race, with them to the grave. Yes, it was quite true that men can't do without their fellow men; that he was as helpless as these unhappy people and he, too, deserved the same faint thrill of pity that he allowed himself once he had left them.

Such, anyhow, were the thoughts that in those endless-seeming weeks ran in the doctor's mind, along with thoughts about his severance from his wife. And such, too, were his friends' thoughts, judging by the look he saw on their faces. But the most dangerous effect of the exhaustion steadily gaining on all engaged in the fight against the epidemic did not consist in their relative indifference to outside events and the feelings of others, but in the slackness and supineness that they allowed to invade their personal lives. They developed a tendency to shirk every movement that didn't seem absolutely necessary or called for efforts that seemed too great to be worth while. Thus these men were led to break, oftener and oftener, the rules of hygiene they themselves had instituted, to omit some of the numerous disinfections they should have practiced, and sometimes to visit the homes of people suffering from pneumonic plague without taking steps to safeguard themselves against infection, because they had been notified only at the last moment and could not be bothered with returning to a sanitary service station, sometimes a considerable distance away, to have the necessary injections. There lay the real danger; for the energy they devoted to fighting the disease made them all the more liable to it. In short, they were gambling on their luck, and luck is not to be coerced.

Only then Rieux turned toward him, raising himself with an effort from the cushion.

"Forgive me, Rambert, only—well, I simply don't know. But stay with us if you want to." A swerve of the car made him break off. Then, looking straight in front of him, he said: "For nothing in the world is it worth turning one's back on what one loves. Yet that is what I'm doing, though why I do not know." He sank back on the cushion. "That's how it is," he added wearily, "and there's nothing to be done about it. So let's recognize the fact and draw the conclusions."

"What conclusions?"

"Ah," Rieux said, "a man can't cure and know at the same time. So let's cure as quickly as we can. That's the more urgent job."

*   *   *

Toward the close of October Castel's anti-plague serum was tried for the first time. Practically speaking, it was Rieux's last card. If it failed, the doctor was convinced the whole town would be at the mercy of the epidemic, which would either continue its ravages for an unpredictable period or perhaps die out abruptly of its own accord.

The day before Castel called on Rieux, M. Othon's son had fallen ill and all the family had to go into quarantine. Thus the mother, who had only recently come out of it, found herself isolated once again. In deference to the official regulations the magistrate had promptly sent for Dr. Rieux the moment he saw symptoms of the disease in his little boy. Mother and father were standing at the bedside when Rieux entered the room. The boy was in the phase of extreme prostration and submitted without a whimper to the doctor's examination. When Rieux raised his eyes he saw the magistrate's gaze intent on him, and, behind, the mother's pale face. She was holding a handkerchief to her mouth, and her big, dilated eyes followed each of the doctor's movements.

"He has it, I suppose?" the magistrate asked in a toneless voice.

"Yes." Rieux gazed down at the child again.

The mother's eyes widened yet more, but she still said nothing. M. Othon, too, kept silent for a while before saying in an even lower tone:

"Well, Doctor, we must do as we are told to do."

Rieux avoided looking at Mme. Othon, who was still holding her handkerchief to her mouth.

"It needn't take long," he said rather awkwardly, "if you'll let me use your phone."

The magistrate said he would take him to the telephone. But before going, the doctor turned toward Mme. Othon.

"I regret very much indeed, but I'm afraid you'll have to get your things ready. You know how it is."

Mme. Othon seemed disconcerted. She was staring at the floor.

Then, "I understand," she murmured, slowly nodding her head. "I'll set about it at once."

Before leaving, Rieux on a sudden impulse asked the Othons if there wasn't anything they'd like him to do for them. The mother gazed at him in silence. And now the magistrate averted his eyes.

"No," he said, then swallowed hard. "But—save my son."

In the early days a mere formality, quarantine had now been reorganized by Rieux and Rambert on very strict lines. In particular they insisted on having members of the family of a patient kept apart. If, unawares, one of them had been infected, the risks of an extension of the infection must not be multiplied. Rieux explained this to the magistrate, who signified his approval of the procedure. Nevertheless, he and his wife exchanged a glance that made it clear to Rieux how keenly they both felt the separation thus imposed on them. Mme. Othon and her little girl could be given rooms in the quarantine hospital under Rambert's charge. For the magistrate, however, no accommodation was available except in an isolation camp the authorities were now installing in the municipal stadium, using tents supplied by the highway department. When Rieux apologized for the poor accommodation, M. Othon replied that there was one rule for all alike, and it was only proper to abide by it.

The boy was taken to the auxiliary hospital and put in a ward of ten beds which had formerly been a classroom. After some twenty hours Rieux became convinced that the case was hopeless. The infection was steadily spreading, and the boy's body was putting up no resistance. Tiny, half-formed, but acutely painful buboes were clogging the joints of the child's puny limbs. Obviously it was a losing fight.

Under the circumstances Rieux had no qualms about testing Castel's serum on the boy. That night, after dinner, they performed the inoculation, a lengthy process, without getting the slightest reaction. At daybreak on the following day they gathered round the bed to observe the effects of this test inoculation on which so much hung.

The child had come out of his extreme prostration and was tossing about convulsively on the bed. From four in the morning Dr. Castel and Tarrou had been keeping watch and noting, stage by stage, the progress and remissions of the malady, Tarrou's bulky form was slightly drooping at the head of the bed, while at its foot, with Rieux standing beside him, Castel was seated, reading, with every appearance of calm, an old leather-bound book. One by one, as the light increased in the former classroom, the others arrived. Paneloux, the first to come, leaned against the wall on the opposite side of the bed to Tarrou. His face was drawn with grief, and the accumulated weariness of many weeks, during which he had never spared himself, had deeply seamed his somewhat prominent forehead. Grand came next. It was seven o'clock, and he apologized for being out of breath; he could only stay a moment, but wanted to know if any definite results had been observed. Without speaking, Rieux pointed to the child. His eyes shut, his teeth clenched, his features frozen in an agonized grimace, he was rolling his head from side to side on the bolster. When there was just light enough to make out the half-obliterated figures of an equation chalked on a blackboard that still hung on the wall at the far end of the room, Rambert entered. Posting himself at the foot of the next bed, he took a package of cigarettes from his pocket. But after his first glance at the child's face he put it back.

From his chair Castel looked at Rieux over his spectacles.

"Any news of his father?"

"No," said Rieux. "He's in the isolation camp."

The doctor's hands were gripping the rail of the bed, his eyes fixed on the small tortured body. Suddenly it stiffened, and seemed to give a little at the waist, as slowly the arms and legs spread out X-wise. From the body, naked under an army blanket, rose a smell of damp wool and stale sweat. The boy had gritted his teeth again. Then very gradually he relaxed, bringing his arms and legs back toward the center of the bed, still without speaking or opening his eyes, and his breathing seemed to quicken. Rieux looked at Tarrou, who hastily lowered his eyes.

They had already seen children die—for many months now death had shown no favoritism—but they had never yet watched a child's agony minute by minute, as they had now been doing since daybreak. Needless to say, the pain inflicted on these innocent victims had always seemed to them to be what in fact it was: an abominable thing. But hitherto they had felt its abomination in, so to speak, an abstract way; they had never had to witness over so long a period the death-throes of an innocent child.

And just then the boy had a sudden spasm, as if something had bitten him in the stomach, and uttered a long, shrill wail. For moments that seemed endless he stayed in a queer, contorted position, his body racked by convulsive tremors; it was as if his frail frame were bending before the fierce breath of the plague, breaking under the reiterated gusts of fever. Then the storm-wind passed, there came a lull, and he relaxed a little; the fever seemed to recede, leaving him gasping for breath on a dank, pestilential shore, lost in a languor that already looked like death. When for the third time the fiery wave broke on him, lifting him a little, the child curled himself up and shrank away to the edge of the bed, as if in terror of the flames advancing on him, licking his limbs. A moment later, after tossing his head wildly to and fro, he flung off the blanket. From between the inflamed eyelids big tears welled up and trickled down the sunken, leaden-hued cheeks. When the spasm had passed, utterly exhausted, tensing his thin legs and arms, on which, within forty-eight hours, the flesh had wasted to the bone, the child lay flat, racked on the rumbled bed, in a grotesque parody of crucifixion.

Bending, Tarrou gently stroked with his big paw the small face stained with tears and sweat. Castel had closed his book a few moments before, and his eyes were now fixed on the child. He began to speak, but had to give a cough before continuing, because his voice rang out so harshly.

"There wasn't any remission this morning, was there, Rieux?"

Rieux shook his head, adding, however, that the child was putting up more resistance than one would have expected. Paneloux, who was slumped against the wall, said in a low voice:

"So if he is to die, he will have suffered longer."

Light was increasing in the ward. The occupants of the other nine beds were tossing about and groaning, but in tones that seemed deliberately subdued. Only one, at the far end of the ward, was screaming, or rather uttering little exclamations at regular intervals, which seemed to convey surprise more than pain. Indeed, one had the impression that even for the sufferers the frantic terror of the early phase had passed, and there was a sort of mournful resignation in their present attitude toward the disease. Only the child went on fighting with all his little might. Now and then Rieux took his pulse—less because this served any purpose than as an escape from his utter helplessness—and when he closed his eyes, he seemed to feel its tumult mingling with the fever of his own blood. And then, at one with the tortured child, he struggled to sustain him with all the remaining strength of his own body. But, linked for a few moments, the rhythms of their heartbeats soon fell apart, the child escaped him, and again he knew his impotence. Then he released the small, thin wrist and moved back to his place.

The light on the whitewashed walls was changing from pink to yellow. The first waves of another day of heat were beating on the windows. They hardly heard Grand saying he would come back as he turned to go. All were waiting. The child, his eyes still closed, seemed to grow a little calmer. His clawlike fingers were feebly plucking at the sides of the bed. Then they rose, scratched at the blanket over his knees, and suddenly he doubled up his limbs, bringing his thighs above his stomach, and remained quite still. For the first time he opened his eyes and gazed at Rieux, who was standing immediately in front of him. In the small face, rigid as a mask of grayish clay, slowly the lips parted and from them rose a long, incessant scream, hardly varying with his respiration, and filling the ward with a fierce, indignant protest, so little childish that it seemed like a collective voice issuing from all the sufferers there. Rieux clenched his jaws, Tarrou looked away. Rambert went and stood beside Castel, who closed the book lying on his knees. Paneloux gazed down at the small mouth, fouled with the sores of the plague and pouring out the angry death-cry that has sounded through the ages of mankind. He sank on his knees, and all present found it natural to hear him say in a voice hoarse but clearly audible across that nameless, never ending wail:

"My God, spare this child!"

But the wail continued without cease and the other sufferers began to grow restless. The patient at the far end of the ward, whose little broken cries had gone on without a break, now quickened their tempo so that they flowed together in one unbroken cry, while the others' groans grew louder. A gust of sobs swept through the room, drowning Paneloux's prayer, and Rieux, who was still tightly gripping the rail of the bed, shut his eyes, dazed with exhaustion and disgust.

When he opened them again, Tarrou was at his side.

"I must go," Rieux said. "I can't bear to hear them any longer."

But then, suddenly, the other sufferers fell silent. And now the doctor grew aware that the child's wail, after weakening more and more, had fluttered out into silence. Around him the groans began again, but more faintly, like a far echo of the fight that now was over. For it was over. Castel had moved round to the other side of the bed and said the end had come. His mouth still gaping, but silent now, the child was lying among the tumbled blankets, a small, shrunken form, with the tears still wet on his cheeks.

Paneloux went up to the bed and made the sign of benediction. Then gathering up his cassock, he walked out by the passage between the beds.

"Will you have to start it all over again?" Tarrou asked Castel.

The old doctor nodded slowly, with a twisted smile.

"Perhaps. After all, he put up a surprisingly long resistance."

Rieux was already on his way out, walking so quickly and with such a strange look on his face that Paneloux put out an arm to check him when he was about to pass him in the doorway.

"Come, Doctor," he began.

Rieux swung round on him fiercely.

"Ah! That child, anyhow, was innocent, and you know it as well as I do!"

He strode on, brushing past Paneloux, and walked across the school playground. Sitting on a wooden bench under the dingy, stunted trees, he wiped off the sweat that was beginning to run into his eyes. He felt like shouting imprecations—anything to loosen the stranglehold lashing his heart with steel. Heat was flooding down between the branches of the fig trees. A white haze, spreading rapidly over the blue of the morning sky, made the air yet more stifling. Rieux lay back wearily on the bench. Gazing up at the ragged branches, the shimmering sky, he slowly got back his breath and fought down his fatigue.

He heard a voice behind him. "Why was there that anger in your voice just now? What we'd been seeing was as unbearable to me as it was to you."

Rieux turned toward Paneloux.

"I know. I'm sorry. But weariness is a kind of madness. And there are times when the only feeling I have is one of mad revolt."

"I understand," Paneloux said in a low voice. "That sort of thing is revolting because it passes our human understanding. But perhaps we should love what we cannot understand."

Rieux straightened up slowly. He gazed at Paneloux, summoning to his gaze all the strength and fervor he could muster against his weariness. Then he shook his head.

"No, Father, I've a very different idea of love. And until my dying day I shall refuse to love a scheme of things in which children are put to torture."

F. SCOTT FITZGERALD
Tender Is the Night

—◦⤨◦—

F. SCOTT FITZGERALD (1896-1940) never received the full measure of critical recognition due him until after his death. He is regarded as the symbolic literary figure of the Jazz Age, but his stories and novels are read today not just as a reflection of a colorful decade but as superb examples of a major novelist's art. His wife's mental breakdowns provided poignant background material for *Tender is the Night*.

"Then we knew where we stood," said Franz. "Dohmler told Warren we would take the case if he would agree to keep away from his daughter indefinitely, with an absolute minimum of five years. After Warren's first collapse, he seemed chiefly concerned as to whether the story would ever leak back to America.

"We mapped out a routine for her and waited. The prognosis was bad—as you know, the percentage of cures, even so-called social cures, is very low at that age."

"These first letters looked bad," agreed Dick.

"Very bad—very typical. I hesitated about letting the first one get out of the clinic. Then I thought it will be good for Dick to know we're carrying on here. It was generous of you to answer them."

Dick sighed. "She was such a pretty thing—she enclosed a lot of snapshots of herself. And for a month there I didn't have anything to do. All I said in my letters was 'Be a good girl and mind the doctors.' "

"That was enough—it gave her somebody to think of outside. For a while she didn't have anybody—only one sister that she doesn't seem very close to. Besides, reading her letters helped us here—they were a measure of her condition."

"I'm glad."

"You see now what happened? She felt complicity—that's neither here nor there, except as we want to revalue her ultimate stability and strength of character. First came this shock. Then she went off to a boarding-school and heard the girls talking—so from sheer self-protection she developed the idea that she had had no complicity—and from there it was easy to slide into a phantom world where all men, the more you liked them and trusted them, the more evil—"

"Did she ever go into the—horror directly?"

"No, and as a matter of fact when she began to seem normal, about October, we were in a predicament. If she had been thirty years old we would have let her make her own adjustment, but she was so young we were afraid she might harden with it all twisted inside her. So Doctor Dohmler said to her frankly, 'Your duty now is to yourself. This doesn't by any account mean the end of anything for you—your life is just at its beginning,' and so forth and so forth. She really has an excellent mind, so he gave her a little Freud to read, not too much, and she was very interested. In fact, we've made rather a pet of her around here. But she is reticent," he added; he hesitated; "We have wondered if in her recent letters to you which she mailed herself from Zurich, she has said anything that would be illuminating about her state of mind and her plans for the future."

Dick considered.

"Yes and no—I'll bring the letters out here if you want. She seems hopeful and normally hungry for life—even rather romantic. Sometimes she speaks of 'the past' as people speak who have been in prison. But you never know whether they refer to the crime or the imprisonment or the whole experience. After all I'm only a sort of stuffed figure in her life."

"Of course, I understand your position exactly, and I express our gratitude once again. That was why I wanted to see you before you see her."

Dick laughed.

"You think she's going to make a flying leap at my person?"

"No, not that. But I want to ask you to go very gently. You are attractive to women, Dick."

"Then God help me! Well, I'll be gentle and repulsive—I'll chew garlic whenever I'm going to see her and wear a stubble beard. I'll drive her to cover."

"Not garlic!" said Franz, taking him seriously. "You don't want to compromise your career. But you're partly joking."

"—and I can limp a little. And there's no real bathtub where I'm living, anyhow."

"You're entirely joking," Franz relaxed—or rather assumed the posture of one relaxed. "Now tell me about yourself and your plans?"

"I've only got one, Franz, and that's to be a good psychologist—maybe to be the greatest one that ever lived."

Franz laughed pleasantly, but he saw that this time Dick wasn't joking.

"That's very good—and very American," he said. "It's more difficult for us." He got up and went to the French window. "I stand here and I see

Zurich—there is the steeple of the Gross-Münster. In its vault my grand-father is buried. Across the bridge from it lies my ancestor Lavater, who would not be buried in any church. Nearby is the statue of another ancestor, Heinrich Pestalozzi, and one of Doctor Alfred Escher. And over everything there is always Zwingli—I am continually confronted with a pantheon of heroes.''

"Yes, I see." Dick got up. "I was only talking big. Everything's just starting over. Most of the Americans in France are frantic to get home, but not me—I draw military pay all the rest of the year if I only attend lectures at the university. How's that for a government on the grand scale that knows its future great men? Then I'm going home for a month and see my father. Then I'm coming back—I've been offered a job.''

"Where?"

"Your rivals—Gisler's Clinic on Interlacken.''

"Don't touch it," Franz advised him. "They've had a dozen young men there in a year. Gisler's a manic-depressive himself, his wife and her lover run the clinic—of course, you understand that's confidential.''

"How about your old scheme for America?" asked Dick lightly. "We were going to New York and start an up-to-date establishment for billionaires.''

"That was students' talk.''

Dick dined with Franz and his bride and a small dog with a smell of burning rubber, in their cottage on the edge of the grounds. He felt vaguely oppressed, not by the atmosphere of modest retrenchment, nor by Frau Gregorovius, who might have been prophesied, but by the sudden con-tracting of horizons to which Franz seemed so reconciled. For him the boundaries of asceticism were differently marked—he could see it as a means to an end, even as a carrying on with a glory it would itself supply, but it was hard to think of deliberately cutting life down to the scale of an inherited suit. The domestic gestures of Franz and his wife as they turned in a cramped space lacked grace and adventure. The post-war months in France, and the lavish liquidations taking place under the ægis of American splendor, had affected Dick's outlook. Also, men and women had made much of him, and perhaps what had brought him back to the centre of the great Swiss watch, was an intuition that this was not too good for a serious man.

He made Kaethe Gregorovius feel charming, meanwhile becoming increasingly restless at the all-pervading cauliflower—simultaneously hat-ing himself too for this incipience of he knew not what superficiality.

"God, am I like the rest after all?''—So he used to think starting awake at night—"Am I like the rest?''

This was poor material for a socialist but good material for those who do much of the world's rarest work. The truth was that for some months he had been going through that partitioning of the things of youth wherein it is decided whether or not to die for what one no longer believes. In the dead white hours in Zurich staring into a stranger's pantry across the upshine of a street-lamp, he used to think that he wanted to be good, he wanted to be kind, he wanted to be brave and wise, but it was all pretty difficult. He wanted to be loved, too, if he could fit it in.

*   *   *

It was May when he next found her. The luncheon in Zurich was a council of caution; obviously the logic of his life tended away from the girl; yet when a stranger stared at her from a nearby table, eyes burning disturbingly like an uncharted light, he turned to the man with an urbane version of intimidation and broke the regard.

"He was just a peeper," he explained cheerfully. "He was just looking at your clothes. Why do you have so many different clothes?"

"Sister says we're very rich," she offered humbly. "Since Grandmother is dead."

"I forgive you."

He was enough older than Nicole to take pleasure in her youthful vanities and delights, the way she paused fractionally in front of the hall mirror on leaving the restaurant, so that the incorruptible quicksilver could give her back to herself. He delighted in her stretching out her hands to new octaves now that she found herself beautiful and rich. He tried honestly to divorce her from any obsession that he had stitched her together—glad to see her build up happiness and confidence apart from him; the difficulty was that, eventually, Nicole brought everything to his feet, gifts of sacrificial ambrosia, of worshipping myrtle.

The first week of summer found Dick re-established in Zurich. He had arranged his pamphlets and what work he had done in the Service into a pattern from which he intended to make his revise of "A Psychology for Psychiatrists." He thought he had a publisher; he had established contact with a poor student who would iron out his errors in German. Franz considered it a rash business, but Dick pointed out the disarming modesty of the theme.

"This is stuff I'll never know so well again," he insisted. "I have a hunch it's a thing that only fails to be basic because it's never had material recognition. The weakness of this profession is its attraction for the man a little crippled and broken. Within the walls of the profession he compensates by tending toward the clinical, the 'practical'—has won his battle without a struggle.

"On the contrary, you are a good man, Franz, because fate selected you for your profession before you were born. You better thank God you had no 'bent'—I got to be a psychiatrist because there was a girl at St. Hilda's in Oxford that went to the same lectures. Maybe I'm getting trite but I don't want to let my current ideas slide away with a few dozen glasses of beer."

"All right," Franz answered. "You are an American. You can do this without professional harm. I do not like these generalities. Soon you will be writing little books called 'Deep Thoughts for the Layman,' so simplified that they are positively guaranteed not to cause thinking. If my father were alive he would look at you and grunt, Dick. He would take his napkin and fold it so, and hold his napkin ring, this very one—"and he would say, 'Well my impression is—' then he would look at you and think suddenly 'What is the use?' then he would stop and grunt again; then we would be at the end of dinner."

"I am alone to-day," said Dick testily. "But I may not be alone to-morrow. After that I'll fold up my napkin like your father and grunt."

Franz waited a moment.

"How about our patient?" he asked.

"I don't know."

"Well, you should know about her by now."

"I like her. She's attractive. What do you want me to do—take her up in the edelweiss?"

"No, I thought since you go in for scientific books you might have an idea."

"—devote my life to her?"

Franz called his wife in the kitchen: "Du lieber Gott! Bitte, bringe Dick noch ein Glas-Bier."

"I don't want any more if I've got to see Dohmler."

"We think it's best to have a program. Four weeks have passed away—apparently the girl is in love with you. That's not our business if we were in the world, but here in the clinic we have a stake in the matter."

"I'll do whatever Doctor Dohmler says," Dick agreed.

But he had little faith that Dohmler would throw much light on the matter; he himself was the incalculable element involved. By no conscious volition of his own, the thing had drifted into his hands. It reminded him of a scene in his childhood when everyone in the house was looking for the lost key to the silver closet, Dick knowing he had hid it under the handkerchiefs in his mother's top drawer; at that time he had experienced a philosophical detachment, and this was repeated now when he and Franz went together to Professor Dohmler's office.

The professor, his face beautiful under straight whiskers, like a vine-overgrown veranda of some fine old house, disarmed him. Dick knew some individuals with more talent, but no person of a class qualitatively superior to Dohmler.

—Six months later he thought the same way when he saw Dohmler dead, the light out on the veranda, the vines of his whiskers tickling his stiff white collar, the many battles that had swayed before the chink-like eyes stilled forever under the frail delicate lids—

". . . Good morning, sir." He stood formally, thrown back to the army.

Professor Dohmler interlaced his tranquil fingers. Franz spoke in terms half of liaison officer, half of secretary, till his senior cut through him in mid-sentence.

"We have gone a certain way," he said mildly. "It's you, Doctor Diver, who can best help us now."

Routed out, Dick confessed: "I'm not so straight on it myself."

"I have nothing to do with your personal reactions," said Dohmler. "But I have much to do with the fact that this so-called 'transference,' " he darted a short ironic look at Franz which the latter returned in kind, "must be terminated. Miss Nicole does well indeed, but she is in no condition to survive what she might interpret as a tragedy."

Again Franz began to speak, but Doctor Dohmler motioned him silent.

"I realize that your position has been difficult."

"Yes, it has."

Now the professor sat back and laughed, saying on the last syllable of his laughter, with his sharp little gray eyes shining through: "Perhaps you have got sentimentally involved yourself."

Aware that he was being drawn on, Dick, too, laughed.

"She's a pretty girl—anybody responds to that to a certain extent. I have no intention—"

Again Franz tried to speak—again Dohmler stopped him with a question directed pointedly at Dick. "Have you thought of going away?"

"I can't go away."

Doctor Dohmler turned to Franz: "Then we can send Miss Warren away."

"As you think best, Professor Dohmler," Dick conceded. "It's certainly a situation."

Professor Dohmler raised himself like a legless man mounting a pair of crutches.

"But it is a professional situation," he cried quietly.

He sighed himself back into his chair, waiting for the reverberating thunder to die out about the room. Dick saw that Dohmler had reached his climax, and he was not sure that he himself had survived it. When the thunder had diminished Franz managed to get his word in.

"Doctor Diver is a man of fine character," he said. "I feel he only has to appreciate the situation in order to deal correctly with it. In my opinion Dick can co-operate right here, without any one going away."

"How do you feel about that?" Professor Dohmler asked Dick.

Dick felt churlish in the face of the situation; at the same time he realized in the silence after Dohmler's pronouncement that the state of inanimation could not be indefinitely prolonged; suddenly he spilled everything.

"I'm half in love with her—the question of marrying her has passed through my mind."

"Tch! Tch!" uttered Franz.

"Wait." Dohmler warned him. Franz refused to wait: "What! And devote half your life to being doctor and nurse and all—never! I know what these cases are. One time in twenty it's finished in the first push—better never see her again!"

"What do you think?" Dohmler asked Dick.

"Of course Franz is right."

*   *   *

It was late afternoon when they wound up the discussion as to what Dick should do, he must be most kind and yet eliminate himself. When the doctors stood up at last, Dick's eyes fell outside the window to where a light rain was falling—Nicole was waiting, expectant, somewhere in that rain. When, presently, he went out buttoning his oil-skin at the throat, pulling down the brim of his hat, he came upon her immediately under the roof of the main entrance.

"I know a new place we can go," she said. "When I was ill I didn't mind sitting inside with the others in the evening—what they said seemed like everything else. Naturally now I see them as ill and its—its—"

"You'll be leaving soon."

"Oh, soon. My sister, Beth, but she's always been called Baby, she's coming in a few weeks to take me somewhere; after that I'll be back here for a last month."

"The older sister?"

"Oh, quite a bit older. She's twenty-four—she's very English. She lives in London with my father's sister. She was engaged to an Englishman but he was killed—I never saw him.''

Her face, ivory gold against the blurred sunset that strove through the rain, had a promise Dick had never seen before: the high cheek-bones, the faintly wan quality, cool rather than feverish, was reminiscent of the frame of a promising colt—a creature whose life did not promise to be only a projection of youth upon a grayer screen, but instead, a true growing: the face would be handsome in middle life; it would be handsome in old age: the essential structure and the economy were there.

''What are you looking at?''

''I was just thinking that you're going to be rather happy.''

Nicole was frightened: ''Am I? All right—things couldn't be worse than they have been.''

In the covered woodshed to which she had led him, she sat cross-legged upon her golf shoes, her burberry wound about her and her cheeks stung alive by the damp air. Gravely she returned his gaze, taking in his somewhat proud carriage that never quite yielded to the wooden post against which he leaned; she looked into his face that always tried to discipline itself into molds of attentive seriousness, after excursions into joys and mockeries of its own. That part of him which seemed to fit his reddish Irish coloring she knew least; she was afraid of it, yet more anxious to explore—this was his more masculine side: the other part, the trained part, the consideration in the polite eyes, she expropriated without question, as most women did.

''At least this institution has been good for languages,'' said Nicole. ''I've spoken French with two doctors, and German with the nurses, and Italian, or something like it, with a couple of scrub-women and one of the patients, and I've picked up a lot of Spanish from another.''

''That's fine.''

He tried to arrange an attitude but no logic seemed forthcoming.

''—Music too. Hope you didn't think I was only interested in ragtime. I practise every day—the last few months I've been taking a course in Zurich on the history of music. In fact it was all that kept me going at times—music and the drawing.'' She leaned suddenly and twisted a loose strip from the sole of her shoe, and then looked up. ''I'd like to draw you just the way you are now.''

It made him sad when she brought out her accomplishments for his approval.

''I envy you. At present I don't seem to be interested in anything except my work.''

"Oh, I think that's fine for a man," she said quickly. "But for a girl I think she ought to have lots of minor accomplishments and pass them on to her children."

"I suppose so," said Dick with deliberated indifference.

Nicole sat quiet. Dick wished she would speak so that he could play the easy rôle of wet blanket, but now she sat quiet.

"You're all well," he said. "Try to forget the past; don't overdo things for a year or so. Go back to America and be a débutante and fall in love—and be happy."

"I couldn't fall in love." Her injured shoe scraped a cocoon of dust from the log on which she sat.

"Sure you can," Dick insisted. "Not for a year maybe, but sooner or later." Then he added brutally: "You can have a perfectly normal life with a houseful of beautiful descendants. The very fact that you could make a complete comeback at your age proves that the precipitating factors were pretty near everything. Young woman, you'll be pulling your weight long after your friends are carried off screaming."

—But there was a look of pain in her eyes as she took the rough dose, the harsh reminder.

"I know I wouldn't be fit to marry any one for a long time," she said humbly.

Dick was too upset to say any more. He looked out into the grain field trying to recover his hard brassy attitude.

"You'll be all right—everybody here believes in you. Why, Doctor Gregory is so proud of you that he'll probably—"

"I hate Doctor Gregory."

"Well, you shouldn't."

Nicole's world had fallen to pieces, but it was only a flimsy and scarcely created world; beneath it her emotions and instincts fought on. Was it an hour ago she had waited by the entrance, wearing her hope like a corsage at her belt?

. . . Dress stay crisp for him, button stay put, bloom narcissus—air stay still and sweet.

"It will be nice to have fun again," she fumbled on. For a moment she entertained a desperate idea of telling him how rich she was, what big houses she lived in, that really she was a valuable property—for a moment she made herself into her grandfather, Sid Warren, the horse-trader. But she survived the temptation to confuse all values and shut these matters into their Victorian side-chambers—even though there was no home left to her, save emptiness and pain.

"I have to go back to the clinic. It's not raining now."

Dick walked beside her, feeling her unhappiness, and wanting to drink the rain that touched her cheek.

*   *   *

"Now of course we have lots of connections there—Father controls certain chairs and fellowships and so forth at the University, and I thought if we took Nicole home and threw her with that crowd—you see she's quite musical and speaks all these languages—what could be better in her condition than if she fell in love with some good doctor—"

A burst of hilarity surged up in Dick, the Warrens were going to buy Nicole a doctor—You got a nice doctor you can let us use? There was no use worrying about Nicole when they were in the position of being able to buy her a nice young doctor, the paint scarcely dry on him.

"But how about the doctor?" he said automatically.

"There must be many who'd jump at the chance."

The dancers were back, but Baby whispered quickly:

"This is the sort of thing I mean. Now where is Nicole—she's gone off somewhere. Is she upstairs in her room? What am *I* supposed to do? I never know whether it's something innocent or whether I ought to go find her."

"Perhaps she just wants to be by herself—people living alone get used to loneliness." Seeing that Miss Warren was not listening he stopped, "I'll take a look around."

For a moment all the outdoors shut in with mist was like spring with the curtains drawn. Life was gathered near the hotel. Dick passed some cellar windows where bus boys sat on bunks and played cards over a litre of Spanish wine. As he approached the promenade, the stars began to come through the white crests of the high Alps. On the horseshoe walk overlooking the lake Nicole was the figure motionless between two lamp stands, and he approached silently across the grass. She turned to him with an expression of: "Here *you* are," and for a moment he was sorry he had come.

"Your sister wondered."

"Oh!" She was accustomed to being watched. With an effort she explained herself: "Sometimes I get a little—it gets a little too much. I've lived so quietly. To-night that music was too much. It made me want to cry—"

"I understand."

"This has been an awfully exciting day."

"I know."

"I don't want to do anything anti-social—I've caused everybody enough trouble. But to-night I wanted to get away."

It occurred to Dick suddenly, as it might occur to a dying man that he had forgotten to tell where his will was, that Nicole had been "re-educated" by Dohmler and the ghostly generations behind him; it occurred to him also that there would be so much she would have to be told. But having recorded this wisdom within himself, he yielded to the insistent face-value of the situation and said:

"You're a nice person—just keep using your own judgment about yourself."

"You like me?"

"Of course."

"Would you—" They were strolling along toward the dim end of the horseshoe, two hundred yards ahead. "If I hadn't been sick would you—I mean, would I have been the sort of girl you might have—oh, slush, you know what I mean."

He was in for it now, possessed by a vast irrationality. She was so near that he felt his breathing change but again his training came to his aid in a boy's laugh and a trite remark.

"You're teasing yourself, my dear. Once I knew a man who fell in love with his nurse—" The anecdote rambled on, punctuated by their footsteps. Suddenly Nicole interrupted in succinct Chicagoese: "Bull!"

"That's a very vulgar expression."

"What about it?" she flared up. "You don't think I've got any common sense—before I was sick I didn't have any, but I have now. And if I don't know you're the most attractive man I ever met you must think I'm still crazy. It's my hard luck, all right—but don't pretend I don't *know*—I know everything about you and me."

Dick was at an additional disadvantage. He remembered the statement of the elder Miss Warren as to the young doctors that could be purchased in the intellectual stockyards of the South Side of Chicago, and he hardened for a moment. "You're a fetching kid, but I couldn't fall in love."

"You won't give me a chance."

"*What!*"

The impertinence, the right to invade implied, astounded him. Short of anarchy he could not think of any chance that Nicole Warren deserved.

"Give me a chance now."

The voice fell low, sank into her breast and stretched the tight bodice over her heart as she came up close. He felt the young lips, her body sighing in relief against the arm growing stronger to hold her. There were now no more plans than if Dick had arbitrarily made some indissoluble mixture, with atoms joined and inseparable; you could throw it all out but never again could they fit back into atomic scale. As he held her and tasted her, and as she curved in further and further toward him, with her own lips, new to herself, drowned and engulfed in love, yet solaced and triumphant, he was thankful to have an existence at all, if only as a reflection in her wet eyes.

"My God," he gasped, "you're fun to kiss."

That was talk, but Nicole had a better hold on him now and she held it; she turned coquette and walked away, leaving him as suspended as in the funicular of the afternoon. She felt: There, that'll show him, how conceited; how he could do with me; oh, wasn't it wonderful! I've got him, he's mine. Now in the sequence came flight, but it was all so sweet and new that she dawdled, wanting to draw all of it in.

She shivered suddenly. Two thousand feet below she saw the necklace and bracelet of lights that were Montreux and Vevey, beyond them a dim pendant of Lausanne. From down there somewhere ascended a faint sound of dance music. Nicole was up in her head now, cool as cool, trying to collate the sentimentalities of her childhood, as deliberate as a man getting drunk after battle. But she was still afraid of Dick, who stood near her, leaning, characteristically, against the iron fence that rimmed the horseshoe; and this prompted her to say: "I can remember how I stood waiting for you in the garden—holding all my self in my arms like a basket of flowers. It was that to me anyhow—I thought I was sweet—waiting to hand that basket to you."

He breathed over her shoulder and turned her insistently about; she kissed him several times, her face getting big every time she came close, her hands holding him by the shoulders.

"It's raining hard."

ALBERT SCHWEITZER
Out of My Life and Thought

———————◆◇◆———————

ALBERT SCHWEITZER (1875-1965), Alsatian-born philosopher, physician, and musician, made his career as a medical missionary in Africa a Christian witness to his belief in service to his fellow human beings. He is widely regarded as one of the giant moral figures of the twentieth century. He founded a jungle hospital in Lambarene, Gabon, in what was then French Equatorial Africa, based on his concept of "reverence for life." Those three words were a crystallization of a philosophy that stands out in marked contrast to the dominant violent trends of contemporary society. Some visitors to his hospital have criticized him for his autocratic attitude toward the blacks and for the crude condition of his clinic. Those critics have missed the point. Schweitzer never set out to build a model hospital. All he tried to do was to bear witness to the principle that each individual has both the responsibility and the ability to use his life to moral advantage.

Two perceptions cast their shadows over my existence. One consists in my realization that the world is inexplicably mysterious and full of suffering; the other in the fact that I have been born into a period of spiritual decadence in mankind. I have become familiar with and ready to deal with each, through the thinking which has led me to the ethical and affirmative position of Reverence for Life. In that principle my life has found a firm footing and a clear path to follow.

I therefore stand and work in the world as one who aims at making men less shallow and morally better by making them think.

With the spirit of the age I am in complete disagreement, because it is filled with disdain for thinking. That such is its attitude is, to some extent, to be explained by the fact that thought has never yet reached the goal which it must set before itself. Time after time it was convinced that it had clearly established an attitude toward life which was in accordance with knowledge and ethically satisfactory. But time after time the truth came out that it had not succeeded.

Doubts, therefore, could well arise as to whether thinking would ever be capable of answering current questions about the world and our relation to it in such a way that we could give a meaning and a content to our lives.

But today in addition to that neglect of thought there is also prevalent a mistrust of it. The organized political, social, and religious associations of our time are at work to induce the individual man not to arrive at his convictions by his own thinking but to make his own such convictions as they keep ready made for him. Any man who thinks for himself and at the same time is spiritually free, is to them something inconvenient and even uncanny. He does not offer sufficient guarantee that he will merge himself in their organization in the way they wish. All corporate bodies look today for their strength not so much to the spiritual worth of the ideas which they represent and to that of the people who belong to them, as to the attainment of the highest possible degree of unity and exclusiveness. It is in this that they expect to find their strongest power for offense and defense.

Hence the spirit of the age rejoices, instead of lamenting, that thinking seems to be unequal to its task, and gives it no credit for what, in spite of imperfections, it has already accomplished. It refuses to admit, what is nevertheless the fact, that all spiritual progress up to today has come about through the achievement of thought, or to reflect that thinking may still be able in the future to accomplish what it has not succeeded in accomplishing as yet. Of such considerations the spirit of the age takes no account. Its only concern is to discredit individual thinking in every possible way, and it deals with that on the lines of the saying: "Whosoever hath not, from him shall be taken away even that which he hath."

Thus, his whole life long, the man of today is exposed to influences which are bent on robbing him of all confidence in his own thinking. The spirit of spiritual dependence to which he is called on to surrender is in everything that he hears or reads; it is in the people whom he meets every day; it is in the parties and associations which have claimed him as their own; it pervades all the circumstances of his life.

From every side and in the most varied ways it is dinned into him that the truths and convictions which he needs for life must be taken by him from the associations which have rights over him. The spirit of the age never lets him come to himself. Over and over again convictions are forced upon him in the same way as, by means of the electric advertisements which flare in the streets of every large town, any company which has sufficient capital to get itself securely established, exercises pressure on him at every step he takes to induce him to buy their boot polish or their soup tablets.

By the spirit of the age, then, the man of today is forced into skepticism about his own thinking, in order to make him receptive to truth which comes to him from authority. To all this constant influence he cannot make the resistance that is desirable because he is an overworked and distracted being without power to concentrate. Moreover, the manifold material trammels which are his lot work upon his mentality in such a way that he comes at last to believe himself unqualified even to make any claim to thoughts of his own.

His self-confidence is also diminished through the pressure exercised upon him by the huge and daily increasing mass of knowledge. He is no longer in a position to take in as something which he has grasped all the new discoveries that are constantly announced; he has to accept them as fact although he does not understand them. This being his relation to scientific truth he is tempted to acquiesce in the idea that in matters of thought also his judgment cannot be trusted.

Thus do the circumstances of the age do their best to deliver us up to the spirit of the age.

The seed of skepticism has germinated. In fact, the modern man has no longer any spiritual self-confidence at all. Behind a self-confident exterior he conceals a great inward lack of confidence. In spite of his great capacity in material matters he is an altogether stunted being, because he makes no use of his capacity for thinking. It will ever remain incomprehensible that our generation, which has shown itself so great by its achievements in discovery and invention, could fall so low spiritually as to give up thinking.

In a period which regards as absurd and little worth, as antiquated and long ago left far behind, whatever it feels to be in any way akin to rationalism or free thought, and which even mocks at the vindication of unalienable human rights which was secured in the eighteenth century, I acknowledge myself to be one who places all his confidence in rational thinking. I venture to say to our generation that it must not think it has done with rationalism because the rationalism of the past had to give first place to romanticism, and then to a *Realpolitik* which is coming to dominate the spiritual sphere as well as the material. When it has run the gauntlet of the follies of this universal *Realpolitik* and has thereby got itself into deeper and deeper misery, both spiritual and material, it will discover at last that there is nothing for it to do but trust itself to a new rationalism, deeper and more efficient than the old, and in that seek its salvation.

Renunciation of thinking is a declaration of spiritual bankruptcy. Where there is no longer a conviction that men can get to know the truth by their own thinking, skepticism begins. Those who work to make our age skeptical in this way, do so in the expectation that, as a result of denouncing all hope of self-discovered truth, men will end by accepting as truth what is forced upon them with authority and by propaganda.

But their calculations are wrong. No one who opens the sluices to let a flood of skepticism pour itself over the land must expect to be able to bring it back within its proper bounds. Of those who let themselves get too disheartened to try any longer to discover truth by their own thinking, only a few find a substitute for it in truth taken from others. The mass of people remain skeptical. They lose all feeling for truth, and all sense of need for it as well, finding themselves quite comfortable in a life without thought driven now here, now there, from one opinion to another.

But the acceptance of authoritative truth, even if that truth has both spiritual and ethical content, does not bring skepticism to an end; it merely covers it up. Man's unnatural condition of not believing that any truth is discoverable by himself, continues, and produces its natural results. The city of truth cannot be built on the swampy ground of skepticism. Our spiritual life is rotten throughout because it is permeated through and through with skepticism, and we live in consequence in a world which in every respect is full of falsehood. We are not far from shipwreck on the rock of wanting to have even truth organized.

Truth taken over by skepticism which has become believing has not the spiritual qualities of that which originated in thinking. It has been externalized and rendered torpid. It does obtain influence over a man, but it is not capable of uniting itself with him to the very marrow of his being. Living truth is that alone which has its origin in thinking.

Just as a tree bears year after year the same fruit and yet fruit which is each year new, so must all permanently valuable ideas be continually born again in thought. But our age is bent on trying to make the barren tree of skepticism fruitful by tying fruits of truth on its branches.

It is only by confidence in our ability to reach truth by our own individual thinking, that we are capable of accepting truth from outside. Unfettered thought, provided it be deep, never degenerates into subjectivity. With its own ideas it stirs those within itself which enjoy any traditional credit for being true, and exerts itself to be able to possess them as knowledge.

Not less strong than the will to truth must be the will to sincerity. Only an age which can show the courage of sincerity can possess truth which works as a spiritual force within it.

Sincerity is the foundation of the spiritual life.

With its depreciation of thinking our generation has lost its feeling for sincerity and with it that for truth as well. It can therefore be helped only by its being brought once more on to the road of thinking.

Because I have this certainty I oppose the spirit of the age, and take upon myself with confidence the responsibility of taking my part in the rekindling of the fire of thought.

Thought on the lines of Reverence for Life is by its very nature peculiarly qualified to take up the struggle against skepticism. It is elemental.

Elemental thinking is that which starts from the fundamental questions about the relations of man to the universe, about the meaning of life, and about the nature of goodness. It stands in the most immediate connection with the thinking which impulse stirs in everyone. It enters into that thinking, widening and deepening it.

Such elemental thinking we find in Stoicism. When as a student I began going through the history of philosophy I found it difficult to tear myself away from Stoicism, and to pursue my way through the utterly different thinking which succeeded it. It is true that the results produced by Stoic thought were far from satisfying me, but I had the feeling that this simple kind of philosophizing was the right one, and I could not understand how people had come to abandon it.

Stoicism seemed to me great in that it goes straight for its goal; that it is universally intelligible, and is at the same time profound; that it makes the best of the truth which it recognizes as such, even if it is unsatisfying; that it puts life into such truth by the earnestness with which it devotes itself to it; that it possesses the spirit of sincerity; that it urges men to collect their thoughts, and to become more inward; and that it arouses in them the sense of responsibility. I felt, too, that the fundamental thought of Stoicism is true, namely that man must bring himself into a spiritual relation with the world, and become one with it. In its essence Stoicism is a nature philosophy which ends in mysticism.

Just as I felt Stoic thinking to be elemental, so I felt that of Lao-tse to be the same, when I became acquainted with his Tao-te-King. For him, too, the important thing is that man shall come, by simple thinking, into a spiritual relation to the world, and prove his unity with it by his life.

There is, therefore, an essential relationship between Greek Stoicism and Chinese. The only distinction between them is that the former had its origin in well-developed, logical thinking, the latter in intuitive thinking which was undeveloped and yet marvelously profound.

This elemental thinking, however, which emerges in European as in extra-European philosophy, is unable to retain the leadership it has won; it must resign that position to the unelemental. It proves a failure because its results are not satisfying. It cannot see any meaning in the impulse to activity and to ethical deeds which is contained in the will-to-live of the spiritually developed man. Hence Greek Stoicism gets no further than the ideal of resignation, Lao-tse no further than the kindly inactivity which to us Europeans seems so curious.

The ultimate explanation of the history of philosophy is that the ideas based on ethical acceptance of the world which are natural to man can never acquiesce contentedly in the results of simple logical thinking about man and his relation to the universe, because they cannot fit themselves into it properly. They therefore compel thinking to take a roundabout way, along which they hope to reach their goal. Thus there arises side by side with elemental thinking an unelemental, in various forms, which grows up round the other and often entirely conceals it.

These roundabout roads which thinking takes lead especially in the direction of attempted explanation of the world which shall represent the will to ethical activity in the world as purposive. In the late Stoicism of an Epictetus and a Marcus Aurelius, in the Rationalism of the eighteenth century, and in that of Kung-tse (Confucius), Mengtse (Mencius), Mi-tse (Micius), and other Chinese thinkers, the philosophy which starts from the elemental problem of the relation of man to the world reaches a theory of ethical world acceptance by tracing the course of world events back to a world-will with ethical aims, and claiming man for service to it. In the thinking of Brahmanism, and of the Buddha, as in the Indian systems generally, and in the philosophy of Schopenhauer, the opposite explanation of the world is put forward, namely that the Life which runs its course in space and time is purposeless, and must be brought to an end. The sensible attitude of man to the world is therefore to die to the world and to life.

Side by side with this form of thinking which, so far, at any rate, as its starting point and its interests are concerned, has remained elemental, there enters the field, especially in European philosophy, another form which is completely unelemental in that it no longer has as its central point the question of man's relation to the world. It busies itself with the problem of the nature of knowledge, with logical speculations, with natural science, with psychology, with sociology, and with other things, as if philosophy were really concerned with the solution of all these questions for their own sake, or as if itself consisted merely in the sifting and systematizing of the results of the various sciences. Instead of urging man to constant meditation on himself and his relation to the world, this philosophy presents him with results of epistemology, of logical speculation, of natural science, of psychology, or of sociology, as matters according to which alone he is to shape his view of his life and his relation to the world. On all these things it discourses to him as if he were not a being who is in the world and lives his life in it, but one who is stationed near it, and contemplates it from the outside.

Because it approaches the problem of the relation of man to the universe from some arbitrarily chosen standpoint, or perhaps passes it by altogether, this unelemental European philosophy lacks unity and consistency, and shows itself more or less restless, artificial, eccentric, and fragmentary. At the same time, it is the richest and most universal. In its systems, half-systems, and no-systems, which succeed and interpenetrate each other, it is able to contemplate the problem of a philosophy of civilization from every side, and in every possible perspective. It is also the most practical in that it deals with the natural sciences, history, and ethical questions more profoundly than the others do.

The world philosophy of the future will owe its origin less to efforts to reconcile European and non-European thought than to those made to reconcile elemental and unelemental thinking.

From the intellectual life of our time mysticism stands aside. It is in essence a form of elemental thinking, because it is directly occupied in enabling the individual man to put himself into a spiritual relation with the world. It despairs, however, of this being possible by means of logical thinking, and falls back on intuition, within which imagination can be active. In a certain sense, then, the mysticism also of the past goes back to a mode of thinking which tries roundabout routes. Since with us only that knowledge which is a result of logical thinking is accepted as truth, the convictions which make up the mysticism above described, cannot become our spiritual possession in the form in which they are expressed and declared to be proved. Moreover, they are not in themselves satisfying. Of all the mysticism of the past it must be said that its ethical content is too slight. It puts men on the road of inwardness, but not on that of a living ethic. The truth of a view of the world must be proved by the fact that the spiritual relation to life and the universe into which that view brings us makes us into inward men with an active ethic.

Against the lack of thought, then, which characterizes our age nothing effective can be done either by the unelemental thinking which takes the roundabout route in the explanation of the world, or by mystical intuition. Power over skepticism is given only to that elemental thinking which takes up and develops the simple thinking which is natural in all men. The unelemental thinking on the other hand, which sets before men certain results of thinking at which it has in one way or another arrived, is not in a position to sustain their own thinking, but takes it from them in order to put another kind in its place. This acceptance of another kind of thinking means a disturbance and weakening of one's own. It is a step towards the acceptance of truth from outside, and thus a step toward skepticism. It was in this way that the great systems of German philosophy which when they appeared were taken up with such enthusiasm, prepared at the beginning of the nineteenth century the ground upon which later on skepticism developed.

To make men thinking beings once more, then, means to make them resort to their own way of thinking that they may try to secure that knowledge which they need for living. In the thinking which starts from Reverence for Life there is to be found a renewal of elemental thinking. The stream which has been flowing for a long distance underground comes again to the surface.

The belief that elemental thinking is now arriving at an ethical and affirmative attitude toward the world and life, which it has hitherto vainly striven to reach, is no self-deception, but is connected with the fact that thinking has become thoroughly realistic.

It used to deal with the world as being only a totality of happenings. With this totality of happenings the only spiritual relation which man can reach is one in which, acknowledging his own natural subordination to it, he secures a spiritual position under it by resignation. To attribute any meaning and purpose to his own activities is impossible with such a conception of the world. He cannot possibly place himself at the service of this totality of happenings which crushes him. His way to acceptance of the world and to ethics is barred.

It thereupon attempts, but in vain, to grasp by means of some sort of explanation of the world what elemental thinking, hindered by this lifeless and incomplete representation of the world, cannot reach in the natural way. This thinking is like a river which on its way to the sea is held up by a range of mountains. Its waters try to find a passage to the sea by roundabout ways. In vain. They only pour themselves into other valleys and fill them. Then, centuries later, the dammed up waters manage to break through.

The world does not consist of happenings only; it contains life as well, and to the life in the world, so far as it comes within my reach, I have to be in a relation which is not only passive but active. By placing myself in the service of that which lives I reach an activity, exerted, upon the world which has meaning and purpose.

However simple and obvious a proceeding it may seem to be when once accomplished, to replace that lifeless idea of the world by a real world which is full of life, a long period of evolution was needed, nevertheless, before it became possible. Just as the solid rock of a mountain range which has risen from the sea first becomes visible when the layers of chalk which covered it have been eroded and washed away by the rain, so, in questions of philosophy, is realistic thinking overlaid by unrealistic.

The idea of Reverence for Life offers itself as the realistic answer to the realistic question of how man and the world are related to each other. Of the world man knows only that everything which exists is, like himself, a manifestation of the Will-to-Live. With this world he stands in a relation of passivity and of activity. On the one hand he is subordinate to the course of events which is given in this totality of life; on the other hand he is capable of affecting the life which comes within his reach by hampering or promoting it, by destroying or maintaining it.

The one possible way of giving meaning to his existence is that of raising his natural relation to the world to a spiritual one. As a being in a passive relation to the world he comes into a spiritual relation to it by resignation. True resignation consists in this: that man, feeling his subordination to the course of world happenings, wins his way to inward freedom from the fortunes which shape the outside of his existence. Inward freedom means that he finds strength to deal with everything that is hard in his lot, in such a way that it all helps to make him a deeper and more inward person, to purify him, and to keep him calm and peaceful. Resignation, therefore, is the spiritual and ethical affirmation of one's own existence. Only he who has gone through the stage of resignation is capable of accepting the world.

As a being in an active relation to the world he comes into a spiritual relation with it by not living for himself alone, but feeling himself one with all life that comes within his reach. He will feel all that life's experiences as his own, he will give it all the help that he possibly can, and will feel all the saving and promotion of life that he has been able to effect as the deepest happiness that can ever fall to his lot.

Let a man once begin to think about the mystery of his life and the links which connect him with the life that fills the world, and he cannot but bring to bear upon his own life and all other life that comes within his reach the principle of Reverence for Life, and manifest this principle by ethical affirmation of life. Existence will thereby become harder for him in every respect than it would be if he lived for himself, but at the same time it will be richer, more beautiful, and happier. It will become, instead of mere living, a real experience of life.

Beginning to think about life and the world leads a man directly and almost irresistibly to Reverence for Life. Such thinking leads to no conclusions which could point in any other direction.

If the man who has once begun to think wishes to persist in his mere living he can do so only by surrendering himself, whenever this idea takes possession of him, to thoughtlessness, and stupefying himself therein. If he perseveres with thinking he can come to no other result than Reverence for Life.

Any thinking by which men assert that they are reaching skepticism or life without ethical ideals, is not thinking but thoughtlessness which poses as thinking, and it proves itself to be such by the fact that it is unconcerned about the mystery of life and the world.

Reverence for Life contains in itself resignation, an affirmative attitude toward the world, and ethics—the three essential elements in a philosophy of life, as mutually interrelated results of thinking.

Up to now there have been systems of thought based on resignation, others based on an affirmative view of the world and still others that sought to satisfy ethics. Not one has there been, however, which has been able to combine the three elements. That is possible only on condition that all three are conceived as essentially products of the universal conviction of Reverence for Life, and are recognized as being one and all contained in it. Resignation and an affirmative view of the world have no separate existence of their own by the side of ethics; they are its lower octaves.

Having its origin in realistic thinking, the ethic of Reverence for Life is realistic, and brings man to a realistic and steady facing of reality.

It may seem, at first glance, as if Reverence for Life were something too general and too lifeless to provide the content of a living ethic. But thinking has no need to trouble as to whether its expressions sound living enough, so long as they hit the mark and have life in them. Anyone who comes under the influence of the ethic of Reverence for Life will very soon be able to detect, thanks to what that ethic demands from him, what fire glows in the lifeless expression. The ethic of Reverence for Life is the ethic of Love widened into universality. It is the ethic of Jesus, now recognized as a logical consequence of thought.

Objection is made to this ethic that it sets too high a value on natural life. To this it can retort that the mistake made by all previous systems of ethics has been the failure to recognize that life as such is the mysterious value with which they have to deal. All spiritual life meets us within natural life. Reverence for Life, therefore, is applied to natural life and spiritual life alike. In the parable of Jesus, the shepherd saves not merely the soul of the lost sheep but the whole animal. The stronger the reverence for natural life, the stronger grows also that for spiritual life.

The ethic of Reverence for Life is found particularly strange because it establishes no dividing line between higher and lower, between more valuable and less valuable life. For this omission it has its reasons.

To undertake to lay down universally valid distinctions of value between different kinds of life will end in judging them by the greater or lesser distance at which they seem to stand from us human beings—as we ourselves judge. But that is a purely subjective criterion. Who among us knows what significance any other kind of life has in itself, and as a part of the universe?

Following on such a distinction there comes next the view that there can be life which is worthless, injury to which or destruction of which does not matter. Then in the category of worthless life we come to include, according to circumstances, different kinds of insects, or primitive peoples.

To the man who is truly ethical all life is sacred, including that which from the human point of view seems lower in the scale. He makes distinctions only as each case comes before him, and under the pressure of necessity, as, for example, when it falls to him to decide which of two lives he must sacrifice in order to preserve the other. But all through this series of decisions he is conscious of acting on subjective grounds and arbitrarily, and knows that he bears the responsibility for the life which is sacrificed.

I rejoice over the new remedies for sleeping sickness, which enable me to preserve life, whereas I had previously to watch a painful disease. But every time I have under the microscope the germs which cause the disease, I cannot but reflect that I have to sacrifice this life in order to save other life.

I buy from natives a young fish eagle, which they have caught on a sandbank, in order to rescue it from their cruel hands. But now I have to decide whether I shall let it starve, or kill every day a number of small fishes, in order to keep it alive. I decide on the latter course, but every day I feel it hard that this life must be sacrificed for the other on my responsibility.

Standing, as he does, with the whole body of living creatures under the law of this dilemma (*Selbstentzweiung*) in the will-to-live, man comes again and again into the position of being able to preserve his own life and life generally only at the cost of other life. If he has been touched by the ethic of Reverence for Life, he injures and destroys life only under a necessity which he cannot avoid, and never from thoughtlessness. So far as he is a free man he uses every opportunity of tasting the blessedness of being able to assist life and avert from it suffering and destruction.

Devoted as I was from boyhood to the cause of the protection of animal life, it is a special joy to me that the universal ethic of Reverence for Life shows the sympathy with .animals which is so often represented as sentimentality, to be a duty which no thinking man can escape. Hitherto ethics have faced the problem of man and beast either uncomprehending or helpless. Even when sympathy with the animal creation was felt to be right, it could not be brought within the scope of ethics, because ethics were really focused only on the behavior of man to man.

When will the time come when public opinion will tolerate no longer any popular amusements which depend on the ill-treatment of animals!

The ethic, then, which originates in thinking is not "according to reason," but nonrational and enthusiastic. It marks off no skillfully defined circle of duties, but lays upon each individual the responsibility for all life within his reach, and compels him to devote himself to helping it.

Any profound view of the world is mysticism, in that it brings men into a spiritual relation with the Infinite. The view of Reverence for Life is ethical mysticism. It allows union with the infinite to be realized by ethical action. This ethical mysticism originates in logical thinking. If our will-to-live begins to think about itself and the world, we come to experience the life of the world, so far as it comes within our reach, in our own life, and to devote our will-to-live to the infinite will-to-live through the deeds we do. Rational thinking, if it goes deep, ends of necessity in the nonrational of mysticism. It has, of course, to deal with life and the world, both of which are nonrational entities.

In the world the infinite will-to-live reveals itself to us as will-to-create, and this is full of dark and painful riddles for us; in ourselves it is revealed as will-to-love, which will through us remove the dilemma (*Selbstentzweiung*) of the will-to-live.

The concept of Reverence for Life has, therefore, a religious character. The man who avows his belief in it, and acts upon the belief, shows a piety which is elemental.

SIR WALTER SCOTT
The Talisman

———⌁———

SIR WALTER SCOTT (1771-1832) was well-acquainted with medical practice, having been crippled by infantile paralysis and having suffered other major illnesses throughout his life. His reputation as a novelist was based largely on the Waverley Novels, including *The Talisman,* but his exhaustive biographies of Dryden, Swift, and Napoleon are tributes to his literary scholarship.

The celebrated Master of the Templars was a tall, thin, war-worn man, with a slow yet penetrating eye, and a brow on which a thousand dark intrigues had stamped a portion of their obscurity. At the head of that singular body, to whom their Order was everything and their individuality nothing—seeking the advancement of its power, even at the hazard of that very religion which the fraternity were originally associated to protect—accused of heresy and witchcraft, although by their character Christian priests—suspected of secret league with the Soldan, though by oath devoted to the protection of the Holy Temple, or its recovery—the whole Order, and the whole personal character of its commander, or Grand Master, was a riddle, at the exposition of which most men shuddered. The Grand Master was dressed in his white robes of solemnity, and he bare the *abacus,* a mystic staff of office, the peculiar form of which has given rise to such singular conjectures and commentaries, leading to suspicions that this celebrated fraternity of Christian knights were embodied under the foulest symbols of paganism.

Conrade of Montserrat had a much more pleasing exterior than the dark and mysterious priest-soldier by whom he was accompanied. He was a handsome man, of middle age, or something past that term, bold in the field, sagacious in council, gay and gallant in times of festivity; but, on the other hand, he was generally accused of versatility, of a narrow and selfish ambition, of a desire to extend his own principality, without regard to the weal of the Latin kingdom of Palestine, and of seeking his own interest, by private negotiations with Saladin, to the prejudice of the Christian leaguers.

When the usual salutations had been made by these dignitaries, and courteously returned by King Richard, the Marquis of Montserrat commenced an explanation of the motives of their visit, sent, as he said they were, by the anxious kings and princes who composed the Council of the Crusaders, "to inquire into the health of their magnanimous ally, the valiant King of England."

"We know the importance in which the princes of the Council hold our health," replied the English King, "and are well aware how much they must have suffered by suppressing all curiosity concerning it for fourteen days, for fear, doubtless, of aggravating our disorder, by showing their anxiety regarding the event."

The flow of the Marquis's eloquence being checked, and he himself thrown into some confusion, by this reply, his more austere companion took up the thread of the conversation, and, with as much dry and brief gravity as was consistent with the presence which he addressed, informed the King that they came from the Council, to pray, in the name of Christendom, "that he would not suffer his health to be tampered with by an infidel physician, said to be despatched by Saladin, until the Council had taken measures to remove or confirm the suspicion which they at present conceived did attach itself to the mission of such a person."

"Grand Master of the holy and valiant Order of Knights Templars, and you, most noble Marquis of Montserrat," replied Richard, "if it please you to retire into the adjoining pavilion, you shall presently see what account we make of the tender remonstrances of our royal and princely colleagues in this religious warfare."

The Marquis and Grand Master retired accordingly; nor had they been many minutes in the outward pavilion when the Eastern physician arrived, accompanied by the Baron of Gilsland and Kenneth of Scotland. The baron, however, was a little later of entering the tent than the other two, stopping, perchance, to issue some orders to the warders without.

As the Arabian physician entered, he made his obeisance, after the Oriental fashion, to the Marquis and Grand Master, whose dignity was apparent, both from their appearance and their bearing. The Grand Master returned the salutation with an expression of disdainful coldness; the Marquis, with the popular courtesy which he habitually practised to men of every rank and nation. There was a pause; for the Scottish knight, waiting for the arrival of De Vaux, presumed not, of his own authority, to enter the tent of the King of England, and, during this interval, the Grand Master sternly demanded of the Moslem, "Infidel, hast thou the courage to practise thine art upon the person of an anointed sovereign of the Christian host?"

"The sun of Allah," answered the sage, "shines on the Nazarene as well as on the true believer, and his servant dare make no distinction betwixt them, when called on to exercise the art of healing."

"Misbelieving Hakim," said the Grand Master, "or whatsoever they call thee for an unbaptised slave of darkness, dost thou well know that thou shalt be torn asunder by wild horses should King Richard die under thy charge?"

"That were hard justice," answered the physician, "seeing that I can but use human means, and that the issue is written in the book of light."

"Nay, reverend and valiant Grand Master," said the Marquis of Montserrat, "consider that this learned man is not acquainted with our Christian Order, adopted in the fear of God, and for the safety of his anointed. Be it known to thee, grave physician, whose skill we doubt not, that your wisest course is to repair to the presence of the illustrious Council of our Holy League, and there to give account and reckoning to such wise and learned leeches as they shall nominate concerning your means of process and cure of this illustrious patient; so shall you escape all the danger which, rashly taking such a high matter upon your sole answer, you may else most likely incur."

"My lords," said El Hakim, "I understand you well. But knowledge hath its champions as well as your military art—nay, hath sometimes had its martyrs as well as religion. I have the command of my sovereign, the Soldan Saladin, to heal this Nazarene king, and, with the blessing of the Prophet, I will obey his commands. If I fail, ye wear swords thirsting for the blood of the faithful, and I proffer my body to your weapons. But I will not reason with one uncircumcised upon the virtue of the medicines of which I have obtained knowledge through the grace of the Prophet, and I pray you interpose no delay between me and my office."

"Who talks of delay?" said the Baron de Vaux, hastily entering the tent. "We have had but too much already. I salute you, my Lord of Montserrat, and you, valiant Grand Master. But I must presently pass with this learned physician to the bedside of my master."

"My lord," said the Marquis, in Norman-French, or the language of Quie, as it was then called, "are you well advised that we came to expostulate, on the part of the Council of the monarchs and princes of the Crusade, against the risk of permitting an infidel and Eastern physician to tamper with a health so valuable as that of your master King Richard?"

"Noble lord Marquis," replied the Englishman, bluntly, "I can neither use many words, nor do I delight in listening to them—moreover, I am much more ready to believe what my eyes have seen than what my ears have heard. I am satisfied that this heathen can cure the sickness of King

Richard, and I believe and trust he will labour to do so. Time is precious. If Mohammed—may God's curse be on him!—stood at the door of the tent, with such fair purpose as this Adonbec el Hakim entertains, I would hold it sin to delay him for a minute. So, give ye God'en, my lords."

"Nay, but," said Conrade of Montserrat, "the King himself said we should be present when this same physician dealt upon him."

The baron whispered the chamberlain, probably to know whether the Marquis spoke truly, and then replied, "My lords, if you will hold your patience, you are welcome to enter with us; but if you interrupt, by action or threat, this accomplished physician in his duty, be it known that, without respect to your high quality, I will enforce your absence from Richard's tent; for know, I am so well satisfied of the virtue of this man's medicines, that were Richard himself to refuse them, by Our Lady of Lanercost, I think I could find in my heart to force him to take the means of his cure whether he would or no. Move onward, El Hakim."

The last word was spoken in the *lingua franca,* and instantly obeyed by the physician. The Grand Master looked grimly on the unceremonious old soldier, but, on exchanging a glance with the Marquis, smoothed his frowning brow as well as he could, and both followed De Vaux and the Arabian into the inner tent, where Richard lay expecting them, with that impatience with which the sick man watches the step of his physician. Sir Kenneth, whose attendance seemed neither asked nor prohibited, felt himself, by the circumstances in which he stood, entitled to follow these high dignitaries, but, concious of his inferior power and rank, remained aloof during the scene which took place.

Richard, when they entered his apartment, immediately exclaimed, "So ho! a goodly fellowship come to see Richard take his leap in the dark. My noble allies, I greet you as the representatives of our assembled league; Richard will again be amongst you in his former fashion, or ye shall bear to the grave what is left of him. De Vaux, lives he or dies he, thou hast the thanks of thy prince. There is yet another—but this fever hath wasted my eyesight! What, the bold Scot, who would climb heaven without a ladder? He is welcome too. Come, Sir Hakim, to the work, to the work!"

The physician, who had already informed himself of the various symptoms of the King's illness, now felt his pulse for a long time, with deep attention, while all around stood silent, and in breathless expectation. The sage next filled a cup with spring water, and dipped into it the small red purse, which, as formerly, he took from his bosom. When he seemed to think it sufficiently medicated, he was about to offer it to the sovereign, who prevented him, by saying, "Hold an instant! Thou hast felt my pulse—let me lay my finger on thine. I too, as becomes a good knight, know something of thine art.''

The Arabian yielded his hand without hesitation, and his long slender dark fingers were, for an instant, enclosed, and almost buried, in the large enfoldment of King Richard's hand.

''His blood beats calm as an infant's,'' said the King; ''so throb not theirs who poison princes. De Vaux, whether we live or die, dismiss this Hakim with honour and safety. Commend us, friend, to the noble Saladin. Should I die, it is without doubt of his faith—should I live, it will be to thank him as a warrior would desire to be thanked.''

He then raised himself in bed, took the cup in his hand, and, turning to the Marquis and the Grand Master, ''Mark what I say, and let my royal brethren pledge me in Cyprus wine—'To the immortal honour of the first Crusader who shall strike lance or sword on the gate of Jerusalem; and to the shame and eternal infamy of whomsoever shall turn back from the plough on which he hath laid his hand!' ''

He drained the cup to the bottom, resigned it to the Arabian, and sank back, as if exhausted, upon the cushions which were arranged to receive him. The physician, then, with silent but expressive signs, directed that all should leave the tent excepting himself and De Vaux, whom no remonstrance could induce to withdraw. The apartment was cleared accordingly.

WILLIAM SHAKESPEARE
Cymbeline

WILLIAM SHAKESPEARE (1564-1616) achieved pre-eminence not solely
because of the majesty of his poetry and his plays but because of his
insight into the human situation. His works take in the full range of
human nobility and frailty. His power derives from his use of language
and his ability to orchestrate the varieties of human experience.
experience.

ACT ONE, SCENE V. *Britain. A room in* CYMBELINE'S *palace.*

Enter Queen, Ladies, *and* CORNELIUS.

Queen. Whiles yet the dew's on ground, gather those flowers;
Make haste: who has the note of them?
  First Lady.   I, madam.
  Queen. Dispatch.   *[Exeunt Ladies.*
Now, master doctor, have you brought those drugs?
  Cor. Pleaseth your highness, ay: here they are, madam:
                        [Presenting a small box.
But I beseech your grace, without offence,—
My conscience bids me ask,—wherefore you have
Commanded of me these most poisonous compounds,
Which are the movers of a languishing death;
But, though slow, deadly?
  Queen.   I wonder, doctor,
Thou ask'st me such a question. Have I not been
Thy pupil long? Hast thou not learn'd me how
To make perfumes? distil? preserve? yea, so
That our great king himself doth woo me oft
For my confections? Having thus far proceeded,—
Unless thou think'st me devilish,—is't not meet
That I did amplify my judgment in
Other conclusions? I will try the forces
Of these thy compounds on such creatures as

73

We count not worth the hanging; but none human,
To try the vigour of them and apply
Allayments to their act, and by them gather
Their several virtues and effects.
    Cor.   Your highness
Shall from this practice but make hard your heart:
Besides, the seeing these effects will be
But noisome and infectious.
    Queen.
[*Aside*] Here comes a flattering rascal; upon him
Will I first work; he's for his master,
And enemy to my son.

Enter PISANIO.

                 How now, Pisanio!
Doctor, your service for this time is ended;
Take your own way.
    Cor. [*Aside*] I do suspect you, madam;
But you shall do no harm.
    Queen. [*To Pisanio*]   Hark thee, a word.
    Cor. [*Aside*] I do not like her. She doth think she has
Strange lingering poisons: I do know her spirit,
And will not trust one of her malice with
A drug of such damn'd nature. Those she has
Will stupefy and dull the sense awhile;
Which first, perchance, she'll prove on cats and dogs,
Then afterward up higher: but there is
No danger in what show of death it makes,
More than the locking-up the spirits a time,
To be more fresh, reviving. She is fool'd
With a most false effect; and I the truer,
So to be false with her.

Cor.   I humbly take my leave. [*Exit.*

*   *   *

ACT V, SCENE V. *Enter* CORNELIUS *and* Ladies.

Enter CORNELIUS *and* Ladies.

Cym.
There's business in these faces. Why so sadly
Greet you our victory? you look like Romans,
And not o' the court of Britain.
  Cor.   Hail, great king!
To sour your happiness, I must report
The queen is dead.
  Cym.   Who worse than a physician
Would this report become? But I consider
By medicine life may be prolong'd, yet death
Will seize the doctor too. How ended she?
  Cor. With horror, madly dying, like her life
Which, being cruel to the world, concluded
Most cruel to herself. What she confess'd
I will report, so please you: these her women
Can trip me, if I err: who with wet cheeks
Were present when she finish'd.
  Cym.   Prithee, say.
  Cor. First, she confess'd she never loved you; only
Affected greatness got by you, not you:
Married your royalty, was wife to your place;
Abhorr'd your person.
  Cym.   She alone knew this;
And, but she spoke it dying, I would not
Believe her lips in opening it. Proceed.
  Cor. Your daughter, whom she bore in hand to love
With such integrity, she did confess
Was as a scorpion to her sight; whose life,
But that her flight prevented it, she had
Ta'en off by poison.
  Cym.   O most delicate fiend!
Who is't can read a woman? Is there more?
  Cor. More, sir, and worse. She did confess she had
For you a mortal mineral; which, being took,
Should by the minute feed on life, and lingering
By inches waste you: in which time she purposed,

By watching, weeping, tendance, kissing, to
O'ercome you with her show, and in time,
When she had fitted you with her craft, to work
Her son into the adoption of the crown:
But, failing of her end by his strange absence,
Grew shameless-desperate; open'd, in despite
Of heaven and men, her purposes; repented
The evils she hatch'd were not effected; so
Despairing died.
    Cym.   Heard you all this, her women?
    First Lady.   We did, so please your highness.
    Cym.   Mine eyes
Were not in fault, for she was beautiful;
Mine ears, that heard her flattery; not my heart,
That thought her like her seeming; it had been vicious
To have mistrusted her: yet, O my daughter!
That it was folly in me, thou mayst say,
And prove it in thy feeling. Heaven mend all!

     Enter LUCIUS, IACHIMO, *the* Soothsayer, *and other* Roman Prisoners,
          guarded; POSTHUMUS *behind, and* IMOGEN.

Thou comest not, Caius, now for tribute; that
The Britons have razed out, though with the loss
Of many a bold one; whose kinsmen have made suit
That their good souls may be appeased with slaughter
Of you their captives, which ourself have granted:
So think of your estate.
    Luc. Consider, sir, the chance of war: the day
Was yours by accident; had it gone with us,
We should not, when the blood was cool, have threaten'd
Our prisoners with the sword. But since the gods
Will have it thus, that nothing but our lives
May be call'd ransom, let it come: sufficeth
A Roman with a Roman's heart can suffer:
Augustus lives to think on't: and so much
For my peculiar care. This one thing only
I will entreat; my boy, a Briton born,
Let him be ransom'd: never master had
A page so kind, so duteous, diligent,

So tender over his occasions, true,
So feat, so nurse-like: let his virtue join
With my request, which I'll make bold your highness
Cannot deny; he hath done no Briton harm,
Though he hath served a Roman: save him, sir,
And spare no blood beside.
    Cym.   I have surely seen him:
His favour is familiar to me
Boy, thou hast look'd thyself into my grace,
And art mine own. I know not why, nor wherefore,
To say "Live, boy:" ne'er thank thy master; live:
And ask of Cymbeline what boon thou wilt,
Fitting my bounty and thy state, I'll give it;
Yea, though thou do demand a prisoner,
The noblest ta'en.
    Imo.   I humbly thank your highness.
    Luc. I do not bid thee beg my life, good lad;
And yet I know thou wilt.
    Imo.   No, no: alack,
There's other work in hand: I see a thing
Bitter to me as death: your life, good master,
Must shuffle for itself.

*   *   *

    Post. A sacrilegious thief, to do't: the temple
Of virtue was she; yea, and she herself.
Spit, and throw stones, cast mire upon me, set
The dogs o' the street to bay me: every villain
Be call'd Posthumus Leonatus; and
Be villany less than 'twas! O Imogen!
My queen, my life, my wife! O Imogen,
Imogen, Imogen!
    Imo.   Peace, my lord; hear, hear—
    Post. Shall's have a play of this? Thou scornful page,
There lie thy part.   *[Striking her: she falls.*
    Pis.   O, gentlemen, help!
Mine and your mistress! O, my lord Posthumus!
You ne'er kill'd Imogen till now. Help, help!—
Mine honour'd lady!

Cym.   Does the world go round?
Post. How come these staggers on me?
Pis.   Wake, my mistress!
Cym. If this be so, the gods do mean to strike me
To death with mortal joy.
Pis.   How fares my mistress?
Imo. O, get thee from my sight;
Thou gavest me poison: dangerous fellow, hence!
Breathe not where princes are.
Cym.   The tune of Imogen!
Pis. Lady,
The gods throw stones of sulphur on me, if
That box I gave you was not thought by me
A precious thing; I had it from the queen.
Cym.   New matter still?
Imo.   It poison'd me.
Cor.   O gods!
I left out one thing which the queen confess'd,
Which must approve thee honest: "If Pisanio
Have," said she, "given his mistress that confection
Which I gave him for cordial, she is served
As I would serve a rat."
Cym.   What's this, Cornelius?
Cor. The queen, sir, very oft importuned me
To temper poisons for her; still pretending
The satisfaction of her knowledge only
In killing creatures vile, as cats and dogs,
Of no esteem: I, dreading that her purpose
Was of more danger, did compound for her
A certain stuff, which, being ta'en, would cease
The present power of life, but in short time
All offices of nature should again
Do their due functions. Have you ta'en of it?
Imo. Most like I did, for I was dead.

GEORGE BERNARD SHAW
A Word First

━━━━━━━━✦━━━━

GEORGE BERNARD SHAW (1856-1940), considered by many to be the foremost literary figure of his time, wrote plays of biting social commentary in high comedy style. He was an active Fabian Socialist whose satirical barbs were most often directed at middle-class morality. Two doctor friends of his family instilled a life-long interest in medical science. Students in the health sciences may find his play, *The Doctor's Dilemma,* as well as some of his prefaces, of particular interest. His lances were tilted in many directions but none with more devastating effect than in the direction of the medical profession.

Please do not class me as one who "doesn't believe in doctors." One of our most pressing social needs is a national staff of doctors whom we can believe in, and whose prosperity shall depend not on the nation's sickness but on its health. There should be no such thing as a poor doctor and no such thing as an ignorant one. The great majority of our doctors today are both poor and ignorant with the conceited ignorance of obsolete or spurious knowledge. Our surgeons obtain the highest official qualifications without having had a single hour of specific manual training; they have to pick up the art of carving us as paterfamilias picks up the art of carving a goose. The general education of our citizens (the patients) leaves them so credulous and gullible, that the doctor, to whom they attribute magical powers over life and death, is forced to treat them according to their folly lest he starve. Those to whom these menacing facts are known, and who are capable of understanding their gravity (including all our really able doctors), will not mistake my aim nor wish me anything but a sympathetic hearing. As for the simpletons (bless their anything-but-sacred simplicity!), if they don't like it, why, they must lump it.

Our mechanist-surgeons and chemist-physicians must, however, forgive me for differing fundamentally and flatly from the scientific basis (if it can be called scientific) of their crude practices. In my view surgeons and physicians should be primarily biologists. To tackle a damaged living organism with the outlook of a repairing plumber and joiner, or to treat an acid stomach by pouring an alkali into it, is to behave like a highly unintelligent artisan, and should entail instant and ignominious dis-qualification by the Privy Council. There are many unlearned amateur pathologists and hygienists, from Mary Baker Eddy to George Hack-enschmidt, who are safer guides than the Harley Street celebrities who laugh at them, their secret being simply that they have had the gumption to guess that it is the mind that makes the body and not the body the mind.

I also expect a doctor to be an evolutionist, and, as such, regard all habits as acquired habits, a man being nothing but amoeba with acquirements. Any doctor found parroting the obsolete nineteenth century cackle about non-acquired heritable habits and non-heritable acquired habits should be removed to the nearest museum of quaint antiquities.

I hope this is clear. If not, please read the preface to my Back to Methuselah until it *is* clear.

1931.

IVAN TURGENEV
The District Doctor

———◦◦◦———

IVAN TURGENEV (1818-1883) belonged to the great Russian literary trinity of which Tolstoy and Dostoevski were other members. Like Tolstoy, he had an aristocratic background but became caught up in social issues. He was unpopular at home but widely read throughout Western Europe and particularly in France, where he lived.

One day in the autumn on my way from a remote part of the country I caught cold and fell ill. Fortunately the fever attacked me in the district town at the inn; I sent for the doctor. In half-an-hour the district doctor appeared, a thin dark-haired man of middle height. He prescribed me the usual sudorific, ordered a mustard-plaster to be put on, very deftly slid a five-rouble note up his sleeve, coughing dryly and looking away as he did so, and then was getting up to go home, but somehow fell into talk and remained. I was exhausted with feverishness; I foresaw a sleepless night, and was glad of a little chat with a pleasant companion. Tea was served. My doctor began to converse freely. He was a sensible fellow, and expressed himself with vigour and some humour. Queer things happen in the world; you may live a long while with some people, and be on friendly terms with them, and never once speak openly with them from your soul; with others you have scarcely time to get acquainted, and all at once you are pouring out to him—or he to you—all your secrets, as though you were at confession. I don't know how I gained the confidence of my new friend—anyway, with nothing to lead up to it, he told me a rather curious incident; and here I will report his tale for the information of the indulgent reader. I will try to tell it in the doctor's own words.

'You don't happen to know,' he began in a weak and quavering voice [the common result of the use of unmixed Berezov snuff], 'you don't happen to know the judge here, Mylov, Pavel Lukitch? . . . You don't happen to know him? . . . Well, it's all the same. [He cleared his throat and rubbed his eyes.] Well, you see, the thing happened, to tell you exactly without mistake, in Lent, at the very time of the thaws. I was sitting at his house—our judge's, you know—playing preference. Suddenly [the doctor made frequent use of this word, suddenly] they tell me, "There's a servant

81

asking for you." I say, "What does he want?" They say, "He has brought a note—it must be from a patient." "Give me the note," I say. So it is from a patient—well and good—you understand—it's our bread and butter. . . . But this is how it was: a lady, a widow, writes to me; she says, "My daughter is dying. Come, for God's sake!" she says; "and the horses have been sent for you." . . . Well, that's all right. But she was twenty miles from the town, and it was midnight out of doors, and the roads in such a state, my word! And as she was poor herself, one could not expect more than two silver roubles, and even that problematic; and perhaps it might only be a matter of a roll of linen and a sack of oatmeal in payment. However, duty, you know, before everything; a fellow creature may be dying. I hand over my cards at once to Kalliopin, the member of the provincial commission, and return home. I look; a wretched little trap was standing at the steps, with peasant's horses, fat—too fat—and their coat as shaggy as felt; and the coachman sitting with his cap off out of respect. Well, I think to myself, "It's clear, my friend, these patients aren't rolling in riches." . . . You smile; but I tell you, a poor man like me has to take everything into consideration. . . . If the coachman sits like a prince, and doesn't touch his cap, and even sneers at you behind his beard, and flicks his whip—then you may bet on six roubles. But this case, I saw, had a very different air. However, I think there's no help for it; duty before everything. I snatch up the most necessary drugs, and set off. Will you believe it? I only just managed to get there at all. The road was infernal: streams, snow, watercourses, and the dyke had suddenly burst there—that was the worst of it! However, I arrived at last. It was a little thatched house. There was a light in the windows; that meant they expected me. I was met by an old lady, very venerable, in a cap. "Save her!" she says; "she is dying." I say, "Pray don't distress yourself—Where is the invalid?" "Come this way." I see a clean little room, a lamp in the corner; on the bed a girl of twenty, unconscious. She was in a burning heat, and breathing heavily—it was fever. There were two other girls, her sisters, scared and in tears. "Yesterday," they tell me, "she was perfectly well and had a good appetite; this morning she complained of her head, and this evening, suddenly, you see, like this." I say again: "Pray don't be uneasy." It's a doctor's duty, you know—and I went up to her and bled her, told them to put on a mustard-plaster, and prescribed a mixture. Meantime I looked at her; I looked at her, you know—there, by God! I had never seen such a face!—she was a beauty, in a word! I felt quite shaken with pity. Such lovely features; such eyes!. . . But, thank God! she became easier; she fell into perspiration, seemed to come to her senses, looked round, smiled, and

passed her hand over her face. . . . Her sisters bent over her. They ask,
"How are you?" "All right," she says, and turns away. I looked at her; she
had fallen asleep. "Well," I say, "now the patient should be left alone." So
we all went out on tiptoe; only a maid remained, in case she was wanted. In
the parlour there was a samovar standing on the table, and a bottle of rum;
in our profession we can't get on without it. They gave me tea; asked me to
stop the night. . . . I consented: where could I go, indeed, at that time of
night? The old lady kept groaning. "What is it?" I say; "she will live; don't
worry yourself; you had better take a little rest yourself; it is about two
o'clock." "But will you send to wake me if anything happens?" "Yes,
yes." The old lady went away, and the girls too went to their own room;
they made up a bed for me in the parlour. Well, I went to bed—but I could
not get to sleep, for a wonder! for in reality I was very tired. I could not get
my patient out of my head. At last I could not put up with it any longer; I got
up suddenly; I think to myself, "I will go and see how the patient is getting
on." Her bedroom was next to the parlour. Well, I got up, and gently
opened the door—how my heart beat! I looked in: the servant was asleep,
her mouth wide open, and even snoring, the wretch! but the patient lay with
her face towards me, and her arms flung wide apart, poor girl! I went up to
her . . . when suddenly, she opened her eyes and stared at me! "Who is it?
who is it?" I was in confusion. "Don't be alarmed, madam," I say; "I am
the doctor; I have come to see how you feel." "You the doctor?" "Yes, the
doctor; your mother sent for me from the town; we have bled you, madam;
now pray go to sleep, and in a day or two, please God! we will set you on
your feet again." "Ah, yes, yes, doctor, don't let me die . . . please,
please." "Why do you talk like that? God bless you!" She is in a fever
again, I think to myself; I felt her pulse; yes, she was feverish. She looked at
me, and then took me by the hand. "I will tell you why I don't want to die; I
will tell you. . . . Now we are alone; and only, please don't you . . . not to
any one . . . Listen . . ." I bent down; she moved her lips quite to my ear;
she touched my cheeks with her hair—I confess my head went round—and
began to whisper . . . I could make out nothing of it. . . . Ah, she was
delicious! . . . She whispered and whispered, but so quickly, and as if it
were not in Russian; at last she finished, and shivering dropped her head on
the pillow, and threatened me with her finger: "Remember, doctor, to no
one." I calmed her somehow, gave her something to drink, waked the
servant, and went away.'

At this point the doctor again took snuff with exasperated energy, and for
a moment seemed stupefied by its effects.

'However,' he continued, 'the next day, contrary to my expectations, the patient was no better. I thought and thought, and suddenly decided to remain there, even though my other patients were expecting me. . . . And you know one can't afford to disregard that; one's practice suffers if one does. But, in the first place, the patient was really in danger; and secondly, to tell the truth, I felt strongly drawn to her. Besides, I liked the whole family. Though they were really badly off, they were singularly, I may say, cultivated people. . . . Their father had been a learned man, an author; he died, of course, in poverty, but he had managed before he died to give his children an excellent education; he left a lot of books too. Either because I looked after the invalid very carefully, or for some other reason; any way, I can venture to say all the household loved me as if I were one of the family. . . . Meantime the roads were in a worse state than ever; all communications, so to say, were cut off completely; even medicine could with difficulty be got from the town . . . The sick girl was not getting better . . . Day after day, and day after day . . . but . . . here . . . [The doctor made a brief pause.] I declare I don't know how to tell you. . . . [He again took snuff, coughed, and swallowed a little tea.] I will tell you without beating about the bush. My patient . . . how shall I say? . . . Well she had fallen in love with me . . . or, no, it was not that she was in love . . . however . . . really, how should one say? [The doctor looked down and grew red.] No,' he went on quickly, 'in love, indeed! A man should not over-estimate himself. She was an educated girl, clever, and well-read, and I had even forgotten my Latin, one may say, completely. As to appearance [the doctor looked himself over with a smile] I am nothing to boast of there either. But God Almighty did not make me a fool; I don't take black for white; I know a thing or two; I could see very clearly, for instance that Alexandra Andreevna—that was her name—did not feel love for me, but had a friendly, so to say, inclination—a respect or something for me. Though she herself perhaps mistook this sentiment, anyway this was her attitude; you may form your own judgment of it. But,' added the doctor, who had brought out all these disconnected sentences without taking breath, and with obvious embarrassment, 'I seem to be wandering rather—you won't understand anything like this . . . There, with your leave, I will relate it in order.'

He drank off a glass of tea, and began in a calmer voice.

'Well, then. My patient kept getting worse and worse. You are not a doctor, my good sir; you cannot understand what passes in a poor fellow's heart, especially at first, when he begins to suspect that the disease is getting the upper hand of him. What becomes of his belief in himself? You suddenly grow so timid; it's indescribable. You fancy then that you have forgotten everything you knew, and that the patient has no faith in you, and that other people begin to notice how distracted you are, and tell you the symptoms with reluctance; that they are looking at you suspiciously, whispering . . . Ah! it's horrid! There must be a remedy, you think, for this disease, if one could find it. Isn't this it? You try—no, that's not it! You don't allow the medicine the necessary time to do good . . . You clutch at one thing, then at another. Sometimes you take up a book of medical prescriptions—here it is, you think! Sometimes, by Jove, you pick one out by chance, thinking to leave it to fate . . . But meantime a fellow-creature's dying, and another doctor would have saved him. "We must have a consultation," you say; "I will not take the responsibility on myself." And what a fool you look at such times! Well, in time you learn to bear it; it's nothing to you. A man has died—but it's not your fault; you treated him by the rules. But what's still more torture to you is to see blind faith in you, and to feel yourself that you are not able to be of use. Well, it was just this blind faith that the whole of Alexandra Andreevna's family had in me; they had forgotten to think that their daughter was in danger. I, too, on my side assure them that it's nothing, but meantime my heart sinks in my boots. To add to our troubles, the roads were in such a state that the coachman was gone for whole days together to get medicine. And I never left the patient's room; I could not tear myself away; I tell her amusing stories, you know, and play cards with her. I watch by her side at night. The old mother thanks me with tears in her eyes; but I think to myself, "I don't deserve your gratitude." I frankly confess to you—there is no object in concealing it now—I was in love with my patient. And Alexandra Andreevna had grown fond of me; she would not sometimes let any one be in her room but me. She began to talk to me, to ask me questions; where I had studied, how I lived, who are my people, whom I go to see. I feel that she ought not to talk; but to forbid her to—to forbid her resolutely, you know—I could not. Sometimes I held my head in my hands, and asked myself, "What are you doing, villain?" . . . And she would take my hand and hold it, give me a long, long look, and turn away, sigh, and say, "How good you are!" Her hands were so feverish, her eyes so large and languid. . . . "Yes," she says, "you are a good, kind man; you are not like our neighbours . . . No, you are not like that . . . Why did I not know you till now!" "Alexandra Andreevna, calm yourself," I would say . . . "I feel, believe me, I don't know how I have gained . . . but there, calm yourself . . . All will be right; you will be well again." And meanwhile I must tell you,' continued the doctor, bending forward and raising his eyebrows, 'that they associated very little with the neighbours, because the smaller people were not on their level, and pride hindered them from being friendly with the rich. I tell you, they were an exceptionally cultivated family; so you know it was gratifying for me. She would only take her medicine from my hands . . . she would lift herself up, poor girl, with my aid, take it, and gaze at me . . . My heart felt as if it were bursting. And meanwhile she was growing worse and worse, worse and worse, all the time; she will die, I think to myself; she must die. Believe me, I would sooner have gone to the grave myself; and here were her mother and sisters watching me, looking into my eyes . . . and their faith in me was wearing away. "Well? how is she?" "Oh, all right, all right!" All right, indeed! My mind was failing me. Well, I was sitting one night alone again by my patient. The maid was sitting there too, and snoring away in full swing; I can't find fault with the poor girl, though; she was worn out too. Alexandra Andreevna had felt very unwell all the evening; she was very feverish. Until midnight she kept tossing about; at last she seemed to fall asleep; at least, she lay still without stirring. The lamp was burning in the corner before the holy image. I sat there, you know, with my head bent; I even dozed a little. Suddenly it seemed as though some one touched me in the side; I turned around . . . Good God! Alexandra Andreevna was gazing with intent eyes at me . . . her lips parted, her cheeks seemed burning. "What is it?" "Doctor shall I die?" "Merciful Heavens!" "No, doctor, no; please don't tell me I shall live . . . don't say so . . . If you knew . . . Listen! for God's sake don't conceal my real position," and her breath came so fast. "If I can know for certain that I must die . . . then I will tell you all—all!" "Alexandra Andreevna, I beg!" "Listen; I have not been asleep at all . . . I have been looking at you for a long while . . . For God's sake! . . . I believe in you; you are a good man, an honest man; I entreat you with all that is sacred in the world—tell me the truth! If you knew how important it is for me . . . Doctor, for God's sake tell me . . . Am I in danger?" "What can I tell you, Alexandra Andreevna, pray?" "For God's sake, I beseech you!" "I can't disguise from you," I say, "Alexandra Andreevna; you are certainly in danger; but God is merciful." "I shall die, I shall die." And it seemed as though she were pleased; her face grew so bright; I was alarmed. "Don't be afraid, don't be afraid! I am not frightened of death at all." She suddenly sat up and leaned on her elbow. "Now . . . yes, now I can tell you that I thank you with my whole heart . . . that you are kind and good—that I love you!" I stare at her, like one possessed; it was terrible for me, you know. "Do you hear, I love you!" "Alexandra Andreevna, how I have deserved—" "No, no, you don't— you don't understand me." . . . And suddenly she stretched out her arms, and taking my head in her hands, she kissed it. . . Believe me, I almost screamed aloud. . . I threw myself on my knees, and buried my head in the pillow. She did not speak; her fingers trembled in my hair; I listen; she is weeping. I began to soothe her, to assure her. . . . I really don't know what I did say to her. "You will wake up the girl," I say to her; "Alexandra Andreevna, I thank you . . . believe me . . . calm yourself." "Enough, enough!" she persisted; "never mind all of them; let them wake, then; let them come in—it does not matter; I am dying, you see . . . And what do you fear? Why are you afraid? Lift up your head . . Or, perhaps, you don't love me; perhaps I am wrong . . . In that case, forgive me." "Alexandra Andreevna, what are you saying! . . . I love you, Alexandra Andreevna." She looked straight into my eyes, and opened her arms wide. "Then take me in your arms." I tell you frankly, I don't know how it was I didn't go mad that night. I feel that my patient is killing herself; I understand, too, that if she did not consider herself on the point of death, she would never have thought of me; and, indeed, say what you will, it's hard to die at twenty without having known love; this was what was torturing her; this was why, in despair, she caught at me—do you understand now? But she held me in her arms, and would not let me go. "Have pity on me, Alexandra Andreevna, and have pity on yourself," I say. "Why," she says; "what is there to think of? You know I must die." . . . This she repeated incessantly . . . "If I knew that I should return to life, and be a proper young lady again, I should be ashamed . . . of course, ashamed . . . but why now?" "But who has said you will die?" "Oh, no, leave off! You will not deceive me; you don't know how to lie—look at your face" . . . "You shall live, Alexandra Andreevna; I will cure you; we will ask your mother's blessing . . . we will be united—we will be happy." "No, no, I have your word! I must die . . . you have promised me . . . you have told me." . . . It was cruel for me—cruel for many reasons. And see what trifling things can do sometimes; it seems nothing at all, but it's painful. It occurred to her to ask me, what is my name; not my surname, but my first name. I must needs be so unlucky as to be called Trifon. Yes, indeed; Trifon Ivanitch. Every one in the house called me Doctor. However, there's no help for it. I say, "Trifon, madam." She frowned, shook her head, and muttered something in French—ah, something unpleasant, of course!—and then she laughed disagreeably too. Well, I spent the whole night with her in this way. Before morning I went away, feeling as though I were mad. When I went again into her room it was day-time, after morning tea. Good God! I could scarcely recognize her; people are laid in their grave looking better than that. I swear to you, on my honour, I don't understand—I absolutely don't understand—now, how I lived through that experience. Three days and nights my patient lingered on. And what nights! What things she said to me! And on the last night—only imagine to yourself—I was sitting near her, and kept praying to God for one thing only: "Take her," I said, "quickly, and me with her." Suddenly the old mother comes unexpectedly into the room. I had already the evening before told her—the mother—there was little hope, and it would be well to send for a priest. When the sick girl saw her mother she said: "It's very well you have come; look at us, we love one another—we have given each other our word." "What does she say, doctor? what does she say?" I turned livid. "She is wandering." I say: "the fever." But she: "Hush, hush, you told me something quite different just now, and have taken my ring. Why do you pretend? My mother is good—she will forgive—she will understand—and I am dying . . . I have no need to tell lies; give me your hand." I jumped up and ran out of the room. The old lady, of course, guessed how it was.

'I will not, however, weary you any longer, and to me, too, of course, it's painful to recall all this. My patient passed away the next day. God rest her soul!' the doctor added, speaking quickly and with a sigh. 'Before her death she asked her family to go out and leave me alone with her.'

' "Forgive me," she said; "I am perhaps to blame towards you . . . my illness . . . but believe me, I have loved no one more than you . . . do not forget me . . . keep my ring:" '

The doctor turned away; I took his hand.

'Ah!' he said, 'let us talk of something else, or would you care to play preference for a small stake? It's not for people like me to give way to exalted emotions. There's only one thing for me to think of; how to keep the children from crying and the wife from scolding. Since then, you know, I have had time to enter into lawful wedlock, as they say . . . Oh . . . I took a merchant's daughter—seven thousand for her dowry. Her name's Akulina; it goes well with Trifon. She is an ill-tempered woman, I must tell you, but luckily she's asleep all day. . . . Well, shall it be preference?'

We sat down to preference for halfpenny points. Trifon Ivanitch won two roubles and a half from me, and went home late, well pleased with his success.

HANS ZINSSER
As I Remember Him

———————◇◇◇◇———————

To return to the matter of frankness with a patient about his own illness, no rules can be set down. Those who have tried to do this have dismally failed. A well-known American physician who was at the same time—to my mind—a canting moralist held on occasion that absolute, uncompromising truthfulness is the only justifiable position, however cruel. That principle may lead to the sort of situation that once occurred in the practice of one of his colleagues who adopted his views. An old lady had what is known as an "epithelioma" of the lip, a growth occurring in the aged which has all the structural earmarks of cancer, but represents a variety that never extends to other organs and usually yields to appropriate treatment. To tell this poor soul, for the sake of one's distorted conscience, that she was suffering from "cancer," planting this spectre in her sensitive old mind, was—however well meant—inhumanly stupid.

*　　*　　*

One must pick one's situations and one's cases, and adjust the truth to the judgment of wise kindness. But one must not "exaggerate" the truth without purpose.

GODS
AND
DEMONS

———◆◇◆———

For many centuries, disease was regarded as a form of punishment. Thus Ivan Ilych writhes not only in the agony of his illness but in his soliloquies with the Deity; what were his wrongdoings that dictated the present punishment? Subconsciously or otherwise, the patient expects the physician not just to provide the best that science has to offer but to act as a surrogate for the Deity in furnishing metaphysical answers. Since the doctor is a prime symbol of life, it is natural that he or she should be invested with godly attributes. When the life force fails, therefore, the doctor is often held accountable. The misperceptions about the powers of the physician have made for strained relations at times between the patient and the physician—and the writer has found this situation rich with dramatic possibilities.

THOMAS DE QUINCEY
Murder as a Fine Art

———◦◦◦———

THOMAS DeQUINCEY (1785-1859) drew on his experience of twenty
years of visions as an opium addict with its innate fantasy world for his
fiction. Body snatchers, or Resurrectionists, were active during his
lifetime, providing physicians with cadavers.

A good many years ago, the reader may remember that I came forward in
the character of a *dilettante* in murder. Perhaps *dilettante* is too strong a
word. *Connoisseur* is better suited to the scruples and infirmity of public
taste. I suppose there is no harm in *that,* at least. A man is not bound to put
his eyes, ears, and understanding into his breeches pocket when he meets
with a murder. If he is not in a downright comatose state, I suppose that he
must see that one murder is better or worse than another, in point of good
taste. Murders have their little differences and shades of merit, as well as
statues, pictures, oratorios, cameos, intaglios, or what not. You may be
angry with the man for talking too much, or too publicly (as to the too much,
that I deny—a man can never cultivate his taste too highly); but you must
allow him to think, at any rate. Well, would you believe it? all my
neighbours came to hear of that little aesthetic essay which I had published;
and, unfortunately, hearing at the very same time of a club that I was
connected with, and a dinner at which I presided—both tending to the same
little object as the essay, viz., the diffusion of a just taste among Her
Majesty's subjects[1]—they got up the most barbarous calumnies against
me. In particular, they said that I, or that the club (which comes to the same
thing), had offered bounties on well-conducted homicides—with a scale of
drawbacks, in case of any one defect or flaw, according to a table issued to
private friends. Now, let me tell the whole truth about the dinner and the
club, and it will be seen how malicious the world is. But, first, confidentially, allow me to say what my real principles are upon the matter in
question.

---

[1]*Her* Majesty:—In the lecture, having occasion to refer to the reigning sovereign, I said
"*His* Majesty"; for at that time William IV was on the throne; but between the lecture and this
supplement had occurred the accession of our present Queen.

As to murder, I never committed one in my life. It's a well-known thing amongst all my friends. I can get a paper to certify as much, signed by lots of people. Indeed, if you come to that, I doubt whether many people could produce as strong a certificate. Mine would be as big as a breakfast tablecloth. There is indeed one member of the club who pretends to say he caught me once making too free with his throat on a club night, after everybody else had retired. But, observe, he shuffles in his story according to his state of civilation. When not far gone, he contents himself with saying that he caught me ogling his throat, and that I was melancholy for some weeks after, and that my voice sounded in a way expressing, to the nice ear of a connoisseur, *the sense of opportunities lost;* but the club all know that he is a disappointed man himself, and that he speaks querulously at times about the fatal neglect of a man's coming abroad without his tools. Besides, all this is an affair between two amateurs, and everybody makes allowances for little asperities and fibs in such a case. "But," say you, "if no murderer, you may have encouraged, or even have bespoken, a murder." No, upon my honour—no. And that was the very point I wished to argue for your satisfaction. The truth is, I am a very particular man in everything relating to murder; and perhaps I carry my delicacy too far. The Stagirite most justly, and possibly with a view to my case, placed virtue in the το μεσον, or middle point between two extremes. A golden mean is certainly what every man should aim at.

The next toast was—"The sublime epoch of Burkism and Harism!"
This was drunk with enthusiasm; and one of the members who spoke to the question made a very curious communication to the company:— "Gentlemen, we fancy Burkism to be a pure invention of our own times; and in fact no Pancirollus has ever enumerated this branch of art when writing *de rebus deperditis.* Still, I have ascertained that the essential principle of this variety in the art *was* known to the ancients; although, like the art of painting upon glass, of making the myrrhine cups, etc., it was lost in the dark ages for want of encouragement. In the famous collection of Greek epigrams made by Planudes is one upon a very fascinating case of Burkism: it is a perfect little gem of art. The epigram itself I cannot lay my hand upon at this moment; but the following is an abstract of it by Salmasius, as I find it in his notes on Vopiscus: 'Est et elegans epigramma Lucilii,[1] ubi medicus et pollinctor de compacto sic egerunt ut medicus

---

[1] The epigram, which had been preserved by Planudes in its Greek form, is here attributed by Salmasius to the Latin satirical poet, Caius Lucilius, who was born about B.C. 148, and died about B.C. 103. It is not found, however, among the preserved fragments of Lucilius; and the Greek form of the epigram is anonymous.

ægros omnes curæ suæ commissos occideret.' This was the basis of the contract, you see,—that on the one part the doctor, for himself and his assigns, doth undertake and contract duly and truly to murder all the patients committed to his charge: but why? There lies the beauty of the case—'Et ut pollinctori amico suo traderet pollingendos.' The *pollinctor,* you are aware, was a person whose business it was to dress and prepare dead bodies for burial. The original ground of the transaction appears to have been sentimental: 'He was my friend,' says the murderous doctor,—'he was dear to me,'—in speaking of the pollinctor. But the law, gentlemen, is stern and harsh: the law will not hear of these tender motives: to sustain a contract of this nature in law, it is essential that a 'considera- tion' should be given. Now, what *was* the consideration? For thus far all is on the side of the pollinctor: he will be well paid for his services; but meantime the generous, the noble-minded doctor gets nothing. What *was* the equivalent, again I ask, which the law would insist on the doctor's taking, in order to establish that 'consideration' without which the contract had no force? You shall hear: 'Et ut pollinctor vicissim τελαμωνας quos furabatur de pollinctione mortuorum medico mitteret donis ad 'alliganda vulnera eorum quos curabat'; *i.e.,* and that reciprocally the pollinctor should transmit to the physician, as free gifts for the binding up of wounds in those whom he treated medically, the belts or trusses (τελαμωνας) which he had succeeded in purloining in the course of his functions about the corpses.

"Now the case is clear: the whole went on a principle of reciprocity which would have kept up the trade for ever." The doctor was also a surgeon: he could not murder *all* his patients: some of the patients must be retained intact. For these he wanted linen bandages. But, unhappily, the Romans wore woollen; on which account it was that they bathed so often. Meantime, there *was* linen to be had in Rome; but it was monstrously dear; and the τελαμωνας, or linen swathing bandages, in which superstition obliged them to bind up corpses, would answer capitally for the surgeon. The doctor, therefore, contracts to furnish his friend with a constant succession of corpses,—provided, and be it understood always, that his sad friend, in return, should supply him with one-half of the articles he would receive from the friends of the parties murdered or to be murdered. The doctor invariably recommended his invaluable friend the pollinctor (whom let us call the undertaker); the undertaker, with equal regard to the sacred rights of friendship, uniformly recommended the doctor. Like Pylades and Orestes, they were models of a perfect friendship: in their lives they were lovely; and on the gallows, it is to be hoped, they were not divided.

"Gentlemen, it makes me laugh horribly when I think of those two friends drawing and re-drawing on each other: 'Pollinctor in account with Doctor, debtor by sixteen corpses: creditor by forty-five bandages, two of which damaged.' Their names unfortunately are lost; but I conceive they must have been Quintus Burkius and Publius Harius. By the way, gentlemen, has anybody heard lately of Hare? I understand he is comfortably settled in Ireland, considerably to the west, and does a little business now and then; but, as he observes with a sigh, only as a retailer—nothing like the fine thriving wholesale concern so carelessly blown up at Edinburgh. 'You see what comes of neglecting business'—is the chief moral, the ἐπιμύθιον, as Æsop would say, which Hare draws from his past experience."

At length came the toast of the day—*Thugdom in all its branches*.

The speeches *attempted* at this crisis of the dinner were past all counting. But the applause was so furious, the music so stormy, and the crashing of glasses so incessant, from the general resolution never again to drink an inferior toast from the same glass, that I am unequal to the task of reporting. Besides which, Toad-in-the-hole now became ungovernable. He kept firing pistols in every direction; sent his servant for a blunderbuss, and talked of loading with ball-cartridge. We conceived that his former madness had returned at the mention of Burke and Hare; or that, being again weary of life, he had resolved to go off in a general massacre. This we could not think of allowing; it became indispensable, therefore, to kick him out; which we did with universal consent, the whole company lending their toes *uno pede*, as I may say, though pitying his gray hairs and his angelic smile. During the operation the orchestra poured in their old chorus. The universal company sang, and (what surprised us most of all) Toad-in-the-hole joined us furiously in singing—

"Et interrogatum est ab omnibus—Ubi est ille Toad-in-the-hole?
Et responsum est ab omnibus—*Non est inventus*."

JOHANN WOLFGANG VON GOETHE
Faust

———❦———

JOHANN WOLFGANG VON GOETHE (1749-1832) studied both medicine and law—he discovered a new bone in the skull, the intermaxillary—before becoming one of the giants in world literature. Goethe was one of the first and most influential of the romantic poets; his *Sorrows of Young Werther* touched off a wave of suicides throughout Europe. In this selection from *Faust,* the scholar, like Goethe himself, desires mastery of all facets of knowledge and of life.

FAUST

O if you could but read my heart and see
How little father and son
Have merited such eulogy!
My father was an honest sombre man,
Who with fantastic zeal, and methods homely-rude,
In earnest quest of truth, on Nature's plan
And on her sacred zones would brood.
In his dark den with close-barred door
He sate with others of his craft,
And studying recipes galore
Concocted many a fatal draught.
There a red lion, a suitor dread,
In the warm bath was mated to a lily,
And both from bridal-bed to bridal-bed
With naked flames were hurried willy-nilly!
And if, in garish colours glassed,
The youthful queen was finally revealed,
The medicine was there! The patients perished fast,
And no one asked, 'But who was healed?'
Thus with our devilish drugs and pills
Here on these valleys, in these hills
We raged far worse than any pest:
Myself to many thousands dared to give
The fatal dose: they died, and I must live
To hear the shameless murderers blessed.

WAGNER

Such fancies are not worth a frown;
What can an honest man do better
Than practise even to the letter
The arts his sires have handed down?
If you revere your father as a youth
You take his teaching with a right good will:
If, as a man, you loose the bonds of truth,
Your son is sure to make them looser still.

FAUST

O happy he who still can hope
To rise from error's dark unfathomed sea!
The knowledge we could use outlies our scope,
And that we have seems mere futility!
But let not such dark fancies scare away
The spirit of this hour serene!

BEN JONSON
Sejanus

————◁✦▷————

BEN JONSON (1573-1637) was a noted dramatist and poet, whose brilliant though somewhat florid style makes better reading than performance drama. No doubt the deaths of several of his children and the primitive state of Elizabethan medical practice colored his portrait of Dr. Empirick. In *Sejanus,* the degenerate physician symbolizes decadent Rome.

Satrius
It is Eudemus, the physician
To Livia, Drusus' wife.
  Sejanus. On with your suit.
Would buy, you said—
  Satrius. A tribune's place, my lord.
  Sejanus. What will he give?
  Satrius. Fifty sestertia.
  Sejanus. Livia's physician, say you, is that fellow?
  Satrius. It is, my lord. Your lordship's answer.
  Sejanus. To what?
  Satrius. The place, my lord. 'Tis for a gentleman
Your lordship will well like of, when you see him,
And one that you may make yours, by the grant.
  Sejanus. Well, let him bring his money, and his name.
  Satrius. 'Thank your lordship. He shall, my lord.
  Sejanus. Come hither.
Know you this same Eudemus? is he learned?
  Satrius. Reputed so, my lord, and of deep practice.
  Sejanus. Bring him in to me, in the gallery;
And take you cause to leave us there together:
I would confer with him, about a grief—
On.   [*Exeunt* SEJANUS, SATRIUS, TERENTIUS, &c.
  Arruntius. So! yet another? yet? O desperate state
Of grovelling honour! seest thou this, O sun,
And do we see thee after? Methinks, day
Should lose his light, when men do lose their shames,

And for the empty circumstance of life,
Betray their cause of living.
    Silius. Nothing so.
Sejanus can repair, if Jove should ruin.
He is now the court god; and well applied
With sacrifice of knees, of crooks, and cringes;
He will do more than all the house of heaven
Can for a thousand hecatombs. 'Tis he
Makes us our day, or night; hell and elysium
Are in his look: we talk of Rhadamanth,
Furies, and firebrands; but it is his frown
That is all these; where, on the adverse part,
His smile is more than e'er yet poets feigned
Of bliss, and shades, nectar—
    Arruntius. A serving boy!
I knew him, at Caius' trencher, when for hire
He prostituted his abused body
To that great gormond, fat Apicius:
And was the noted pathic of the time.
    Sabinus. And, now, the second face of the whole world!
The partner of the empire, hath his image
Reared equal with Tiberius, born in ensigns;
Commands, disposes every dignity.
Centurions, tribunes, heads of provinces,
Prætors, and consuls; all that heretofore
Rome's general suffrage gave, is now his sale.
The gain, or rather spoil of all the earth,
One, and his house, receives.
    Silius. He hath of late
Made him a strength too, strangely, by reducing
All the prætorian bands into one camp,
Which he commands: pretending that the soldiers,
By living loose and scattered, fell to riot;
And that if any sudden enterprise
Should be attempted, their united strength
Would be far more than severed; and their life
More strict, if from the city more removed.
    Sabinus. Where now he builds what kind of forts he please,
Is heard to court the soldier by his name,
Woos, feasts the chiefest men of action,
Whose wants, nor loves, compel them to be his.

And though he ne'er were liberal by kind,
Yet to his own dark ends, he's most profuse,
Lavish, and letting fly, he cares not what
To his ambition.
    Arruntius. Yet, hath he ambition?
Is there that step in state can make him higher,
Or more, or anything he is, but less?
    Silius. Nothing but emperor.
    Arruntius. The name Tiberius,
I hope, will keep, howe'er he hath foregone
The dignity and power.
    Silius. Sure, while he lives.
    Arruntius. And dead, it comes to Drusus. Should he fail,
To the brave issue of Germanicus;
And they are three: too many—ha? for him
To have a plot upon?
    Silius. I do not know
The heart of his designs; but sure their face
Looks farther than the present.
    Arruntius. By the gods,
If I could guess he had but such a thought,
My sword should cleave him down from head to heart,
But I would find it out: and with my hand
I'd hurl his panting brain about the air
In mites as small as atomi, to undo
The knotted bed—
    Sabinus. You are observed, Arruntius.
    Arruntius [*turns to* Natta, Terentius, &c.]. Death!
      I dare tell him so; and all his spies:
You sir, I would, do you look? and you.
    Sabinus. Forbear.

Scene ii—*The former Scene continued*

A Gallery discovered opening into the State Room.

Enter Satrius *with* Eudemus.

    Satrius. Here he will instant be; let's walk a turn;
You're in a muse, Eudemus?
    Eudemus. Not I, sir.

I wonder he should mark me out so! well,
Jove and Apollo form it for the best.   [*Aside*.
   Satrius. Your fortune's made unto you now, Eudemus,
If you can but lay hold upon the means;
Do but observe his humour, and—believe it—
He is the noblest Roman, where he takes—

Enter SEJANUS.

Here comes his lordship.
   Sejanus. Now, good Satrius.
   Satrius. This is the gentleman, my lord.
   Sejanus. Is this?
Give me your hand, we must be more acquainted.
Report, sir, hath spoke out your art and learning:
And I am glad I have so needful cause,
However in itself painful and hard,
To make me known to so great virtue—Look,
Who is that, Satrius? [*Exit* SATRIUS] I have a grief, sir,
That will desire your help. Your name's Eudemus?
   Eudemus. Yes.
   Sejanus. Sir?
   Eudemus. It is, my lord.
   Sejanus. I hear you are
Physician to Livia, the princess.
   Eudemus. I minister unto her, my good lord.
   Sejanus. You minister to a royal lady, then.
   Eudemus. She is, my lord, and fair.
   Sejanus. That's understood
Of all their sex, who are or would be so;
And those that would be, physic soon can make them:
For those that are, their beauties fear no colours.
   Eudemus. Your lordship is conceited.
   Sejanus. Sir, you know it,
And can, if need be, read a learned lecture
On this, and other secrets. 'Pray you, tell me,
What more of ladies, besides Livia,
Have you your patients?
   Eudemus. Many, my good lord.
The great Augusta, Urgulania,
Mutilia Prisca, and Plancina: divers—

Sejanus. And, all these tell you the particulars
Of every several grief? how first it grew,
And then increased; what action caused that;
What passion that; and answer to each point
That you will put them?
 Eudemus. Else, my lord, we know not
How to prescribe the remedies.
 Sejanus. Go to,
You are a subtile nation, you physicians!
And grown the only cabinets in court,
To ladies' privacies. Faith, which of these
Is the most pleasant lady in her physic?
Come, you are modest now.
 Eudemus. 'Tis fit, my lord.
 Sejanus. Why, sir, I do not ask you of their urines,
Whose smell's most violet, or whose siege is best,
Or who makes hardest faces on her stool?
Which lady sleeps with her own face a nights?
Which puts her teeth off, with her clothes, in court?
Or, which her hair, which her complexion,
And, in which box she puts it? These were questions
That might, perhaps, have put your gravity
To some defence of blush. But, I inquired,
Which was the wittiest, merriest, wantonest?
Harmless interrogatories, but conceits.—
Methinks Augusta should be most perverse,
And froward in her fit.
 Eudemus. She's so, my lord.
 Sejanus. I knew it: and Mutilia the most jocund.
 Eudemus. 'Tis very true, my lord.
 Sejanus. And why would you
Conceal this from me, now? Come, what is Livia?
I know she's quick and quaintly spirited,
And will have strange thoughts, when she is at leisure:
She tells them all to you.
 Eudemus. My noblest lord,
He breathes not in the Empire, or on earth,
Whom I would be ambitious to serve
In any act, that may preserve mine honour,
Before your lordship.
 Sejanus: Sir, you can lose no honour,

By trusting aught to me. The coarsest act
Done to my service, I can so requite,
As all the world shall style it honourable:
Your idle, virtuous definitions,
Keep honour poor, and are as scorned as vain:
Those deeds breathe honour that do suck in gain.
    Eudemus. But, good my lord, if I should thus betray
The counsels of my patient, and a lady's
Of her high place and worth; what might your lordship,
Who presently are to trust me with your own,
Judge of my faith?
    Sejanus. Only the best, I swear.
Say now that I should utter you my grief,
And with it the true cause; that it were love,
And love to Livia, you should tell her this:
Should she suspect your faith? I would you could
Tell me as much from her; see if my brain
Could be turned jealous.
    Eudemus. Happily, my lord,
I could in time tell you as much and more;
So I might safely promise but the first
To her from you.
    Sejanus. As safely, my Eudemus,
I now dare call thee so, as I have put
The secret into thee.
    Eudemus. My lord—
    Sejanus. Protest not,
Thy looks are vows to me; use only speed,
And but affect her with Sejanus' love,
Thou art a man, made to make consuls. Go.
    Eudemus. My lord, I'll promise you a private meeting
This day together.
    Sejanus. Canst thou?
    Eudemus. Yes.
    Sejanus. The place?
    Eudemus. My gardens, whither I shall fetch your lordship.
    Sejanus. Let me adore my Æsculapius.
Why, this indeed is physic! and outspeaks
The knowledge of cheap drugs, or any use
Can be made out of it! more comforting

Than all your opiates, juleps, apozems,
Magistral syrups, or—Begone, my friend,
Not barely styled, but created so;
Expect things greater than thy largest hopes,
To overtake thee: Fortune shall be taught
To know how ill she hath deserved thus long,
To come behind thy wishes. Go, and speed.

[*Exit* EUDEMUS.

Ambition makes more trusty slaves than need.
These fellows, by the favour of their art,
Have still the means to tempt; oft-times the power.
If Livia will be now corrupted, then
Thou hast the way, Sejanus, to work out
His secrets, who, thou know'st, endures thee not,
Her husband, Drusus: and to work against them.
Prosper it, Pallas, thou that betterest wit;
For Venus hath the smallest share in it.

*　　*　　*

SEJANUS. Physician, thou art worthy of a province,
For the great favours done unto our loves;
And, but that greatest Livia bears a part
In the requital of thy services,
I should alone despair of aught, like means,
To give them worthy satisfaction.
　Livia. Eudemus, I will see it, shall receive
A fit and full reward for his large merit.—
But for this portion we intend to Drusus,
No more our husband now, whom shall we choose
As the most apt and abled instrument,
To minister it to him?
　Eudemus. I say, Lygdus.
　Sejanus. Lygdus? what's he?
　Livia. An eunuch Drusus loves.
　Eudemus. Ay, and his cup-bearer.
　Sejanus. Name not a second.
If Drusus love him, and he have that place,
We cannot think a fitter.
　Eudemus. True, my Lord.

For free access and trust are two main aids.
    Sejanus. Skilful physician!
    Livia. But he must be wrought
To the undertaking, with some laboured art.
    Sejanus. Is he ambitious?
    Livia. No.
    Sejanus. Or covetous?
    Livia. Neither.
    Eudemus. Yet, gold is a good general charm.
    Sejanus. What is he, then?
    Livia. Faith, only wanton, light.
    Sejanus. How! is he young and fair?
    Eudemus. A delicate youth.
    Sejanus. Send him to me, I'll work him.—Royal lady,
Though I have loved you long, and with that height
Of zeal and duty, like the fire, which more
It mounts it trembles, thinking nought could add
Unto the fervour which your eye had kindled;
Yet, now I see your wisdom, judgment, strength,
Quickness, and will, to apprehend the means
To your own good and greatness, I protest
Myself through rarified, and turned all flame
In your affection: such a spirit as yours,
Was not created for the idle second
To a poor flash, as Drusus; but to shine
Bright as the moon among the lesser lights,
And share the sov'reignty of all the world.
Then Livia triumphs in her proper sphere,
When she and her Sejanus shall divide
The name of Cæsar, and Augusta's star
Be dimmed with glory of a brighter beam:
When Agrippina's fires are quite extinct,
And the scarce-seen Tiberius borrows all
His little light from us, whose folded arms
Shall make our perfect orb. [*Knocking within.*] Who's that?
    Eudemus,
Look. [Exit EUDEMUS.] 'Tis not Drusus, lady, do not fear.
    Livia. Not I, my lord: my fear and love of him
Left me at once.
    Sejanus. Illustrious lady, stay—
    Eudemus [*within*]. I'll tell his lordship.

Re-enter EUDEMUS.

Sejanus. Who is it, Eudemus?
Eudemus. One of your lordship's servants brings you word
The emperor hath sent for you.
Sejanus. O! where is he?
With your fair leave, dear princess, I'll but ask
A question, and return.   [*Exit.*
Eudemus. Fortunate princess!
How are you blest in the fruition
Of this unequalled man, the soul of Rome,
The Empire's life, and voice of Cæsar's world!
Livia. So blessed, my Eudemus, as to know
The bliss I have, with what I ought to owe
The means that wrought it. How do I look to-day?
Eudemus. Excellent clear, believe it. This same focus
Was well laid on.
Livia. Methinks 'tis here not white.
Eudemus. Lend me your scarlet, lady. 'Tis the sun,
Hath giv'n some little taint unto the ceruse;
You should have used of the white oil I gave you.
Sejanus, for your love! his very name
Commandeth above Cupid or his shafts—

                                          [*Paints her cheek.*

Livia. Nay, now you've made it worse.
Eudemus. I'll help it straight—
And but pronounced, is a sufficient charm
Against all rumour; and of absolute power
To satisfy for any lady's honour.
Livia. What do you now, Eudemus?
Eudemus. Make a light focus,
To touch you o'er withal. Honoured Sejanus!
What act, though ne'er so strange and insolent,
But that addition will at least bear out,
If't do not expiate?
Livia. Here, good physician.
Eudemus. I like this study to preserve the love
Of such a man, that comes not every hour
To greet the world.—'Tis now well, lady, you should
Use of the dentifrice I prescribed you too,
To clear your teeth, and the prepared pomatum,

To smooth the skin:—A lady cannot be
Too curious of her form, that still would hold
The heart of such a person, made her captive,
As you have his: who, to endear him more
In your clear eye, hath put away his wife,
The trouble of his bed, and your delights,
Fair Apicata, and made spacious room
To your new pleasures.
    Livia. Have not we returned
That with our hate to Drusus, and discovery
Of all his counsels?
    Eudemus. Yes, and wisely, lady.
The ages that succeed, and stand far off
To gaze at your high prudence, shall admire,
And reckon it an act without your sex:
It hath that rare appearance. Some will think
Your fortune could not yield a deeper sound,
Than mixed with Drusus; but, when they shall hear
That, and the thunder of Sejanus meet,
Sejanus, whose high name doth strike the stars,
And rings about the concave; great Sejanus,
Whose glories, style, and titles are himself,
The often iterating of Sejanus:
They then will lose their thoughts, and be ashamed
To take acquaintance of them.

Re-enter SEJANUS.

    Sejanus. I must make
A rude departure, lady; Cæsar sends
With all his haste both of command and prayer.
Be resolute in our plot; you have my soul,
As certain yours as it is my body's.
And, wise physician, so prepare the poison,
As you may lay the subtile operation
Upon some natural disease of his:
Your eunuch send to me. I kiss your hands,
Glory of ladies, and commend my love
To your best faith and memory.
    Livia. My lord.

I shall but change your words. Farewell. Yet, this
Remember for your heed, he loves you not;
You know what I have told you; his designs
Are full of grudge and danger; we must use
More than a common speed.

    Sejanus. Excellent lady,
How you do fire my blood!

    Livia. Well, you must go?
The thoughts be best, are least set forth to show.

                         [*Exit* SEJANUS.

    Eudemus. When will you take some physic, lady?

    Livia. When
I shall, Eudemus: but let Drusus' drug
Be first prepared.

    Eudemus. Were Lygdus made, that's done;
I have it ready. And, to-morrow morning
I'll send you a perfume, first to resolve
And procure sweat, and then prepare a bath
To cleanse and clear the cutis; against when
I'll have an excellent new fucus made,
Resistive 'gainst the sun, the rain, or wind,
Which you shall lay on with a breath, or oil,
As you best like, and last some fourteen hours.
This change came timely, lady, for your health,
And the restoring of your complexion,
Which Drusus' choler had almost burnt up;
Wherein your fortune hath prescribed you better
Than art could do.

    Livia. Thanks, good physician,
I'll use my fortune, you shall see, with reverence.
Is my coach ready?

    Eudemus. It attends your highness.   [*Exeunt.*

HERMAN MELVILLE
White Jacket

——————◄∞►——————

HERMAN MELVILLE (1819-1891) stands like a colossus over American
literature. His *Moby Dick* is regarded as one of the three or four greatest
American novels. He was obsessed with questions of good and evil. In
White Jacket he wrote about his sea-going days as a sailor aboard the
U.S.S. United States.

*   *   *

THE SURGEON OF THE FLEET.

Cadwallader Cuticle, M.D., and Honorary Member of the most distinguished Colleges of Surgeons both in Europe and America, was our
Surgeon of the Fleet. Nor was he at all blind to the dignity of his position; to
which, indeed, he was rendered peculiarly competent, if the reputation he
enjoyed was deserved. He had the name of being the foremost Surgeon in
the Navy, a gentleman of remarkable science, and a veteran practitioner.

He was a small, withered man, nearly, perhaps quite, sixty years of age.
His chest was shallow, his shoulders bent, his pantaloons hung round
skeleton legs, and his face was singularly attenuated. In truth, the corporeal
vitality of this man seemed, in a good degree, to have died out of him. He
walked abroad, a curious patch-work of life and death, with a wig, one glass
eye, and a set of false teeth, while his voice was husky and thick; but his
mind seemed undebilitated as in youth; it shone out of his remaining eye
with basilisk brilliancy.

Like most old physicians and surgeons who have seen much service, and
have been promoted to high professional place for their scientific attain-
ments, this Cuticle was an enthusiast in his calling. In private, he had once
been heard to say, confidentially, that he would rather cut off a man's arm
than dismember the wing of the most delicate pheasant. In particular, the
department of Morbid Anatomy was his peculiar love; and in his state-room
below he had a most unsightly collection of Parisian casts, in plaster and
wax, representing all imaginable malformations of the human members,
both organic and induced by disease. Chief among these was a cast, often to
be met with in the Anatomical Museums of Europe, and no doubt an
unexaggerated copy of a genuine original; it was the head of an elderly

woman, with an aspect singularly gentle and meek, but at the same time wonderfully expressive of a gnawing sorrow, never to be relieved. You would almost have thought it the face of some abbess, for some unspeakable crime voluntarily sequestered from human society, and leading a life of agonised penitence without hope; so marvellously sad and tearfully pitiable was this head. But when you first beheld it, no such emotions ever crossed your mind. All your eyes and all your horrified soul were fast fascinated and frozen by the sight of a hideous, crumpled horn, like that of a ram, downward growing out from the forehead, and partly shadowing the face; but as you gazed, the freezing fascination of its horribleness gradually waned, and then your whole heart burst with sorrow, as you contemplated those aged features, ashy pale and wan. The horn seemed the mark of a curse for some mysterious sin, conceived and committed before the spirit had entered the flesh. Yet that sin seemed something imposed, and not voluntarily sought; some sin growing out of the heartless necessities of the predestination of things; some sin under which the sinner sank in sinless woe.

But no pang of pain, not the slightest touch of concern, ever crossed the bosom of Cuticle when he looked on this cast. It was immovably fixed to a bracket, against the partition of his state-room, so that it was the first object that greeted his eyes when he opened them from his nightly sleep. Nor was it to hide the face, that upon retiring, he always hung his Navy cap upon the upward curling extremity of the horn, for that obscured it but little.

The Surgeon's cot-boy, the lad who made up his swinging bed and took care of his room, often told us of the horror he sometimes felt when he would find himself alone in his master's retreat. At times he was seized with the idea that Cuticle was a preternatural being; and once entering his room in the middle watch of the night, he started at finding it enveloped in a thick, bluish vapour, and stifling with the odours of brimstone. Upon hearing a low groan from the smoke, with a wild cry he darted from the place, and, rousing the occupants of the neighbouring state-rooms, it was found that the vapour proceeded from smouldering bunches of lucifer matches, which had become ignited through the carelessness of the Surgeon. Cuticle, almost dead, was dragged from the suffocating atmosphere, and it was several days ere he completely recovered from its effects. This accident took place immediately over the powder magazine; but as Cuticle, during his sickness, paid dearly enough for transgressing the laws prohibiting combustibles in the gun-room, the Captain contented himself with privately remonstrating with him.

Well knowing the enthusiasm of the Surgeon for all specimens of morbid anatomy, some of the ward-room officers used to play upon his credulity, though, in every case, Cuticle was not long in discovering their deceptions. Once, when they had some sago pudding for dinner, and Cuticle chanced to be ashore, they made up a neat parcel of this bluish-white, firm, jelly-like preparation, and placing it in a tin box, carefully sealed with wax, they deposited it on the gun-room table, with a note, purporting to come from an eminent physician in Rio, connected with the Grand National Museum on the Praca d' Acclamacao, begging leave to present the scientific Senhor Cuticle—with the donor's compliments—an uncommonly fine specimen of a cancer.

Descending to the ward-room, Cuticle spied the note, and no sooner read it, than, clutching the case, he opened it, and exclaimed, "Beautiful! splendid! I have never seen a finer specimen of this most interesting disease."

"What have you there, Surgeon Cuticle?" said a Lieutenant, advancing.

"Why, sir, look at it; did you ever see anything more exquisite?"

"Very exquisite indeed; let me have a bit of it, will you, Cuticle?"

"Let you have a bit of it!" shrieked the Surgeon, starting back. "Let you have one of my limbs! I wouldn't mar so large a specimen for a hundred dollars; but what can you want of it? You are not making collections!"

"I'm fond of the article," said the Lieutenant; "it's a fine cold relish to bacon or ham. You know, I was in New Zealand last cruise, Cuticle, and got into sad dissipation there among the cannibals; come, let's have a bit, if it's only a mouthful."

"Why, you infernal Feejee!" shouted Cuticle, eyeing the other with a confounded expression; "you don't really mean to eat a piece of this cancer?"

"Hand it to me, and see whether I will not," was the reply.

"In God's name, take it!" cried the Surgeon, putting the case into his hands, and then standing with his own uplifted.

"Steward!" cried the Lieutenant, "the castor—quick! I always use plenty of pepper with this dish, Surgeon; it's oystery. Ah! this is really delicious," he added, smacking his lips over a mouthful. "Try it now, Surgeon, and you'll never keep such a fine dish as this, lying uneaten on your hands, as a mere scientific curiosity."

Cuticle's whole countenance changed; and, slowly walking up to the table, he put his nose close to the tin case, then touched its contents with his finger and tasted it. Enough. Buttoning up his coat, in all the tremblings of an old man's rage he burst from the ward-room, and, calling for a boat, was not seen again for twenty-four hours.

But though, like all other mortals, Cuticle was subject at times to these fits of passion—at least under outrageous provocation—nothing could exceed his coolness when actually employed in his imminent vocation. Surrounded by moans and shrieks, by features distorted with anguish inflicted by himself, he yet maintained a countenance almost supernaturally calm; and unless the intense interest of the operation flushed his wan face with a momentary tinge of professional enthusiasm, he toiled away, untouched by the keenest misery coming under a fleet-surgeon's eye. Indeed, long habituation to the dissecting-room and the amputation-table had made him seemingly impervious to the ordinary emotions of humanity. Yet you could not say that Cuticle was essentially a cruel-hearted man. His apparent heartlessness must have been of a purely scientific origin. It is not to be imagined even that Cuticle would have harmed a fly, unless he could procure a microscope powerful enough to assist him in experimenting on the minute vitals of the creature.

But notwithstanding his marvellous indifference to the sufferings of his patients, and spite even of his enthusiasm in his vocation—not cooled by frosting old age itself—Cuticle, on some occasions, would effect a certain disrelish of his profession, and declaim against the necessity that forced a man of his humanity to perform a surgical operation. Especially was it apt to be thus with him, when the case was one of more than ordinary interest. In discussing it previous to setting about it, he would veil his eagerness under an aspect of great circumspection, curiously marred, however, by continual sallies of unsuppressible impatience. But the knife once in his hand, the compassionless surgeon himself, undisguised, stood before you. Such was Cadwallader Cuticle, our Surgeon of the Fleet.

*   *   *

A CONSULTATION OF MAN-OF-WAR SURGEONS.

It seems customary for the Surgeon of the Fleet, when any important operation in his department is on the anvil, and there is nothing to absorb professional attention from it, to invite his brother surgeons, if at hand at the time, to a ceremonious consultation upon it. And this, in courtesy, his brother surgeons expect.

In pursuance of this custom, then, the surgeons of the neighbouring American ships of war were requested to visit the Neversink in a body, to advise concerning the case of the top-man, whose situation had now become critical. They assembled on the half-deck, and were soon joined by their respected senior, Cuticle. In a body they bowed as he approached, and accosted him with deferential regard.

"Gentlemen," said Cuticle, unostentatiously seating himself on a camp-stool, handed him by his cot-boy, "we have here an extremely interesting case. You have all seen the patient, I believe. At first I had hopes that I should have been able to cut down to the ball, and remove it; but the state of the patient forbade. Since then, the inflammation and sloughing of the part has been attended with a copious suppuration, great loss of substance, extreme debility and emaciation. From this, I am convinced that the ball has shattered and deadened the bone, and now lies impacted in the medullary canal. In fact, there can be no doubt that the wound is incurable, and that amputation is the only resource. But, gentlemen, I find myself placed in a very delicate predicament. I assure you I feel no professional anxiety to perform the operation. I desire your advice, and if you will now again visit the patient with me, we can then return here and decide what is best to be done. Once more, let me say, that I feel no personal anxiety whatever to use the knife."

The assembled surgeons listened to this address with the most serious attention, and, in accordance with their superior's desire, now descended to the sick-bay, where the patient was languishing. The examination concluded, they returned to the half-deck, and the consultation was renewed.

"Gentlemen," began Cuticle, again seating himself, "you have now just inspected the limb; you have seen that there is no resource but amputation; and now, gentlemen, what do you say? Surgeon Bandage, of the Mohawk, will you express your opinion?"

"The wound is a very serious one," said Bandage—a corpulent man, with a high German forehead—shaking his head solemnly.

"Can anything save him but amputation?" demanded Cuticle.

"His constitutional debility is extreme," observed Bandage, "but I have seen more dangerous cases."

"Surgeon Wedge, of the Malay," said Cuticle, in a pet, "be pleased to give *your* opinion; and let it be definitive, I entreat:" this was said with a severe glance toward Bandage.

"If I thought," began Wedge, a very spare, tall man, elevating himself still higher on his toes, "that the ball had shattered and divided the whole *femur,* including the *Greater* and *Lesser Trochanter* the *Linear aspera* the *Digital fossa,* and the *Intertrochanteric,* I should certainly be in favour of amputation; but that, sir, permit me to observe, is not my opinion."

"Surgeon Sawyer, of the Buccaneer," said Cuticle, drawing in his thin lower lip with vexation, and turning to a round-faced, florid, frank, sensible-looking man, whose uniform coat very handsomely fitted him, and was adorned with an unusual quantity of gold lace; "Surgeon Sawyer, of the Buccaneer, let us now hear *your* opinion, if you please. Is not amputation the only resource, sir?"

"Excuse me," said Sawyer, "I am decidedly opposed to it; for if hitherto the patient has not been strong enough to undergo the extraction of the ball, I do not see how he can be expected to endure a far more severe operation. As there is no immediate danger of mortification, and you say the ball cannot be reached without making large incisions, I should support him, I think, for the present, with tonics, and gentle antiphlogistics, locally applied. On no account would I proceed to amputation until further symptoms are exhibited."

"Surgeon Patella, of the Algerine," said Cuticle, in an ill-suppressed passion, abruptly turning round on the person addressed, "will *you* have the kindness to say whether *you* do not think that amputation is the only resource?"

Now Patella was the youngest of the company, a modest man, filled with a profound reverence for the science of Cuticle, and desirous of gaining his good opinion, yet not wishing to commit himself altogether by a decided reply, though, like Surgeon Sawyer, in his own mind he might have been clearly against the operation.

"What you have remarked, Mr. Surgeon of the Fleet," said Patella, respectfully hemming, "concerning the dangerous condition of the limb, seems obvious enough; amputation would certainly be a cure to the wound; but then, as, notwithstanding his present debility, the patient seems to have a strong constitution, he might rally as it is, and by your scientific treatment, Mr. Surgeon of the Fleet"—bowing—"be entirely made whole, without risking an amputation. Still, it is a very critical case, and amputation may be indispensable; and if it *is* to be performed, there ought to be no delay whatever. That is my view of the case, Mr. Surgeon of the Fleet."

"Surgeon Patella, then, gentlemen," said Cuticle, turning round triumphantly, "is clearly of opinion that amputation should be immediately performed. For my own part—individually, I mean, and without respect to the patient—I am sorry to have it so decided. But this settles the question, gentlemen—in my own mind, however, it was settled before. At ten o'clock to-morrow morning the operation will be performed. I shall be happy to see you all on the occasion, and also your juniors" (alluding to the absent *Assistant Surgeons*). "Good-morning, gentlemen; at ten o'clock, remember."

And Cuticle retreated to the Ward-room.

*   *   *

THE OPERATION

Next morning, at the appointed hour, the surgeons arrived in a body. They were accompanied by their juniors, young men ranging in age from nineteen years to thirty. Like the senior surgeons, these young gentlemen were arrayed in their blue navy uniforms, displaying profusion of bright buttons, and several broad bars of gold lace about the wristbands. As in honour of the occasion, they had put on their best coats; they looked exceedingly brilliant.

The whole party immediately descended to the half-deck, where preparations had been made for the operation. A large garrison-ensign was stretched across the ship by the main-mast, so as completely to screen the space behind. This space included the whole extent aft to the bulk-head of the Commodore's cabin, at the door of which the marine-orderly paced, in plain sight, cutlass in hand.

Upon two gun-carriages, dragged amidships, the Deathboard (used for burials at sea) was horizontally placed, covered with an old royal-stun-sail. Upon this occasion, to do duty as an amputation-table, it was widened by an additional plank. Two match-tubs, near by, placed one upon another, at either end supported another plank, distinct from the table, whereon was exhibited an array of saws and knives of various and peculiar shapes and sizes; also, a sort of steel, something like the dinner-table implement, together with long needles, crooked at the end for taking up the arteries, and large darning-needles, thread and bee's-wax, for sewing up a wound.

At the end nearest the large table was a tin basin of water, surrounded by small sponges, placed at mathematical intervals. From the long horizontal pole of a great-gun rammer—fixed in its usual place overhead—hung a number of towels, with "U.S." marked in the corners.

All these arrangements had been made by the "Surgeon's steward," a person whose important functions in a man-of-war will, in a future chapter, be centered upon at large. Upon the present occasion, he was bustling about, adjusting and readjusting the knives, needles, and carver, like an over-conscientious butler fidgeting over a dinner-table just before the convivialists enter.

But by far the most striking object to be seen behind the ensign was a human skeleton, whose every joint articulated with wires. By a rivet at the apex of the skull, it hung dangling from a hammock-hook fixed in a beam above. Why this object was here, will presently be seen; but why it was placed immediately at the foot of the amputation-table, only Surgeon Cuticle can tell.

While the final preparations were being made, Cuticle stood conversing with the assembled Surgeons and Assistant Surgeons, his invited guests.

"Gentlemen," said he, taking up one of the glittering knives and artistically drawing the steel across it; "Gentlemen, though these scenes are very unpleasant, and in some moods, I may say, repulsive to me—yet how much better for our patient to have the contusions and lacerations of his present wound—with all its dangerous symptoms—converted into a clean incision, free from these objections, and occasioning so much less subsequent anxiety to himself and the Surgeon. Yes," he added, tenderly feeling the edge of his knife, "amputation is our only resource. Is it not so, Surgeon Patella?" turning toward that gentlemen, as if relying upon some sort of an assent, however clogged with conditions.

"Certainly," said Patella, "amputation is your only resource, Mr. Surgeon of the Fleet; that is, I mean, if you are fully persuaded of its necessity."

The other surgeons said nothing, maintaining a somewhat reserved air, as if conscious that they had no positive authority in the case, whatever might be their own private opinions; but they seemed willing to behold, and, if called upon, to assist at the operation, since it could not now be averted.

The young men, their Assistants, looked very eager, and cast frequent glances of awe upon so distinguished a practitioner as the venerable Cuticle.

"They say he can drop a leg in one minute and ten seconds from the moment the knife touches it," whispered one of them to another.

"We shall see," was the reply, and the speaker clapped his hand to his fob to see if his watch would be forthcoming when wanted.

"Are you all ready here?" demanded Cuticle, now advancing to his steward; "have not those fellows got through yet?" pointing to three men of the carpenter's gang, who were placing bits of wood under the gun-carriages supporting the central table.

"They are just through, sir," respectfully answered the steward, touching his hand to his forehead, as if there were a cap-front there.

"Bring up the patient, then," said Cuticle.

"Young gentlemen," he added, turning to the row of Assistant Surgeons, "seeing you here reminds me of the classes of students once under my instruction at the Philadelphia College of Physicians and Surgeons. Ah, those were happy days!'' he sighed, applying the extreme corner of his handkerchief to his glass-eye. "Excuse an old man's emotions, young gentlemen; but when I think of the numerous rare cases that then came under my treatment, I cannot but give way to my feelings. The town, the city, the metropolis, young gentlemen, is the place for you students; at least in these dull times of peace, when the army and navy furnish no inducements for a youth ambitious of rising in our honourable profession. Take an old man's advice, and if the war now threatening between the States and Mexico should break out, exchange your navy commissions for commissions in the army. From having no military marine herself, Mexico has always been backward in furnishing subjects for the amputation-tables of foreign navies. The cause of science has languished in her hands. The army, young gentlemen, is your best school; depend upon it. You will hardly believe it, Surgeon Bandage,'' turning to that gentlemen, "but this is my first important case of surgery in a nearly three years' cruise. I have been almost wholly confined in this ship to doctor's practice—prescribing for fevers and fluxes. True, the other day a man fell from the mizzen-top-sail-yard; but that was merely an aggravated case of dislocations and bones splintered and broken. No one, sir, could have made an amputation of it, without severely contusing his conscience. And mine—I may say it, gentlemen, without ostentation is—peculiarly susceptible.''

And so saying, the knife and carver touchingly dropped to his sides, and he stood for a moment fixed in a tender reverie. But a commotion being heard beyond the curtain, he started, and, briskly crossing and recrossing the knife and carver, exclaimed, "Ah, here comes our patient; surgeons, this side of the table, if you please; young gentlemen, a little further off, I beg. Steward, take off my coat—so; my neckerchief now; I must be perfectly unencumbered, Surgeon Patella, or I can do nothing whatever.''

These articles being removed, he snatched off his wig, placing it on the gun-deck capstan; then took out his set of false teeth, and placed it by the side of the wig; and, lastly, putting his forefinger to the inner angle of his blind eye, spirited out the glass optic with professional dexterity, and deposited that, also, next to the wig and false teeth.

Thus divested of nearly all inorganic appurtenances, what was left of the Surgeon slightly shook itself, to see whether anything more could be spared to advantage.

"Carpenter's mates," he now cried, "will you never get through with that job?''

"Almost through, sir—just through," they replied, staring round in

search of the strange, unearthly voice that addressed them; for the absence
of his teeth had not at all improved the conversational tones of the Surgeon
of the Fleet.

With natural curiosity, these men had purposely been lingering, to see all
they could; but now, having no further excuse, they snatched up their
hammers and chisels, and—like the stage-builders decamping from a public
meeting at the eleventh hour, after just completing the rostrum in time for
the first speaker—the Carpenter's gang withdrew.

The broad ensign now lifted, revealing a glimpse of the crowd of
man-of-war's-men outside, and the patient, borne in the arms of two of his
mess-mates, entered the place. He was much emaciated, weak as an infant,
and every limb visibly trembled, or rather jarred, like the head of a man
with the palsy. As if an organic and involuntary apprehension of death had
seized the wounded leg, its nervous motions were so violent that one of the
mess-mates was obliged to keep his hand upon it.

The top-man was immediately stretched upon the table, the attendants
steadying his limbs, when, slowly opening his eyes, he glanced about at the
glittering knives and saws, the towels and sponges, the armed sentry at the
Commodore's cabin-door, the row of eager-eyed students, the meagre
death's-head of a Cuticle, now with his shirt sleeves rolled up upon his
withered arms, and knife in hand, and, finally, his eyes settled in horror
upon the skeleton, slowly vibrating and jingling before him, with the slow,
slight roll of the frigate in the water.

"I would advise perfect repose of your every limb, my man," said
Cuticle, addressing him; "the precision of an operation is often impaired by
the inconsiderate restlessness of the patient. But if you consider, my good
fellow," he added, in a patronising and almost sympathetic tone, and
slightly pressing his hand on the limb, "if you consider how much better it is
to live with three limbs than to die with four, and especially if you but knew
to what torments both sailors and soldiers were subjected before the time of
Celsus, owing to the lamentable ignorance of surgery then prevailing, you
would certainly thank God from the bottom of your heart that *your*
operation has been postponed to the period of this enlightened age, blessed
with a Bell, a Brodie, and a Lally. My man, before Celsus's time, such was
the general ignorance of our noble science, that, in order to prevent the
excessive effusion of blood, it was deemed indispensable to operate with a
red-hot knife"—making a professional movement toward the thigh—"and
pour scalding oil upon the parts"—elevating his elbow, as if with a tea-pot
in his hand—"still further to sear them, after amputation had been
performed."

"He is fainting!" said one of his mess-mates; "quick! some water!" The steward immediately hurried to the top-man with the basin.

Cuticle took the top-man by the wrist, and feeling it a while, observed, "Don't be alarmed, men," addressing the two mess-mates; "he'll recover presently; this fainting very generally takes place." And he stood for a moment, tranquilly eyeing the patient.

Now the Surgeon of the Fleet and the top-man presented a spectacle which, to a reflecting mind, was better than a church-yard sermon on the mortality of man.

Here was a sailor, who four days previous, had stood erect—a pillar of life—with an arm like a royal-mast and a thigh like a windlass. But the slightest conceivable fingertouch of a bit of crooked trigger had eventuated in stretching him out, more helpless than an hour-old babe, with a blasted thigh, utterly drained of its brawn. And who was it that now stood over him like a superior being, and, as if clothed himself with the attributes of immortality, indifferently discoursed of carving up his broken flesh, and thus piecing out his abbreviated days. Who was it, that in capacity of Surgeon, seemed enacting the part of a Regenerator of life? The withered, shrunken, one-eyed, toothless, hairless Cuticle; with a trunk half dead—a *memento mori* to behold!

And while, in those soul-sinking and panic-striking premonitions of speedy death which almost invariably accompany a severe gun-shot wound, even with the most intrepid spirits; while thus drooping and dying, this once robust top-man's eye was now waning in his head like a Lapland moon being eclipsed in clouds—Cuticle, who for years had still lived in his withered tabernacle of a body—Cuticle, no doubt sharing in the common self-delusion of old age—Cuticle must have felt his hold of life as secure as the grim hug of a grizzly bear. Verily, Life is more awful than Death; and let no man, though his live heart beat in him like a cannon—let him not hug his life to himself; for, in the predestinated necessities of things, that bounding life of his is not a whit more secure than the life of a man on his death-bed. To-day we inhale the air with expanding lungs, and life runs through us like a thousand Niles; but to-morrow we may collapse in death, and all our veins be dry as the Brook Kedron in a drought.

"And now, young gentlemen," said Cuticle, turning to the Assistant Surgeons, "while the patient is coming to, permit me to describe to you the highly-interesting operation I am about to perform."

"Mr. Surgeon of the Fleet," said Surgeon Bandage, "if you are about to lecture, permit me to present you with your teeth; they will make your discourse more readily understood." And so saying, Bandage, with a bow, placed the two semicircles of ivory into Cuticle's hands.

"Thank you, Surgeon Bandage," said Cuticle, and slipped the ivory into its place.

"In the first place, now, young gentlemen, let me direct your attention to the excellent preparation before you. I have had it unpacked from its case, and set up here from my state-room, where it occupies the spare berth; and all this for your express benefit, young gentlemen. This skeleton I procured in person from the Hunterian department of the Royal College of Surgeons in London. It is a masterpiece of art. But we have no time to examine it now. Delicacy forbids that I should amplify at a juncture like this"—casting an almost benignant glance toward the patient, now beginning to open his eyes; "but let me point out to you upon this thigh-bone"—disengaging it from the skeleton, with a gentle twist—"the precise place where I propose to perform the operation. *Here,* young gentlemen, *here* is the place. You perceive it is very near the point of articulation with the trunk."

"Yes," interposed Surgeon Wedge, rising on his toes, "yes, young gentlemen, the point of articulation with the *acetabulum* of the *os innominatum.*"

"Where's your Bell on Bones, Dick?" whispered one of the assistants to the student next to him. "Wedge has been spending the whole morning over it, getting out the hard names."

"Surgeon Wedge," said Cuticle, looking round severely, "we will dispense with your commentaries, if you please, at present. Now, young gentlemen, you cannot but perceive, that the point of operation being so near the trunk and the vitals, it becomes an unusually beautiful one, demanding a steady hand and a true eye; and, after all, the patient may die under my hands."

"Quick, Steward! water, water; he's fainting again!" cried the two mess-mates.

"Don't be alarmed for your comrade, men," said Cuticle, turning round. "I tell you it is not an uncommon thing for the patient to betray some emotion upon these occasions—most usually manifested by swooning; it is quite natural it should be so. But we must not delay the operation. Steward, that knife—no, the next one—there, that's it. He is coming to, I think"—feeling the top-man's wrist. "Are you all ready, sir?"

This last observation was addressed to one of the Neversink's assistant surgeons, a tall, lank, cadaverous young man, arrayed in a sort of shroud of white canvas, pinned about his throat, and completely enveloping his person. He was seated on a match-tub—the skeleton swinging near his head—at the foot of the table, in readiness to grasp the limb, as when a plank is being severed by a carpenter and his apprentice.

"The sponges, Steward," said Cuticle, for the last time taking out his teeth, and drawing up his shirt sleeves still further. Then, taking the patient by the wrist, "Stand by, now, you mess-mates; keep hold of his arms; pin him down. Steward, put your hand on the artery; I shall commence as soon as his pulse begins to—*now, now!*" Letting fall the wrist, feeling the thigh carefully, and bowing over it an instant, he drew the fatal knife unerringly across the flesh. As it first touched the part, the row of surgeons simultaneously dropped their eyes to the watches in their hands while the patient lay, with eyes horribly distended, in a kind of waking trance. Not a breath was heard; but as the quivering flesh parted in a long, lingering gash, a spring of blood welled up between the living walls of the wounds, and two thick streams, in opposite directions, coursed down the thigh. The sponges were instantly dipped in the purple pool; every face present was pinched to a point with suspense; the limb writhed; the man shrieked; his mess-mates pinioned him; while round and round the leg went the unpitying cut.

"The saw!" said Cuticle.

Instantly it was in his hand.

Full of the operation, he was about to apply it, when, looking up, and turning to the assistant surgeons, he said, "Would any of you young gentlemen like to apply the saw? A splendid subject!"

Several volunteered; when, selecting one, Cuticle surrendered the instrument to him, saying, "Don't be hurried, now; be steady."

While the rest of the assistants looked upon their comrade with glances of envy, he went rather timidly to work; and Cuticle, who was earnestly regarding him, suddenly snatched the saw from his hand. "Away, butcher! you disgrace the profession. Look at *me!*"

For a few moments the thrilling, rasping sound was heard; and then the top-man seemed parted in twain at the hip, as the leg slowly slid into the arms of the pale, gaunt man in the shroud, who at once made away with it, and tucked it out of sight under one of the guns.

"Surgeon Sawyer," now said Cuticle, courteously turning to the surgeon of the Mohawk, "would you like to take up the arteries? They are quite at your service, sir."

"Do, Sawyer; be prevailed upon," said Surgeon Bandage.

Sawyer complied; and while, with some modesty he was conducting the operation, Cuticle, turning to the row of assistants said, "Young gentlemen, we will now proceed with our illustration. Hand me that bone, Steward." And taking the thigh-bone in his still bloody hands, and holding it conspiciously before his auditors, the Surgeon of the Fleet began:

"Young gentlemen, you will perceive that precisely at this spot— *here*—to which I previously directed your attention—at the corresponding spot precisely—the operation has been performed. About here, young gentlemen, here''—lifting his hand some inches from the bone—''about *here* the great artery was. But you noticed that I did not use the tourniquet; I never do. The forefinger of my steward is far better than a tourniquet, being so much more manageable, and leaving the smaller veins uncompressed. But I have been told, young gentlemen, that a certain Seignior Seignioroni, a surgeon of Seville, has recently invented an admirable substitute for the clumsy, old-fashioned tourniquet. As I understand it, it is something like a pair of *calipers,* working with a small Archimedes screw—a very clever invention, according to all accounts. For the padded points at the end of the arches''—arching his forefinger and thumb—''can be so worked as to approximate in such a way, as to—but you don't attend to me, young gentlemen,'' he added, all at once starting.

Being more interested in the active proceedings of Surgeon Sawyer, who was now threading a needle to sew up the overlapping of the stump, the young gentlemen had not scrupled to turn away their attention altogether from the lecturer.

A few moments more, and the top-man, in a swoon, was removed below into the sick-bay. As the curtain settled again after the patient had disappeared, Cuticle, still holding the thigh-bone of the skeleton in his ensanguined hands, proceeded with his remarks upon it; and having concluded them, added, ''Now, young gentlemen, not the least interesting consequence of this operation will be the finding of the ball, which, in case of non-amputation, might have long eluded the most careful search. That ball, young gentlemen, must have taken a most circuitous route. Nor, in cases where the direction is oblique, is this at all unusual. Indeed, the learned Henner gives us a most remarkable—I had almost said an incredible—case of a soldier's neck, where the bullet, entering at the part called Adam's Apple—''

''Yes,'' said Surgeon Wedge, elevating himself, ''the *pomum Adami.*''

''Entering the point called *Adam's Apple,*'' continued Cuticle, severely emphasising the last two words, ''ran completely around the neck, and, emerging at the same hole it had entered, shot the next man in the ranks. It was afterward extracted, says Henner, from the second man, and pieces of the other's skin were found adhering to it. But examples of foreign substances being received into the body with a ball, young gentlemen, are frequently observed. Being attached to a United States ship at the time, I happened to be near the spot of the battle of Ayacucho, in Peru. The day after the action, I saw in the barracks of the wounded a trooper, who, having been severely injured in the brain, went crazy, and, with his own holster-pistol, committed suicide in the hospital. The ball drove inward a portion of his woollen night-cap——''

"In the form of a *cul-de-sac,* doubtless," said the undaunted Wedge.

"For once, Surgeon Wedge, you use the only term that can be employed; and let me avail myself of this opportunity to say to you, young gentlemen, that a man of true science"—expanding his shallow chest a little—"uses but few hard words, and those only when none other will answer his purpose; whereas the smatterer in science"—slightly glancing toward Wedge—"thinks, that by mouthing hard words, he proves that he understands hard things. Let this sink deep in your minds, young gentlemen; and, Surgeon Wedge"—with a stiff bow—"permit me to submit the reflection to yourself. Well, young gentlemen, the bullet was afterward extracted by pulling upon the external parts of the *cul-de-sac*—a simple, but exceedingly beautiful operation. There is a fine example, somewhat similar, related in Guthrie; but, of course, you must have met with it, in so well-known a work as his Treatise upon Gun-shot Wounds. When, upward of twenty years ago, I was with Lord Cochrane, then Admiral of the fleets of this very country"—pointing shoreward, out of a port-hole—"a sailor of the vessel to which I was attached, during the blockade of Bahia, had his leg——" But by this time the fidgets had completely taken possession of his auditors, especially of the senior surgeons; and turning upon them abruptly, he added, "But I will not detain you longer, gentlemen"—turning round upon all the surgeons—"your dinners must be waiting you on board your respective ships. But, Surgeon Sawyer, perhaps you may desire to wash your hands before you go. There is the basin, sir; you will find a clean towel on the rammer. For myself, I seldom use them"—taking out his handkerchief. "I must leave you now, gentlemen"—bowing. "To-morrow, at ten, the limb will be upon the table, and I shall be happy to see you all upon the occasion. Who's there?" turning to the curtain, which then rustled.

"Please, sir," said the Steward, entering, "the patient is dead."

"The body also, gentlemen, at ten precisely," said Cuticle, once more turning round upon his guests. "I predicted that the operation might prove fatal; he was very much run down. Good-morning;" and Cuticle departed.

"He does not, surely, mean to touch the body?" exclaimed Surgeon Sawyer, with much excitement.

"Oh, no!" said Patella, "that's only his way; he means, doubtless, that it may be inspected previous to being taken ashore for burial."

The assemblage of gold-laced surgeons now ascended to the quarter-deck; the second cutter was called away by the bugler, and, one by one, they were dropped aboard of their respective ships.

The following evening the mess-mates of the top-man rowed his remains ashore, and buried them in the eververnal Protestant cemetery, hard by the Beach of the Flamingoes, in plain sight from the bay.

PINDAR
Pythia III

———∞———

PINDAR (c. 522 B.C.—c. 443 B.C.) anticipated by more than 2500 years the use of poetry in therapy. In this poem he invokes the god of healing to effect a cure through poetry.

His mind was tame: for so he taught
That artisan of cures and strengthened limbs,
Gentle Asclepios
The magnificent who delivered men from all disease.

DYLAN THOMAS
The Doctor and the Devils

———————⊸∞⊶———————

DYLAN THOMAS (1914-1953) said of himself, "I have seen the gates of hell." His extreme sensitivity and Christian guilt caused him great pain and made him view not only himself but the rest of the world as full of hypocrites. "The Doctor and the Devils" is based on a true story.

ROCK. I stand before you, gentlemen, as a lecturer in Anatomy, a scientist, a specialist, a *material* man to whom the heart, for instance, is an elaborate physical organ and not the 'seat of love,' a man to whom the 'soul,' because it has no shape, does not exist.

But paradox is inherent in all dogma, and so I stand before you also as a man of sentiment, of spiritual aspirations, intellectually creative impulses, social convictions, moral passions. And it is in my dual capacity of scientist and sociologist, materialist and moralist, anatomist and artist, that I shall attempt to conduct my lectures, to expound, inform, illustrate, entertain and edify.

Our aim for ever must be the pursuit of the knowledge of Man in his entirety. To study the flesh, the skin, the bones, the organs, the nerves of Man, is to equip our minds with a knowledge that will enable us to search *beyond* the body. The noble profession at whose threshold you stand as neophytes is not an end in itself. The science of Anatomy contributes to the great sum of all Knowledge, which is the Truth: the whole Truth of the Life of Man upon this turning earth. And so: Observe precisely. Record exactly. Neglect nothing. Fear no foe. Never swerve from your purpose. Pay no heed to Safety.

For I believe that all men can be happy and that the good life can be led upon this earth.

I believe that all men must work towards that end.

And I believe that that end justifies any means. . . .

Let no scruples stand in the way of the progress of medical science!

Rock bows: a curt, but studied bow.
The students rise.

And Rock walks off the platform.

The other man on the platform makes a gesture of dismissal to the students, then follows Rock.

And all the students suddenly begin talking as they move down the Lecture Hall.

HALLWAY OF ROCK'S ACADEMY.

Rock and his companion on the platform are walking through the Hallway towards a door under the stairs. They open the door and go through. We follow them, through the open door, into a

SMALL CLOAK-ROOM.

It is a bare, dark room. A few pegs on the wall—Rock's cloak and top-hat hang from one—and a table with a water jug and a basin on it.

Rock rolls up his sleeves, very circumspectly, as his companion pours water into the basin.

We hear, from outside, the noise of the students.

> ROCK. [With a nod towards the noise.] What do they talk about afterwards, I wonder? Do they repeat one's words of golden guidance? Or make disparaging remarks about one's waistcoat? I think when I was a student we used to tell one another stories: they were anatomical, too. Ah, thank you, Murray. . . .

Rock begins to wash his hands in the basin. Murray takes off his coat.

> MURRAY. You agree with all you said?
> ROCK. But naturally.
> MURRAY. 'The end justifies *any* means?' That is—to say the least of it—unscrupulous.
> ROCK. Then do not say 'the least of it.' Say 'the most': that it is *honest*.

And Murray begins to wash his hands.

> ROCK. You're coming to my dinner, of course? I can deplore the sacrilege of digging up the dead for anatomists to dissect.
> FIRST GENTLEMAN. [To no one in particular.] I wish I had retired with the ladies.
> ROCK. I am no platform drummer, no hawker of slogans, but I say that

the Resurrectionists who dig up the dead and sell them to the Anatomical Schools are a direct result of the wrongness of the Law. The Law says that surgeons must possess a high degree of skill. And a surgeon cannot acquire that skill without working upon dead human beings. But the Law also says that the only dead human beings we *can* work upon must come from the public gallows; a very uncertain, and meagre, supply. Legally, the hangman is our one provider. But he would have to hang all the *liars* in the City or all the men who are unfaithful to their wives, before there would be sufficient subjects for us. Therefore, we have to obtain our bodies illegally.

I myself, last term, had to pay out five hundred guineas to the Resurrectionists.

Rock drinks.
Murray passes the port to the Second Gentleman. The Second Gentleman fills his glass.

> SECOND GENTLEMAN. [Aside.] What very good port they provide in a mortuary these days . . .

But Rock now has the attention of the whole table.

> ROCK. Do not suppose for a moment that, even after dinner and in one of those mellow, argumentative moods in which one would try to prove that black is white or that politicians are incorruptible, I regard the Resurrectionists as anything but the vicious human vermin of the gutters of the city; in fact, a pack of devils.
>
> But as the Law says 'No' to our need, to the need of progressive science, so up crawl these creatures to satisfy that need *against* the Law. The same applies to every city, though *ours* is rather more fortunate than most; it is *full* of perverted blackguards.
> GREEN. [Provokingly.] If you dislike so much the Law that applies to your own science, Thomas, why did you become an anatomist rather than anything else?
> ROCK. There was more body to it.
> FIRST GENTLEMAN. You would make our City sound to a stranger like Sodom or Gomorrah. . . .
> GREEN. It *is* a seat of learning, after all, Thomas . . .
> ROCK. And the bowels of squalor. Look any night at the streets of this 'cultured city.' Observe, with academic calm, the homeless and the

hopeless and the insane and the wretchedly drunken lying in their rags on the stinking cobbles. Look for yourselves, sirs, at the beggars, and the cripples, and the tainted children, and the pitiful, doomed girls. Write a scholastic pamphlet on the things that prowl in the alleys, afraid to see the light; they were men and women once. Be proud of *that* if you can.

In the silence that follows, Murray rises to his feet.

MURRAY. If you'll excuse me, gentlemen, I must try to brave this—'*terrible* city at night.' You'll excuse me?

At a smiling nod—for Rock has again, suddenly, changed mood—Murray bows and goes out of the room.

ROCK. [At his most jocularly donnish.] And now, gentlemen, no more such talk from me.
SECOND GENTLEMAN. Oh, surely, not a little entertaining gossip about cannibalism, for a change?
ROCK. No, no, no, not another word. Or, as my friend Murray would say, 'Let us change the subject.'

LONG SHOT of the dinner table, Rock at the head, waggishly professional.
They are drinking coffee, but there is a decanter at Rock's elbow. Annabella is frigidly angry.

ANNABELLA. . . . And that is what I *believe,* and that is what is right.
ROCK. [Pointedly to Bennett.] Have some brandy. . . .
ANNABELLA. There can be, and there always has been, only *one* path of virtue.
ROCK. Surprisingly I agree with you, Annabella.
ANNABELLA. Then it is only for the second time in your life.
ROCK. I can't remember the first. But I agree with what you say, not with what you *mean. I believe in the virtue of following no path but your own, wherever it leads. . . .*
ANNABELLA. And that is precisely the sort of statement that antagonizes you to the whole of the profession. . . . For all your great successes and your famous friends, you do not know how many people there are who would be delighted to see you ruined. . . .
ELIZABETH. [To Bennet.] Do you like this City, Mr. Bennet, after the

Continent? I think you were very fortunate to have travelled around
so much with your parents in the holidays. . . .

BENNET. I like France, ma'am, very much indeed. Of course, I like
this City, too. . . .

ANNABELLA. Mr. Bennet, do you, as a student, find that my brother's
language and attitude are congenial to the other students?

ROCK. How d' you find the brandy, Bennet? Not mellow enough for
you?

BENNET. No, sir . . . it's . . . excellent. Yes, Miss Rock, we all find
Doctor Rock's language and . . . er . . . attitude . . . most . . .
congenial and, and . . . and *stimulating*.

ANNABELLA. Like brandy on persons of weak health, physical or
mental.

ELIZABETH. I should very much like to see Paris, Mr. Bennet. . . .

ANNABELLA. My dear Elizabeth, is this a geographical conver-
sazione? I merely wanted to know . . .

ROCK. [To Bennet.] Without embarrassing you further, and allowing
you no opportunity of savouring, let alone swallowing, the brandy
you were kind enough to call excellent, may I explain to you that
what my sister really wishes to know is whether you agree with her
that the medical profession, with some notable exceptions, consider
me a seducer of youth and an atheist? [In another tone.] You have no
need to answer, of course. . . . [Gently.] Has he, Elizabeth, my
dear? I would far prefer to talk about Paris. . . .

BENNET. [In an agony of embarrassment, but still determined to
defend his master.] I can't pretend to know what the medical
profession thinks of Doctor Rock, Miss Rock, but *we* all think that
most of the other doctors and professors are enormously *jealous* of
him. [To Elizabeth.] Jealous because he's a great anatomist, ma'am,
and a great—[He breaks off.]

ROCK. H'm! I know Paris well, especially the cafes. I always used to
wear a yachting cap in France, I can't think why. . . . I wish you'd
been there with me, my dear. . . .

DISSOLVE to

SMALL ROOM IN LODGING/HOUSE.

Nelly, at the fire, is stirring a wooden spoon in a black pot, and something is
being fried. We hear the sizzling.

Kate, with an almost bristleless broom, is brushing the broken glass into a
corner.
The broken table has been laid; there are four pewter mugs on it.
Suddenly there is a noise of singing and stamping from outside.
The door is crashed open and Broom dances in, a bottle under each arm.

> MURRAY. She was murdered by two paid thugs of yours: Fallon and
> Broom. I saw her last night after the theatre. She was well and gay.
> There are no signs of violence upon her body.
> ROCK. Thugs of *mine*, Mr. Murray? Do you remember that you
> yourself paid them for the last *three* subjects?
> MURRAY. She was murdered. I saw her. [Slowly, remembering.] She
> had a red shawl on.
> ROCK. Indisputable evidence that she was murdered. She should have
> worn a white shawl, for purity. And what if she *was* murdered, Mr.
> Murray? We are anatomists, not policemen; we are scientists, not
> moralists. Do *I, I,* care if every lewd and sottish woman of the
> streets has her throat slit from ear to ear? She served no purpose in
> life save the cheapening of physical passion and the petty traffics of
> lust. Let her serve her purpose in death.
> MURRAY. You hired Fallon and Broom to murder her as you hired
> them to murder the others.
> ROCK. I need bodies. They brought bodies. I pay for what I need. I do
> not hire murders . . .

Rock walks over to the door. Murray still has his back to it. Rock stops.
Their eyes meet. Then Murray moves aside. Rock opens the door and
walks out. We see him walking down the Corridor.

CUT. DISSECTING ROOM OF ROCK'S ACADEMY.

Rock walks in.
Students are gathered round the table where Jennie's body lies. We do not
see the body.
The students move aside as Rock enters.
He stands in the middle of the group. For a moment he is silent, his head
held a little to one side, looking down at the unseen body.

> MURRAY'S VOICE. There are no marks of violence upon the body.
> ELIZABETH'S VOICE. . . . . You bear false witness. . . .

MURRAY'S VOICE. I swear that Jennie and Billy are murdered. . . .

ELIZABETH'S VOICE. It is quite easy for you to wreck your life. . . .

And he turns and walks back through the garden towards the Academy.
Now his step is quicker and more purposeful.

ELIZABETH'S ROOM.

Rock, his coat off, but still immaculately dressed, is seated in a deep chair
with his head against the back of it.

Elizabeth is curling what remains of his hair with curling-tongs.

Rock has an air of indolent luxury.

ROCK. [Complacently.] The sensual apotheosis of the intellectual
animal. . . .

ELIZABETH. If you say so, my dear.

ROCK. The mind is relaxed, the body is pleasured and pampered,
rancour has taken a holiday, and I am full of bliss, like a cat on the
tiles of heaven. . . .

ELIZABETH. It must be very nice to talk. . . .

ROCK. It *is* comparable only to the pleasure of not having to think *as*
you talk. . . . [Sighing.] I am a fool to-day.

ELIZABETH. Yes. Thomas . . .

ROCK. [With a change of voice.] But not so much of a fool as some I
know. That rumour-breeder of a Murray!
Falls in love with a pretty face and then won't cut it up once the
little trollop's dead. Says she's murdered. Says, in effect, I murdered her myself.

ELIZABETH. [Mildly.] Oh, Thomas.

ROCK. When *I* take up assassination, I shall start with the surgeons in
this city and work *up* to the gutter. . . . And now, to-day, along he
comes with some fantastic rigmarole about a crippled idiot. Billy
Bedlam. Says *he's* murdered, too. Poor Billy's bed was the cobbles,
rain or snow, and he ate like a rat from the garbage heaps, and
swallowed all the rot-gut he could buy or beg. He was a consumptive
and an epileptic. A wonder he hadn't been found dead years ago.
. . .

ELIZABETH. What did you tell Mr. Murray?

ROCK. I said: 'Mr. Murray, go down and cut up the body and put it in
the brine baths. Be careful you don't fall in yourself—you're
wearing a good suit!'

ELIZABETH. [Casually.] And what did he do?

ROCK. What did he do? Why, what I told him to do, of course. No vicious-minded little prig with emotional adenoids is going to intimidate *me* with his whine and wail of 'Murder! Murder!' He suffers from hallucinations. My hands, to him, are red as Macbeth's.
. . .

Rock raises his very white hands in an elegant gesture, and smoothes the palm of one hand along the back of the other. . . .

Music
Pitch darkness.
Through the darkness, the laughter of Broom.
Then sudden light, and Fallon's hands, palms downwards, fingers stretched and tautened, murdering down the screen.
As the hands move we hear Fallon's voice, blurred in a distorting mirror of sound.

FALLON'S VOICE. There's devil in my hands. Let me go, my hands!

Then, close, from above, the upward-staring faces of old women and children, their eyes wide, their mouths open.

FALLON'S VOICE. Don't be frightened. . . . There's nothing to lose.
. . .

CITY STREET.

We see Fallon and Broom walking, in the slanting snowstorm, by the side of the Porter and his barrow with the tea-chest on it.

INTERIOR OF POLICE STATION.

Mr. and Mrs. Webb are still pleading to the Policeman.

MR. WEBB. No, no, sir, she said she'd come from Donegal when we was all drinkin' together last night. . . .
POLICEMAN. Drinkin'!
MRS. WEBB. Mrs. Flynn her name was, I've told you twenty times. . . .
Mr. Webb, with hesitant, frightened fingers touches his own mouth.
MR. WEBB. And now there's blood all over here. . . .

POLICEMAN. [*Placatingly.*] You sit down now, I'll come with you by
and by. . . .

He turns away from them and moves towards the back of the room.

MRS. WEBB. [*Dully,* as though repeating a lesson.] Mrs. Flynn her
name was. . . . They killed her. . . . Fallon and Broom. . . .

The always shadowy HALL in ROCK'S ACADEMY, with its white secret
witnesses staring from the glass cases.
Rock is mounting the stairs.
We follow him as he climbs, and hear the voice of his mind.

ROCK'S VOICE. Gentlemen. . . . Gentlemen, let us to-day dissect the
human conscience. Lay it on the slab. Open it up.
You see? The liver of the conscience is knobbled by emotional
excesses.
The veins of the conscience are full of bad blood.
The heart of the conscience palpitates like a snared rabbit's. . . .

Now he is walking along the Corridor, opening a door, to the small
Reference Library.

REFERENCE LIBRARY IN ROCK'S ACADEMY.

ROCK'S VOICE. In short, gentlemen, the conscience is a *very* unhealthy
subject. . . .

And, at the end of these words, he is sitting in a chair behind a desk, facing
us.
The room is empty.
And Rock, at the desk, addresses the empty room as though there were a
gathering of students in it, turning from one invisible listener to another.

ROCK. There is right and wrong, gentlemen, just as there is right and
left. Mine is the *right* direction. The fact that the majority would
consider it the *wrong* direction, only substantiates my opinion that I
am right. . . .

There is a knock on the door.

ROCK. Stay out.

Tom comes in.

    ROCK. I see, sir, that to keep you out I should have said, 'Come in.'
    TOM. Fallon and Broom, sir.
    ROCK. Indeed? Must I laugh, weep, tear my hair, swoon for ecstasy!
    TOM. They've brought a body, sir.
    ROCK. I did not expect that they would bring a soul.
    TOM. [Suggestively.] They bring so many subjects, sir . . . sixteen or
        more up till to-day . . . and always fresh. . . .
    ROCK. They are corpse-diviners. Or, as some have green fingers for
        gardening, so they have black fingers for death. Do you expect the
        dead to walk here, Tom? They need assistance. Fallon and Broom
        provide that assistance. Have Mr. Murray pay them.
    TOM. Yes, Sir.

Tom, with a side glance at Rock, goes out.
And Rock, alone, again speaks in a soft voice to his unseen audience.
    ROCK. You see gentlemen? . . .
SMALL ROOM IN LODGING/HOUSE.

We look at the room from above.
In the centre of the room stands the Policeman. Behind him, standing close
    together for protection, are Mr. and Mrs. Webb. Fallon leans against the
    table, facing the Policeman.
And behind him are Kate, Nelly, and Broom.
They are frozen.
As, from above, we move down closer to them, they unfreeze.
    FALLON. [Smiling] And where did the old fools tell ye they saw the
        body, sir?
Mrs. Webb points to the straw.
The Policeman kicks the straw aside. Broom laughs.
    FALLON. Maybe the mice, they dragged it down their little hole. . . .
The Policeman bends down, to stare at the floor-boards.
    POLICEMAN. Blood on the boards.
A moment's silence.
    FALLON. And has there ever been, for the love o' God, a Hallowe'en
        party with no blood spilt? We was all convivial; there was fightin' in
        every room of the house.

POLICEMAN. [In a whisper.] Cold!

Mr. and Mrs. Webb come into the room.

The Policeman nods towards the open tea-chest.

Timidly they move towards it and look down.

MR. WEBB. The old woman.

Mrs. Webb nods and crosses herself.

POLICEMAN. What was her name?

CUT again to CLOSE-UP of Mrs. Flynn's face.

MRS. WEBB'S VOICE. Mrs. Flynn. . . .

REFERENCE LIBRARY IN ROCK'S ACADEMY.

Rock, a sheet of paper in his hand, is walking up and down, in a
　characteristic lecture manner, behind his desk.

Some distance away, the other side of the desk, sits Murray.

> ROCK. [Gesturing with the paper in his hand.] If this does not upset
> some apple-carts, I shall believe that the apples have been glued on
> like the coco-nuts in coco-nut shies; if this does not help to change
> the idiotic laws that apply to our profession, I shall run amok; I shall
> send Doctor Hocking a Christmas Greeting and sign it 'Yours in
> Homage'; I shall place my spiritual welfare in the hands of the
> Reverend Doctor Lever and have my seat *reserved* in hell.
>
> MURRAY. I tell you, this isn't the time to attack.
>
> ROCK. The national anthem of the rabbit world.
>
> MURRAY. If you publish that letter now, attacking the system by which
> the medical schools get their bodies, you'll be raising a question you
> might have some difficulty in answering *yourself*.
>
> ROCK. Am I still a Doctor Bluebeard to you, then, you terrified old
> lady? Do I spend my nights a-murdering?
>
> MURRAY. I do not know, sir, what you do with your nights. I do not
> imagine that you can *sleep*. But I do know that *Fallon* and *Broom* are
> murderers. It is only my respect for you, and my great obligations,
> and my *cowardice,* that have stopped me from running out of this
> murder school and telling the whole city what I know and what I
> guess. . . . Even so, there are rumours. *I* have not spread them. But
> Jennie's death, and Billy's, have passed *quite* unnoticed. Rumours
> are contagious.
>
> ROCK. So are scabies. To destroy them you do not wear the armour of
> defense, you wield the weapon of sulphur ointment. And, by God,
> there's sulphur in this letter. . . .

Tom comes in.

TOM. The police have been here.

ROCK. What is yours, sir? A rum and bitters?

TOM. [Bewildered.] Sir?

ROCK. Since you do not knock before you come in, I must assume that this is a public-house. . . .

TOM. I beg your pardon, sir, but the police came about the new subject. Fallon and Broom, sir.

ROCK. Am I never to hear the end of those men's names?

MURRAY. [Softly.] Never, perhaps. . . .

TOM. And they're taking the subject away. . . .

ROCK. Why didn't you call the police? . . .

TOM. [More bewildered.] Sir, I . . .

ROCK. Go away and lock up the silver. If there isn't any silver, lock up Mr. Mattheson: he has a gold tooth.

And Tom goes out.

MURRAY. Must you antagonize every one?

ROCK. Yes.

MURRAY. You heard? The police.

ROCK. Outside the gates of hell are not the words 'Abandon Hope All Ye Who Enter Here,' but 'I Told You So.'

MURRAY. And if the police ask the questions, as they are bound to do, what shall I say?

ROCK. Say nothing. Squeak. They will recognize the voice of a rat.

Murray goes to the door. As he opens it Rock speaks.

ROCK. You will find cheese in the larder. Leave some for Tom.

The door slams.

CLOSE-UP of Rock. The sardonicism, the mockery, have vanished from his face.

DISSOLVE.

LONG SHOT of LONG CORRIDOR IN ROCK'S ACADEMY.

We see Tom coming up towards us from the end of the Corridor.

We see him open a door, put his head around the door. We hear him speak into the room behind the door, but are too far away to catch the words.

He comes on up the Corridor, opens another door, puts his head round the door. We hear him speak into the room behind the door, but though his voice is louder now, we still cannot catch the words.

He comes on up the Corridor, opens the door of the Reference Library, puts his head round the door. And now we are close enough to hear the words.

> TOM. Fallon and Broom. They've arrested Fallon and Broom. Murder.

He withdraws his head.

From the opposite end of the Corridor we now see, in *LONG SHOT,* Tom padding on, away from camera. . . .

DISSOLVE.

To another CORRIDOR

TRACK UP the empty Corridor.

As we track we hear a mumble of voices growing louder. We read a door marked "Board Room."

The noise rises.

INTERIOR OF BOARD ROOM.

Around the long table are attorneys, counsel, police officials, Hocking, and Green.

> FIRST POLICE OFFICIAL. . . . and if Doctor Rock did not know that these bodies were murdered, he's a far less canny gentleman than I supposed. . . .
>
> FIRST ATTORNEY. He knew. One corpse might pass him by, but Fallon and Broom were in the wholesale trade. . . .
>
> SECOND POLICE OFFICIAL. Indict him as accessory after the fact. . . .
>
> HOCKING. I do not exonerate Doctor Rock, but I will not have the whole medical profession of the City put on trial.
>
> GREEN. Accuse Rock, you accuse the integrity of all the surgeons in the City.

The Chairman (the Lord Chief Justice) nods in agreement.

HOCKING. Oh, more than that. The whole aristocracy of learning that has been so carefully built up would be tumbled to the ground. The stain upon his character would spread across the whole of our culture. There could be no more respect for us. Indictment of Rock would mean *the death of a class.* . . .

PRIVATE SMOKEROOM IN AN INN (as in Sequence 27).

The two old gentlemen are seated there with silver tankards in their hands.

FIRST GENTLEMAN. A great pity his letter appeared in all the newspapers. . . .
SECOND GENTLEMAN. On the very day of the arrest. Your health!
FIRST GENTLEMAN. Health!
SECOND GENTLEMAN. It was so very untactful.

There is a silence during which they drink. They gaze at their tankards.

FIRST GENTLEMAN. 'We must have more bodies,' he said. Dear, dear.
SECOND GENTLEMAN. We must have more *murders*.
FIRST GENTLEMAN. An ugly word, Richard.
SECOND GENTLEMAN. Doctor Rock has endangered the dignity of the higher professions. . . . If he is indicted as accessory after the fact . . .
FIRST GENTLEMAN. No, no, Richard, that must never be. Guilty or not guilty, his part in this affair must be kept in a decent obscurity, or Anarchy will be walking abroad in the land. . . .
SECOND GENTLEMAN. They should all be shot against the wall. . . .
FIRST GENTLEMAN. Who, Richard?

The Second Gentleman makes a vague, sweeping gesture.

SECOND GENTLEMAN. All of 'em. . . .

CLOSE SHOT of two elderly professors in mortar-boards and gowns, against the background of a very large, ornately gold-framed portrait of another old professor.

FIRST PROFESSOR. I agree with you entirely. His whole attitude to society spelt ruin from the first. Attack Tradition, it always bites back; and its teeth are well grounded.

SECOND PROFESSOR. A man who could be so persistently and obnoxiously rude to his elders and intellectual betters would think *nothing* of murdering his *own children* for a penny piece.

FIRST PROFESSOR. That is, perhaps, a little extravagant. We *must* disregard personal prejudice, though I agree that to be called 'anaemic buffoon' could not predispose him in your favour. But Rock is a *symbol*. . . .

SECOND PROFESSOR. I agree. A symbol of scholarship. In a manner of speaking, we could regard ourselves as 'the royal family of the intellect,' and . . .

FIRST PROFESSOR. My dear Fraser! . . .

SECOND PROFESSOR. . . . and if a member of the royal family is accused of a commoner's crime, then it is the *whole family* that is accused. An elaborate simile—but you see my point?

And the two professors wag their chins in complete agreement.

INTERIOR OF BOARD ROOM.

Around the table the attorneys, counsel, police officials, Hocking, and Green.

FIRST ATTORNEY. Perhaps we are forgetting the murder of children and old women in our concern for our sacred society of autocratic schoolmen. . . .

CHAIRMAN. It is a very grave position. . . .

SECOND POLICE OFFICIAL. Rock is guilty of connivance. . . .

FIRST POLICE OFFICIAL. I am afraid we *will* have to use him as a witness, gentlemen. . . .

CHAIRMAN. Oh, certainly, certainly. . . .

The police officials rise.

CHAIRMAN. [In an undertone to Hocking next to him.] But we won't call him, of course.

CORRIDOR IN ROCK'S ACADEMY.

Tom padding up the Corridor.

He stops outside the Reference Library, opens the door.

The students begin to rush down the gallery steps towards the doors and the
   platform, shouting.
Rock stands rigid.
He pales with temper, glaring at the rushing students as though they were
   his enemies.
In its intensity, his dignity is malevolent.

   ROCK. Gentlemen!

Cold, controlled fury stops the rush.
The students stand frozen.
The noise of the crowd is still loud.

> ROCK. I have attempted to teach you the dignity of man; I have
> succeeded in producing the degradation of a *mob*. Because the
> verminous gutter-snipes of the City snarl and gibber in the street,
> because the scum from the brothels and the rot-gut shops howl for
> blood outside my window, must *you* conduct yourselves, in return,
> as though you were born in a quagmire and nurtured on hog-wash?
>
> Take your seats. Pay no attention to *the mob*. The mob can never
> win. Remember that the louder a man shouts, the emptier is his
> argument.
>
> Remember that you are here to study osteology, syndesmology,
> myology, angiology, neurology, splanchnology: not bar-room
> pugilism or the morals of the crapulous bog-trotter and the tosspot.
>
> [In his usual lecturing voice.] The heart, gentlemen, is a four-
> chambered muscular bag which lies in the cavity of the thorax . . .

DISSOLVE to

CITY STREET.

Night.
The noise of the crowd is a distant, insistent background. We see, striding
   in front of us, the black-cloaked top-hatted figure of Rock with his heavy
   stick.

> ROCK. [Suddenly in another mood.] I was successful. I was estab-
> lished, I was standing in the light. . . . Then out of the mud of the
> darkness come two ignorant animals, and slowly, quite unknown to

themselves, they set about the task of bringing my life and my work down, down, into the slime that bred them. . . . Perhaps from the very moment of their monstrous births, it was decreed by some sadistic jack-in-office of the universe, that they should befoul and ruin a fellow creature they had never heard of: a garrulous, over-credulous, conceited little anatomist, in a city they had never seen. . . .

From outside the noise of the crowd rises. And as the noise rises, so the voices of Elizabeth and Rock become quieter and more intimate.

ELIZABETH. Let us go away.
ROCK. No, we must stay for ever.
ELIZABETH. I have never asked you before, Thomas, because I love you. Did you know that the bodies that those men brought you had been murdered?

The noise of the crowd rises. Now it is very loud.
And the night sky beyond the window is glowing.
Elizabeth and Rock turn sharply to look towards the window.

VOICES OF THE CROWD. Rock! Rock!
Hang Rock!
Burn him!
Burn!
Burn!
Rock's the boy who buys the beef. . . .

Annabella comes in. She is palely, composedly angry.

ANNABELLA. Do you know what those hooligans are *doing*, Thomas?

She crosses to the window.

ROCK. I gather that they are not subscribing to a testimonial to me. . . .
ANNABELLA. Look! Look!

COURT-ROOM.

LORD CHIEF JUSTICE. The Lord Justice Clerk and Lord Commissioners of Justiciary in respect of the verdict before recorded, determine and adjudge the said Robert Fallon, to be carried from the bar, and to be fed upon bread and water only until Wednesday, the 28th January, and upon that day to be taken forth to the common place of execution and then and there between the hours of eight and ten o'clock to be hanged by the neck until he be dead. And may Almighty God have mercy on your soul.

DISSOLVE to

Large CLOSE-UP of Rock.

ROCK. I have no need of your sympathy. When I see a tear, I smell a crocodile.

TRACK BACK to show that Rock is standing on the platform of the empty Lecture Hall. Murray, a good distance from Rock, stands at the window, looking out.
Their voices echo in the Hall.

MURRAY. [Turning round.] For God's sake, Thomas, can you do nothing but—stand still and gibe?
ROCK. Would you have me death-dance and *moan,* like a Gaelic dipsomaniac at a distillery fire? Must tragedy go immediately to the feet and the tongue? Because I can observe my history *calmly* as it burns and topples around me, you emotional gluttons think yourselves cheated. 'Oh, he can't *feel* anything,' you say. 'When we told him his life was over, he did not tear the relics of his hair or address the travelling moon in blank verse. He blew his nose and called for Burgundy.'
MURRAY. [Deliberately.] Fallon is to hang.
ROCK. A quick end. If they wished his death to be longer and infinitely more painful, they should marry him to Doctor Hocking's daughter.
MURRAY. Fallon is to hang. Nelly Connor is 'not guilty'! Broom and his woman are free to murder again! And *you*?
ROCK. I shall stay here.
I shall listen to the voices of the crowd outside my window, *inside my head;* it will not be long before they forget me; I shall never forget them.
I shall stay here. The whispers of the slanderer and the backbiter

will always be with me: mice behind the wall. I shall stay here. I shall count my friends on the fingers of one hand, then on one finger, then on none.

Camera Cranes Back, looking down at Rock and Murray all the time, over the empty tiers of the classroom.
Although Rock becomes further and further off, in *LONG SHOT,* the sound, booming hollowly through the empty classroom, remains in full close-up.

> ROCK. My lectures will be very well attended, at the beginning. I shall possess a sinister attraction to the young: dangerous and exciting, like dining with a vampire. But the attendance will diminish.
>
> I shall stay here to see in the eyes of the passing stranger in the street cruelty and contempt; in the eyes of the poor the terrible accusation: 'You killed the lost, the weak, the homeless, the hopeless, the helpless. Murderer of the poor!' God help me, life will go on. . . .

CONDEMNED CELL.

Fallon on a chair in the middle of the cell.
His hair is shaven.
A Phrenologist is measuring his head. He speaks the measurements aloud to an assistant, who writes them down in a book.
Fallon submits, with interest, to the examination.

CLOSE SHOT of Alice and Murray at a table in a TAVERN.
Around them the noise of the Market-place drinking. And pipes in the distance.

> ALICE. Fallon's dead—why isn't the Doctor dead? Nobody remembers Jennie now.
> MURRAY. Oh, there's lots of ways of dying. *I* remember.

CLOSE SHOT of Annabella and Elizabeth; behind them, the window of ELIZABETH'S ROOM looking out on the wintry trees in the garden.

> ANNABELLA. Do you *know* what it is to be lonely? I've always been lonely. I wanted to be mistress of my brother's house, I wanted to

give dinner parties and dances and be charming and admired. I
wanted to marry. But people wouldn't visit us because *you* married
him. It doesn't matter now. Now nobody'll come. . . .

ELIZABETH. I married him because I loved him. But we're only a very
little part of his life, Bella.

   I've been lonely, too.

CLOSE SHOT of Hocking and the Chairman (the Lord Chief Justice,
whom we saw in Sequences 111 and 114) against the background of
imposing bookcases.

CHAIRMAN. So, officially speaking, he's innocent as a lamb, the wolf.

HOCKING. We saved him from a criminal prosecution.

CHAIRMAN. Of course, of course. In order to save the good name of
society. Fallon and Broom could have brought their bodies to *you*,
of course. It just happened it was Rock they chose.

HOCKING. I would have none of their bodies.

CHAIRMAN. No?

HOCKING. But now it's all over. All over. We can speak our minds
now.

CHAIRMAN. We save him from public ruin, so that we can ruin him
privately. H'm, I'm sure he's grateful. . . .

LECTURE HALL OF ROCK'S ACADEMY.

Rock is on the platform.
The auditorium is densely packed.
We see Rock from the back of the Hall, over the heads of the students.
And we move, slowly, over the heads towards him as he speaks.

ROCK. To think, then, is to enter into a perilous country, colder of
welcome than the polar wastes, darker than a Scottish Sunday,
where the hand of the unthinker is always raised against you, where
the wild animals, who go by such names as Envy, Hypocrisy, and
Tradition, are notoriously carnivorous, and *where the parasites
rule*.

   To *think* is dangerous. The majority of men have found it easier to
writhe their way into the parasitical bureaucracy, or to *droop* into
the slack ranks of the ruled. I beg you all to devote your lives to
danger; I pledge you to adventure; I command you to experiment.

[Slowly.] Remember that the practice of Anatomy is absolutely vital to the *progress* of medicine. Remember that the progress of medicine is vital to the progress of mankind. And mankind is worth fighting for: killing and lying and dying for. Forget what you like. Forget all I have ever told you. But remember that. . . .

Now we see Rock in *CLOSE-UP*.
DISSOLVE to

CITY STREET.

Gathering dusk.
We hear the thin, high singing of the wind in the street.
And, in the background, the sound of the voices of children drifting through the dusk.
Rock, from a grey distance, is walking towards us along the street. He is cloaked, top-hatted.
And as he comes closer to us a little girl runs out of the shadows of a side-street, runs barefoot through the wind, her black hair leaping.
She is grimed from the gutters of the city; her dress is thin and ragged; one shoulder is naked.
And she runs at Rock's side, crying out:

GIRL. Give us a penny, mister, give us a penny. . . .

The camera *TRACKS BACK* as Rock, and the little girl running at his side, move on down the street.
The Rock stops, at a corner.
And the little girl stops; she stands still in a shadow at the mouth of a narrow tunnel-like street. She is almost lost in the shadow, her hair is mixed into the darkness, but we see her white face and white, naked shoulder.
Rock stands just outside the shadow.
He puts a penny in her hand.
He looks down at her, and is silent for a moment.

ROCK. It's a bitter cold night to be running about in the streets. You should go home.

The child in the shadows shakes her head.

CHILD. Granny says I can't come home until I got four-pence. . . .

Rock fumbles in his pocket for another coin.
The child holds out her hand from the shadow around her.

> ROCK. What's your name, lassie?
> CHILD. I'm Maggie Bell.
> ROCK. [Almost as though to himself.] I'm Doctor Rock.

And the child runs screaming into the darkness.
And Rock walks on, away from us.

HILL ABOVE THE CITY.

The dusk is deeper. . . .
The wind is blowing wilder. . . .
We look down the hill.
Out of the dusk, a long way off, Rock is climbing up towards us.
And as he climbs, we hear his voice. But it is only the little, wind-blown
   whisper of a voice, and we cannot hear a word of it.
And as he climbs on and up, so the windy whisper loudens and we being to
   hear the words.
We begin to hear the fragments of sentences.
We hear some words and then the wind rises for a second and blows them
   away.
Then we hear more words, from the voice of his mind; the wind again will
   not let the words finish but blows them away.
And again; and again; and again.
Always the voice is the voice of Rock, but it is never twice on the same
   level: it is the voice of Rock young, then old, then gay, then sad; a high
   voice, a low voice.
And the sound of it rises as he climbs.

> ROCK'S VOICE. And the child in the cold runs away from my name. . . .
> My name is a ghost to frighten children. . . .
> Will *my* children cry '*Murder*' and '*Blood*' when I touch them . . . as if
>   my hands were Fallon's hands? . . .
> 'Be good, be good, or the terrible Doctor will come with his knife.'
> Poor Billy! I came to you with my knife.
> Did I *know*, did I *know* from the very beginning?
> Never answer, never answer, even to yourself alone in the night. . . .
> All's over now. . . .
> Oh, Elizabeth, hold my hand. . . .

'Oh, it isn't a hand, it's a pair of scissors! . . .'
Did I set myself up as a little god over death?
Over death. . . .
All over . . . over . . . over . . .
Did I set myself above pity? . . .
Oh, my God, I knew what I was doing!

And he passes us and climbs up the long hill, and his voice climbs with him
   into darkness, into a whisper, into silence, into the climax of
MUSIC.

MARK TWAIN
The Innocents Abroad

———❦———

MARK TWAIN (1835-1910) found in faith healers and Indian doctors
ample material for his satirical writings. His deep interest in medical
matters can be viewed against the background of the tragic deaths of his
brother, daughters, and wife. Like George Bernard Shaw, he had a
strong tongue to put in the cheeks of readers.

Yesterday we met a woman riding on a little jackass, and she had a little
child in her arms; honestly, I thought the child had goggles on as we
approached, and I wondered how its mother could afford so much style.
But when we drew near, we saw that the goggles were nothing but a camp
meeting of flies assembled around each of the child's eyes, and at the same
time there was a detachment prospecting its nose. The flies were happy, the
child was contented, and so the mother did not interfere.

As soon as the tribe found out that we had a doctor in our party, they
began to flock in from all quarters. Dr. B., in the charity of his nature, had
taken a child from a woman who sat nearby and put some sort of a wash
upon its diseased eyes. That woman went off and started the whole nation,
and it was a sight to see them swarm! The lame, the halt, the blind, the
leprous—all the distempers that are bred of indolence, dirt, and
iniquity—were represented in the Congress in ten minutes, and still they
came! Every woman that had a sick baby brought it along, and every
woman that hadn't borrowed one. What reverent and what worshiping
looks they bent upon that dread, mysterious power, the Doctor! They
watched him take his phials out; they watched him measure the particles of
white power; they watched him add drops of one precious liquid and drops
of another; they lost not the slightest movement; their eyes were riveted
upon him with a fascination that nothing could distract. I believe they
thought he was gifted like a god. When each individual got his portion of
medicine, his eyes were radiant with joy—notwithstanding by nature they
are a thankless and impassive race—and upon his face was written the
unquestioning faith that nothing on earth could prevent the patient from
getting well now.

Christ knew how to preach to these simple, superstitious, disease-tortured creatures: He healed the sick. They flocked to our poor human doctor this morning when the fame of what he had done to the sick child went abroad in the land, and they worshiped him with their eyes while they did not know as yet whether there was virtue in his simples or not. The ancestors of these—people precisely like them in color, dress, manners, customs, simplicity—flocked in vast multitudes after Christ, and when they saw him make the afflicted whole with a word, it is no wonder they worshiped him. No wonder his deeds were the talk of the nation. No wonder the multitude that followed him was so great that at one time— thirty miles from here—they had to let a sick man down through the roof because no approach could be made to the door; no wonder his audiences were so great at Galilee that he had to preach from a ship removed a little distance from the shore; no wonder that even in the desert places about Bethsaida, five thousand invaded his solitude, and he had to feed them by a miracle or else see them suffer for their confiding faith and devotion; no wonder when there was a great commotion in a city in those days, one neighbor explained it to another in words to this effect: "They say that Jesus of Nazareth is come!"

QUACKS
AND
CLOWNS

So long as people continue to reach out indiscriminately for solutions to their torment, they are bound to have a rendezvous with error and exploitation. The license to practice medicine provides no ironclad assurance of infallibility or even competence. Not even the finest medical education can protect the public against faulty diagnoses or prognoses—or flights of fancy that are not regarded as such by the practitioner. Authors who write about illness have the advantage of hindsight. They can also use their pens to settle scores or to say things in public that they might be hesitant to say in medical offices.

CHARLES DICKENS
The Pickwick Papers

CHARLES DICKENS (1812-1870) wrote spectacularly popular novels—popular not just in England but in almost every country of the civilized world. His comic characterizations and realistic portrayals of London street life were infused with extreme sympathy for the poor, reflecting Dickens's lifelong bitterness over his experiences in a workhouse as a young boy.

CHAPTER 30

How the Pickwickians made and cultivated the Acquaintance of a couple of nice Young Men belonging to one of the Liberal Professions; how they disported themselves on the Ice; and how their first Visit came to a conclusion

'Well, Sam,' said Mr. Pickwick as that favoured servitor entered his bed-chamber with his warm water, on the morning of Christmas Day, 'Still frosty?'

'Water in the wash-hand basin's a mask o' ice, sir,' responded Sam.

'Severe weather, Sam,' observed Mr. Pickwick.

'Fine time for them as is well wropped up, as the Polar Bear said to himself, ven he was practising his skating,' replied Mr. Weller.

'I shall be down in a quarter of an hour, Sam,' said Mr. Pickwick, untying his nightcap.

'Wery good, sir,' replied Sam. 'There's a couple o' Sawbones down stairs.'

'A couple of what!' exclaimed Mr. Pickwick, sitting up in bed.

'A couple o' Sawbones,' said Sam.

'What's a Sawbones?' inquired Mr. Pickwick, not quite certain whether it was a live animal, or something to eat.

'What! Don't you know what a Sawbones is, sir?' inquired Mr. Weller. 'I thought everybody know'd as a Sawbones was a Surgeon.'

'Oh, a Surgeon, eh?' said Mr. Pickwick, with a smile.

'Just that, sir,' replied Sam. 'These here ones as is below, though, aint reg'lar thorough-bred Sawbones; they're only in trainin'.'

153

'In other words they're Medical Students, I suppose?' said Mr. Pickwick.

Sam Weller nodded assent.

'I am glad of it,' said Mr. Pickwick, casting his nightcap energetically on the counterpane, 'They are fine fellows; very fine fellows; with judgments matured by observation and reflection; tastes refined by reading and study. I am very glad of it.'

'They're a smokin' cigars by the kitchen fire,' said Sam.

'Ah!' observed Mr. Pickwick, rubbing his hands, 'overflowing with kindly feelings and animal spirits. Just what I like to see.'

'And one on 'em,' said Sam, not noticing his master's interruption, 'one on 'em's got his legs on the table, and is a drinkin' brandy neat, vile the tother one—him in the barnacles—has got a barrel o' oysters atween his knees, wich he's a openin' like steam, and as fast as he eats 'em, he takes a aim vith the shells at young dropsy, who's a sittin' down fast asleep, in the chimbley corner.'

'Eccentricities of genius, Sam,' said Mr. Pickwick. 'You may retire.'

Sam did retire accordingly; Mr. Pickwick, at the expiration of the quarter of an hour, went down to breakfast.

'Here he is at last!' said old Mr. Wardle. 'Pickwick, this is Miss Allen's brother, Mr. Benjamin Allen. Ben we call him, and so may you if you like. This gentleman is his very particular friend, Mr. —'

'Mr. Bob Sawyer,' interposed Mr. Benjamin Allen; whereupon Mr. Bob Sawyer and Mr. Benjamin Allen laughed in concert.

Mr. Pickwick bowed to Bob Sawyer, and Bob Sawyer bowed to Mr. Pickwick; Bob and his very particular friend then applied themselves most assiduously to the eatables before them; and Mr. Pickwick had an opportunity of glancing at them both.

Mr. Benjamin Allen was a coarse, stout, thick-set young man, with black hair cut rather short, and a white face cut rather long. He was embellished with spectacles, and wore a white neckerchief. Below his single-breasted black surtout, which was buttoned up to his chin, appeared the usual number of pepper-and-salt coloured legs, terminating in a pair of imperfectly polished boots. Although his coat was short in the sleeves it disclosed no vestige of a linen wristband; and although there was quite enough of his face to admit of the encroachment of a shirt collar, it was not graced by the smallest approach to that appendage. He presented, altogether, rather a mildewy appearance, and emitted a fragrant odour of full-flavoured Cubas.

Mr. Bob Sawyer, who was habited in a coarse blue coat, which, without being either a great-coat or a surtout, partook of the nature and qualities of both, had about him that sort of slovenly smartness, and swaggering gait, which is peculiar to young gentlemen who smoke in the streets by day, shout and scream in the same by night, call waiters by their Christian names, and do various other acts and deeds of an equally facetious description. He wore a pair of plaid trousers, and a large rough double-breasted waistcoat; out of doors, he carried a thick stick with a big top. He eschewed gloves, and looked, upon the whole, something like a dissipated Robinson Crusoe.

Such were the two worthies to whom Mr. Pickwick was introduced, as he took his seat at the breakfast table on Christmas morning.

'Splendid morning, gentlemen,' said Mr. Pickwick.

Mr. Bob Sawyer slightly nodded his assent to the proposition, and asked Mr. Benjamin Allen for the mustard.

'Have you come far this morning, gentlemen?' inquired Mr. Pickwick.

'Blue Lion at Muggleton,' briefly responded Mr. Allen.

'You should have joined us last night,' said Mr. Pickwick.

'So we should,' replied Bob Sawyer, 'but the brandy was too good to leave in a hurry; wasn't it, Ben?'

'Certainly,' said Mr. Benjamin Allen; 'and the cigars were not bad, or the pork chops either; were they, Bob?'

'Decidedly not,' said Bob. The particular friends resumed their attack upon the breakfast, more freely than before, as if the recollection of last night's supper had imparted a new relish to the meal.

'Peg away, Bob,' said Mr. Allen to his companion, encouragingly.

'So I do,' replied Bob Sawyer. And so, to do him justice, he did.

'Nothing like dissecting, to give one an appetite,' said Mr. Bob Sawyer, looking round the table.

Mr. Pickwick slightly shuddered.

'By the bye, Bob,' said Mr. Allen, 'have you finished that leg yet?'

'Nearly,' replied Sawyer, helping himself to half a fowl as he spoke. 'It's a very muscular one for a child's.'

'Is it?' inquired Mr. Allen, carelessly.

'Very,' said Bob Sawyer, with his mouth full.

'I've put my name down for an arm, at our place,' said Mr. Allen. 'We're clubbing for a subject, and the list is nearly full, only we can't get hold of any fellow that wants a head. I wish you'd take it.'

'No,' replied Bob Sawyer; 'can't afford expensive luxuries.'

'Nonsense!' said Allen.

'Can't indeed,' rejoined Bob Sawyer. 'I wouldn't mind a brain, but I couldn't stand a whole head.'

'Hush, hush, gentlemen, pray,' said Mr. Pickwick, 'I hear the ladies.'

*   *   *

'And a very snug little business you have, no doubt?' said Mr. Winkle, knowingly.

'Very,' replied Bob Sawyer. 'So snug, that at the end of a few years you might put all the profits in a wine glass, and cover 'em over with a gooseberry leaf.'

'You cannot surely mean that?' said Mr. Winkle. 'The stock itself—'

'Dummies, my dear boy,' said Bob Sawyer; 'half the drawers have nothing in 'em, and the other half don't open.'

'Nonsense!' said Mr. Winkle.

'Fact—honor!' returned Bob Sawyer, stepping out into the shop, and demonstrating the veracity of the assertion by divers hard pulls at the little gilt knobs on the counterfeit drawers. 'Hardly anything real in the shop but the leeches, and *they* are second-hand.'

'I shouldn't have thought it!' exclaimed Mr. Winkle, much surprised.

'I hope not,' replied Bob Sawyer, 'else where's the use of appearances, eh? But what will you take? Do as we do? That's right. Ben, my fine fellow, put your hand into the cupboard, and bring out the patent digester.'

Mr. Benjamin Allen smiled his readiness, and produced from the closet at his elbow a black bottle half full of brandy.

'You don't take water, of course?' said Bob Sawyer.

'Thank you,' replied Mr. Winkle. 'It's *rather* early. I should like to qualify it, if you have no objection.'

'None in the least, if you can reconcile it to your conscience,' replied Bob Sawyer; tossing off, as he spoke, a glass of the liquor with great relish. 'Ben, the pipkin!'

Mr. Benjamin Allen drew forth, from the same hiding-place, a small brass pipkin, which Bob Sawyer observed he prided himself upon, particularly because it looked so business-like. The water in the professional pipkin having been made to boil, in course of time, by various little shovelsful of coal, which Mr. Bob Sawyer took out of a practicable window-seat, labelled 'Soda Water,' Mr. Winkle adulterated his brandy; and the conversation was becoming general, when it was interrupted by the entrance into the shop of a boy, in a sober grey livery and a gold-laced hat, with a small covered basket under his arm: whom Mr. Bob Sawyer immediately hailed with, 'Tom, you vagabond, come here.'

The boy presented himself accordingly.

'You've been stopping to over all the posts in Bristol, you idle young scamp!' said Mr. Bob Sawyer.

'No, sir, I haven't,' replied the boy.

'You had better not!' said Mr. Bob Sawyer, with a threatening aspect. 'Who do you suppose will ever employ a professional man, when they see his boy playing at marbles in the gutter, or flying the garter in the horse-road? Have you no feeling for your profession, you groveller? Did you leave all the medicine?'

'Yes, sir.'

'The powders for the child, at the large house with the new family, and the pills to be taken four times a day at the ill-tempered old gentleman's with the gouty leg?'

'Yes, sir.'

'Then shut the door, and mind the shop.'

'Come,' said Mr. Winkle, as the boy retired, 'things are not quite so bad as you would have me believe, either. There is *some* medicine to be sent out.'

Mr. Bob Sawyer peeped into the shop to see that no stranger was within hearing, and leaning forward to Mr. Winkle, said, in a low tone:

'He leaves it all, at the wrong houses.'

Mr. Winkle looked perplexed, and Bob Sawyer and his friend laughed.

'Don't you see?' said Bob. 'He goes up to a house, rings the area bell, pokes a packet of medicine without a direction into the servant's hand, and walks off. Servant takes it into the dining-parlour; master opens it, and reads the label: "Draught to be taken at bed-time—pills as before—lotion as usual—*the* powder. From Sawyer's, late Nockemorf's. Physicians' prescriptions carefully prepared," and all the rest of it. Shows it to his wife—*she* reads the label; it goes down to the servants—*they* read the label. Next day, boy calls: "Very sorry—his mistake—immense business—great many parcels to deliver—Mr. Sawyer's compliments—late Nockemorf." The name gets known, and that's the thing, my boy, in the medical way. Bless your heart, old fellow, it's better than all the advertising in the world. We have got one four-ounce bottle that's been to half the houses in Bristol, and hasn't done yet.'

'Dear me, I see,' observed Mr. Winkle; 'what an excellent plan!'

'Oh, Ben and I have hit upon a dozen such,' replied Bob Sawyer, with great glee. 'The lamplighter has eighteenpence a week to pull the night-bell for ten minutes every time he comes round; and my boy always rushes into church, just before the psalms, when the people have got nothing to do but look about 'em, and calls me out, with horror and dismay depicted on his countenance. "Bless my soul," everybody says, "somebody taken suddenly ill! Sawyer, late Nockemorf, sent for. What a business that young man has!" '

At the termination of this disclosure of some of the mysteries of medicine, Mr. Bob Sawyer and his friend, Ben Allen, threw themselves back in their respective chairs, and laughed boisterously. When they had enjoyed the joke to their hearts' content, the discourse changed to topics in which Mr. Winkle was more immediately interested.

We think we have hinted elsewhere, that Mr. Benjamin Allen had a way of becoming sentimental after brandy. The case is not a peculiar one, as we ourself can testify: having, on a few occasions, had to deal with patients who have been afflicted in a similar manner. At this precise period of his existence, Mr. Benjamin Allen had perhaps a greater predisposition to maudlinism than he had ever known before; the cause of which malady was briefly this. He had been staying nearly three weeks with Mr. Bob Sawyer; Mr. Bob Sawyer was not remarkable for temperance, nor was Mr. Benjamin Allen for the ownership of a very strong head; the consequence was, that, during the whole space of time just mentioned, Mr. Benjamin Allen had been wavering between intoxication partial, and intoxication complete.

'My dear friend,' said Mr. Ben Allen, taking advantage of Mr. Bob Sawyer's temporary absence behind the counter, whither he had retired to dispense some of the second-hand leeches, previously referred to: 'my dear friend, I am very miserable.'

Mr. Winkle professed his heartfelt regret to hear it, and begged to know whether he could do anything to alleviate the sorrows of the suffering student.

'Nothing, my dear boy, nothing,' said Ben. 'You recollect Arabella, Winkle? My sister Arabella—a little girl, Winkle, with black eyes—when we were down at Wardle's? I don't know whether you happened to notice her, a nice little girl, Winkle. Perhaps my features may recall her countenance to your recollection?'

Mr. Winkle required nothing to recall the charming Arabella to his mind; and it was rather fortunate he did not, for the features of her brother Benjamin would unquestionably have proved but an indifferent refresher to his memory. He answered, with as much calmness as he could assume, that he perfectly remembered the young lady referred to, and sincerely trusted she was in good health.

'Our friend Bob is a delightful fellow, Winkle,' was the only reply of Mr. Ben Allen.

'Very,' said Mr. Winkle; not much relishing this close connexion of the two names.

'I designed 'em for each other; they were made for each other, sent into the world for each other, born for each other. Winkle,' said Mr. Ben Allen, setting down his glass with emphasis. 'There's a special destiny in the matter, my dear sir; there's only five years' difference between 'em, and both their birthdays are in August.'

Mr. Winkle was too anxious to hear what was to follow, to express much wonderment at this extraordinary coincidence, marvelous as it was; so Mr. Ben Allen, after a tear or two, went on to say, that, notwithstanding all his esteem and respect and veneration for his friend, Arabella had unaccountably and undutifully evinced the most determined antipathy to his person.

'And I think,' said Mr. Ben Allen, in conclusion, '*I* think there's a prior attachment.'

'Have you any idea who the object of it might be?' asked Mr. Winkle, with great trepidation.

Mr. Ben Allen seized the poker, flourished it in a warlike manner above his head, inflicted a savage blow on an imaginary skull, and wound up by saying, in a very expressive manner, that he only wished he could guess; that was all.

'I'd show him what I thought of him,' said Mr. Ben Allen. And round went the poker again, more fiercely than before.

All this was, of course, very soothing to the feelings of Mr. Winkle, who remained silent for a few minutes; but at length mustered up resolution to inquire whether Miss Allen was in Kent.

'No, no,' said Mr. Ben Allen, laying aside the poker, and looking very cunning; 'I didn't think Wardle's exactly the place for a headstrong girl; so, as I am her natural protector and guardian, our parents being dead, I have brought her down into this part of the country to spend a few months at an old aunt's, in a nice dull close place. I think that will cure her, my boy. If it doesn't, I'll take her abroad for a little while, and see what that'll do.'

'Oh, the aunt's is in Bristol, is it?' faltered Mr. Winkle.

'No, no, not in Bristol,' replied Mr. Ben Allen, jerking his thumb over his right shoulder: 'over that way; down there. But, hush, here's Bob. Not a word, my dear friend, not a word.'

Short as this conversation was, it roused in Mr. Winkle the highest degree of excitement and anxiety. The suspected prior attachment rankled in his heart. Could he be the object of it? Could it be for him that the fair Arabella had looked scornfully on the sprightly Bob Sawyer, or had he a successful rival? He determined to see her, cost what it might; but here an insurmountable objection presented itself, for whether the explanatory 'over that way,' and 'down there,' of Mr. Ben Allen, meant three miles off, or thirty, or three hundred, he could in no wise guess.

But he had no opportunity of pondering over his love just then, for Bob Sawyer's return was the immediate precursor of the arrival of a meat pie from the baker's, of which that gentleman insisted on his staying to partake. The cloth was laid by an occasional charwoman, who officiated in the capacity of Mr. Bob Sawyer's housekeeper; and a third knife and fork having been borrowed from the mother of the boy in the grey livery (for Mr. Sawyer's domestic arrangements were as yet conducted on a limited scale), they sat down to dinner; the beer being served up, as Mr. Sawyer remarked, 'in its native pewter.'

After dinner, Mr. Bob Sawyer ordered in the largest mortar in the shop, and proceeded to brew a reeking jorum of rum-punch therein: stirring up and amalgamating the materials with a pestle in a very creditable and apothecary-like manner. Mr. Sawyer, being a bachelor, had only one tumbler in the house, which was assigned to Mr. Winkle as a compliment to the visitor: Mr. Ben Allen being accommodated with a funnel with a cork in the narrow end: and Bob Sawyer contented himself with one of those wide-lipped crystal vessels inscribed with a variety of cabalistic characters, in which chemists are wont to measure out their liquid drugs in compounding prescriptions. These preliminaries adjusted, the punch was tasted, and pronounced excellent; and it having been arranged that Bob Sawyer and Ben Allen should be considered at liberty to fill twice to Mr. Winkle's once, they started fair, with great satisfaction and good-fellowship.

There was no singing, because Mr. Bob Sawyer said it wouldn't look professional; but to make amends for this deprivation there was so much talking and laughing that it might have been heard, and very likely was, at the end of the street. Which conversation materially lightened the hours and improved the mind of Mr. Bob Sawyer's boy, who, instead of devoting the evening to his ordinary occupation of writing his name on the counter, and rubbing it out again, peeped through the glass door, and thus listened and looked on at the same time.

The mirth of Mr. Bob Sawyer was rapidly ripening into the furious; Mr. Ben Allen was fast relapsing into the sentimental, and the punch had well-nigh disappeared altogether, when the boy hastily running in, announced that a young woman had just come over, to say that Sawyer late Nockemorf was wanted directly, a couple of streets off. This broke up the party. Mr. Bob Sawyer, understanding the message, after some twenty repetitions, tied a wet cloth round his head to sober himself, and, having partially succeeded, put on his green spectacles and issued forth. Resisting all entreaties to stay till he came back, and finding it quite impossible to engage Mr. Ben Allen in any intelligible conversation on the subject nearest his heart, or indeed on any other, Mr. Winkle took his departure, and returned to the Bush.

GUSTAVE FLAUBERT
Madame Bovary

———— ❧ ————

GUSTAVE FLAUBERT (1821-1880) suffered from lifelong bouts of depression. His precise, objective prose style expresses his realistic, yet downbeat outlook on life. Flaubert's father was a doctor, the director of the Rouen city hospital. *Madame Bovary* contains some of the sharpest insights into the mind of doctors to be found anywhere in literature.

He had recently read an article praising a new method of curing clubfoot, and since he was all for progress he conceived the patriotic idea that, "to keep up with the times," Yonville ought to be the scene of operations for "talipes, commonly known as clubfoot."

"After all, what's there to lose?" he said to Emma. "And look at what's to be gained!" He enumerated on his fingers the advantages of the attempt: "Almost certain success, cure and improved appearance for the patient, swift fame for the surgeon. Why shouldn't your husband, for example, relieve poor Hippolyte, at the Lion d'Or? He'd be sure to talk about this cure to every traveler at the inn, and then" (Homais lowered his voice and looked around) "what's to stop me from sending a little article about it to the newspaper? And when the article gets around! People talk about it and it builds up like a snowball rolling down a hill! After that, who knows? Who knows?"

Emma was convinced: Charles had a good chance of succeeding; she had no reason to doubt his skill, and what a satisfaction it would be for her to have persuaded him to take a step that would enhance his reputation and add to his fortune! She was eager to have something more solid than love to lean on.

Urged on by the apothecary and Emma, Charles agreed to go through with it. He sent to Rouen for Dr. Duval's book and buried himself in it every night, holding his head between his hands.

While Charles was studying talipes equinus, talipes varus and talipes valgus, in other words, *strephocatopodia, strephendopodia* and *strephexopodia* (or, to put it more clearly, deviations of the foot downward, inward or outward), along with *strephypopodia* and *strephanopodia*

162

(downward or upward torsion), Monsieur Homais was using every possible argument to talk the stableboy into consenting to the operation:

"You'll feel nothing more than a slight pain at the very most; it's just a prick, like a little bloodletting, less painful than the removal of some kinds of corns."

Hippolyte thought it over, stupidly rolling his eyes.

"Look, it means nothing to me," the pharmacist went on, "I'm only trying to convince you for your own sake, out of pure humanity! I'd like to see you get rid of that hideous limp, my friend, and that swaying of the lumbar region—it must hinder you considerably in your work, no matter what you claim."

Homais then described how much more vigorous and active he would feel, and even gave him to understand that he would be more successful with women, which made the stableboy smile foolishly. After that, Homais appealed to his pride:

"Are you a man or not? What would have happened if you'd been called to the colors, to go out and defend our country against her enemies? . . . Ah, Hippolyte!"

And Homais walked away, declaring that he was totally unable to understand how anyone could so stubbornly refuse the benefits of science.

Poor Hippolyte eventually gave in, for there was a veritable conspiracy against him. Binet, who never meddled in other people's affairs, Madame Lefrançois, Artémise, the neighbors, even the mayor, Monsieur Tuvache—everyone urged him, preached to him, shamed him; but what finally decided him was the fact that it would cost him nothing. Bovary even agreed to furnish the apparatus for the operation. This generosity had been Emma's idea, and he had accepted it, inwardly telling himself that his wife was an angel.

Following the pharmacist's advice he managed, after two failures, to have the cabinetmaker and the locksmith construct a kind of box weighing about eight pounds, using generous quantities of iron, wood, tin, leather, screws and nuts.

Meanwhile, in order to know which of Hippolyte's tendons to cut, he had to determine which kind of clubfoot he had.

The foot formed almost a straight line with the leg, although it also turned inward, so that it was an equinus mingled with a little varus, or perhaps a slight varus with a strong admixture of equinus. But with his equinus—which actually was as wide as a horse's hoof, with rough skin, hard tendons and huge toes whose black nails were like the nails of a horseshoe—the taliped galloped like a deer from morning to night. He was constantly seen in the square, hopping around the carts, thrusting his crippled leg forward. In fact, this leg seemed to be more vigorous than the other. Through long use it had taken on what might almost be called moral qualities of patience and determination, and Hippolyte preferred to rest his weight on it whenever he was given heavy work to do.

Since it was an equinus, Charles would have to cut the Achilles tendon, leaving the anterior tibial muscle to be taken care of later, to cure the varus, for he was afraid to risk two operations at once, and he was already trembling at the thought of getting into some important region he knew nothing about.

Ambrose Paré applying a ligature directly to an artery for the first time since Celsus had done it fifteen centuries before, Dupuytren about to cut into an abscess through a thick layer of the brain, Gensoul wh... he performed the first resection of the upper maxillary—none of these men had such a pounding heart, such trembling hands or such a tense mind as Monsieur Bovary when he approached Hippolyte with his tenotomy knife in his hand. And, as in a hospital, beside him on a table lay a pile of lint, waxed thread and a great many bandages—a whole pyramid of bandages, the apothecary's entire stock. It was Monsieur Homais who, beginning early in the morning, had organized all these preparations, as much to dazzle the multitude as to delude himself. Charles pierced the skin; there was a sharp snap: the tendon was cut, the operation was over. Hippolyte was overcome with surprise; he bent over Bovary's hands and covered them with kisses.

"Come now, be calm," said the apothecary. "You can express your gratitude to your benefactor later."

And he went downstairs to announce the result to the five or six curious souls who were standing in the courtyard, expecting to see Hippolyte walk out without a limp. Charles buckled his patient into the apparatus and went home, where Emma was anxiously waiting for him at the door. She threw her arms around his neck; they sat down to table; he ate heartily and even asked for a cup of coffee with his dessert, a dissolute pleasure which he usually allowed himself only on Sundays when there was company.

They spent a delightful evening, full of intimate talk and shared dreams. They spoke of their future fortune, of the improvements they would make in their house. He saw his fame spreading, his prosperity growing, his wife loving him forever; and she was happy to refresh herself with a new, healthier, more commendable feeling: she now had a little affection for the poor man who loved her so. The thought of Rodolphe came into her mind for a moment, but then her eyes turned back to Charles and she noticed with surprise that his teeth were not at all bad-looking.

They were in bed when Monsieur Homais suddenly came into their bedroom, despite the cook's objections. He was holding a newly written sheet of paper in his hand: it was the article he had composed for the *Fanal de Rouen*. He had brought it for them to read.

"Read it to us," said Bovary.

He read:

" 'Despite the prejudices that still cover part of the face of Europe like a net, enlightenment is beginning to penetrate our rural areas. Thus on Tuesday our little town of Yonville was the scene of a surgical experiment that was also an act of lofty philanthropy. Monsieur Bovary, one of our most distinguished practitioners . . .' "

"Oh, that's too much, too much!" said Charles, choked with emotion.

"No, it's not! Not at all! Don't be too modest. '. . . operated on a clubfoot . . .' I didn't use the scientific term, because in a newspaper, you know . . . everyone might not understand; the masses must be . . ."

"Yes, you're right," said Bovary. "Go on."

"I'll take it up where I left off," said the pharmacist.

" 'Monsieur Bovary, one of our most distinguished practitioners, operated on a clubfoot. The patient was Hippolyte Tautain, stableboy for the past twenty-five years at the Lion d'Or inn, under the management of Madame Lefrançois, on the Place d'Armes. The novelty of the undertaking and the interest taken in the patient had drawn such a large gathering of people that there was a veritable crush in front of the establishment. The operation went off as though by magic, and only a few drops of blood appeared on the skin, as if to announce that the rebellious tendon had at last yielded to the surgeon's art. The patient, strangely enough (we report this from first-hand observation), gave no indication of pain. So far his condition leaves nothing to be desired. All evidence points to a short convalescence, and who knows?—perhaps at the next village festival we shall see our good Hippolyte taking part in Bacchic dances amid a chorus of joyous companions, thus proving to one and all, by his high spirits and his capers, that he has been completely cured. Hail to our magnanimous men of science! Hail to those tireless spirits who work day and night for the improvement or the relief of mankind! Hail, all hail! May we not now proclaim that the blind shall see, the deaf shall hear and the lame shall walk? What fanaticism promised to the elect in days gone by, science is now achieving for all men! We shall keep our readers informed about the successive phases of this remarkable cure.' "

Five days later, however, Madame Lefrançois rushed in panic-stricken and cried, "Help! He's dying! It's driving me out of my mind!"

Charles immediately headed for the Lion d'Or, and the pharmacist, seeing him hurry across the square without a hat, abandoned his pharmacy. He too went to the inn; he arrived panting, flushed and worried, and he asked all the people he saw climbing the stairs, "What's wrong with our interesting taliped?"

The taliped was writhing in terrible convulsions; the apparatus enclosing his leg was pounding against the wall so violently that it threatened to break through.

Taking every precaution to avoid disturbing the position of the leg, Charles and the pharmacist took off the box and saw a horrible sight: the foot was a shapeless mass, so swollen that the entire skin seemed ready to burst, and it was covered with black and blue marks caused by the famous apparatus. Hippolyte had previously complained that it was hurting him, but no one had paid any attention to him; it was now obvious that his complaints had not been entirely unjustified, and he was allowed to keep his foot out of the box for several hours. But as soon as the swelling had gone down a little the two experts deemed it advisable to put the apparatus back on, and they fastened it more tightly than before, in order to speed things up. Finally, three days later, when Hippolyte could stand it no longer, they removed the box once again and were amazed at what they saw. A livid tumescence ran up the leg, and scattered over it were pustules from which a black liquid was oozing. The case had taken a serious turn. Hippolyte was beginning to despair, and Madame Lefrançois had him moved the little dining room beside the kitchen, so that he would at least have some distraction.

But the tax collector, who ate dinner there every day, complained bitterly about such company. Hippolyte was then carried into the billiard room.

He lay there groaning under his heavy blankets, pale, unshaven and hollow-eyed, occasionally turning his sweaty head on the dirty pillow while flies swooped down on it from all sides. Madame Bovary came to see him now and then. She brought him linen for his poultices, comforted and encouraged him. He had no lack of company, especially on market-days, when peasants gathered around him to play billiards, fence with the cues, smoke, drink, sing and shout.

"How are you coming along?" they would ask, clapping him on the shoulder. "You don't look as if you're in very good shape. But it's your own fault! You should have . . ." And they would tell him stories about people who had been cured by remedies other than his; then, by way of consolation, they would add, "You're coddling yourself! Why don't you get up? You're pampering yourself like a king! Well, one thing is sure, you old rascal: you don't smell good!"

It was true: gangrene was mounting higher and higher. It made Bovary feel sick himself. He came in every hour, every few minutes. Hippolyte would look at him with eyes full of terror, sobbing and stammering, "When will I be well again? Oh, save me! I'm so miserable! So miserable!"

And the doctor always went away telling him to eat lightly.

"Don't listen to him, my boy," Madame Lefrançois would say. "They've made you suffer enough already! You mustn't get any weaker than you are now. Here, swallow this."

And she would give him some good bouillon, a slice of mutton or a piece of bacon, and sometimes a little glass of brandy, although he could not muster up enough strength to raise it to his lips.

Father Bournisien, having learned that he was getting worse, came and asked to see him. He began by telling him how sorry he was about his condition, but then he told him he ought to rejoice over it, since it was the Lord's will, and quickly take advantage of this opportunity to become reconciled with heaven.

LUIGI PIRANDELLO
Henry IV

———∽∞∾———

LUIGI PIRANDELLO (1867-1936) turned theatre into psychological catharsis. His exploration of the meaning of sanity in "Henry IV" is based on his own tragedy of living with an insane wife.

Belcredi [*suddenly*]. I say, I've never understood why they take degrees in medicine.

Di Nolli [*amazed*]. Who?

Belcredi. The alienists!

Di Nolli. What ought they to take degrees in, then?

Frida. If they are alienists, in what else should they take degrees?

Belcredi. In law, of course! All a matter of talk! The more they talk, the more highly they are considered. "Analogous elasticity," "the sensation of distance in time!" And the first thing they tell you is that they don't work miracles—when a miracle's just what is wanted! But they know that the more they say they are not miracle-workers, the more folk believe in their seriousness!

GEORGE BERNARD SHAW
Doctors' Delusions

AN IMPROBABLE FICTION
From Time and Tide, 22 February 1929

Once upon a time, in the country of the Half Mad, which was cut off from the western end of Europe in prehistoric times to prevent the inhabitants from injuring any but themselves, the King fell ill. As he had always been well spoke of, and had established very kindly relations with his subjects, his illness caused a great increase of their affection for him and for his family. All the married women saw in the Queen a wife anxious about her husband, with a sick-bed to provide for. All the men saw in the King a fellow-man suffering as they themselves had suffered or might at any moment have to suffer. For sickness is a Great Leveller, and consequently a great breeder of sympathy, unlike that Impostor Death, who gives a pompous eminence to even the humblest. And thus, with sympathy added to loyalty, the nation was in such a state of concern about the King as had never before arisen within living memory. Naturally, the case being one of dangerous illness, it was to the doctors that the nation turned for help and reassurance.

Now in the country of the Half Mad the doctors had long before this taken the place of the medieval Church. There was a law that when a man was ill he must on pain of punishment send for his parish priest; but this law had been so long disregarded that only a few specialists in Church history knew of its existence. Its place had been taken by a law that when there was sickness in the house the doctor must be sent for, and that if the doctor said that any part of a sick child's body must be cut out its parents must have that done at once whether they approved or not, or else be haled before a magistrate and heavily fined, or, should the child have died, committed for trial for having killed it.

To such powers as this were added extraordinary privileges. For instance, doctors were licensed to commit murder with impunity, provided they did it either by administering poison or by using knives of a particular shape in such a manner that the victim did not die until he or she had been put to bed. Not only was no inquest held and no indictment brought against the doctor, but he was actually paid for his labor, and sometimes invited to the funeral.

169

As the Half Mad were so jealous of their liberties that a priest could not even order a father to have his child baptized, it will be seen that this strange people, though half sane on the subject of priests, were wholly mad on the subject of doctors, willingly granting them powers which they had denied to their Kings at the cost of revolution and civil war.

Now the doctors, being no worse than other people, did their best to prove worthy of their extraordinary trust by using it for the relief of the sick, and making it impossible for anyone to become a doctor except by years of study to qualify him for his duties. But as the Half Mad, whilst bowing down with the deepest reverence to the condition of omniscience which they supposed these studies to confer, would not pay a doctor anything until they were actually ill and threatened with death, the doctors were mostly poor, and would have starved altogether if the nation had been in a reasonably healthy condition. Thus their duty to themselves and their wives and children was to keep their patients ill as long and as often as possible; to persuade them that they were dangerously ill when there was nothing the matter with them that their own recuperative powers could not cure; and even to deprive them of as many of their limbs and organs as they could without killing the goose that laid the golden eggs. On the other hand, their duty to their patients and their country was to do exactly the contrary, and strive to their utmost to produce a state of things in which doctors would starve.

Now in the kingdom of the Half Mad, people always ended by believing what they wanted to believe, no matter how much it might be contradicted by facts; and so it had come about that the doctors, though they were as kindly and honorable as could reasonably be expected, and sometimes very clever, had built up an elaborately reasoned and ingenious series of mechanical explanations of all the diseases, giving them impressive names, and setting forth the treatments and operations and medicines proper to them, until at last they could do almost anything with a patient except cure him or even allow him a fair chance of curing himself. Thus the calling of a doctor to the sick-bed was rather a pious ceremony enforced by law than a proceeding from which any relief to the patient could be expected. But the doctors were wonderfully accurate in predicting the time at which the patient would die in their hands; and this was very necessary for the settlement of the affairs of patients who had any affairs to settle.

With a Faith (for such it was) in this condition, naturally there were Heresies in all directions. New methods of treating disease were discovered; but the doctors took so long to learn the old ones that they had no time for the new ones. Even the surgeons had to do without any manual training, and picked up their art as the father of a family picks up the art of carving a turkey. So, instead of adopting the new methods, they excommunicated the new practitioners and all their accomplices. Only, as the heretics either cured their patients or at least did not kill them by obsolete and barbarous treatments, the doctors, when they were ill themselves, often resorted to the heretics for treatment.

This was the state of things when the King fell ill. He had twelve doctors to attend him; and when there was no sign of his being cured, his people became anxious, and said, "A single doctor is generally sufficient to kill one of us, so how can the King survive twelve doctors?"

Then the King's son, who was at the other side of the world among the black savages (for he was very tired of the white ones), came flying, sailing, and express-training at an amazing speed back to his father, and spoke with the King's chief physician, who was so delightful a person that his patients were often cured by his mere appearance in the bedroom. The Prince knew that his father's case must be most serious since it resisted the presence of this great healer and the influence of the King's faith in him. And the Prince said to him: "Doc, the King my father does not seem to be getting any better. Is it not possible to get a move on?"

"In what direction, sir?" replied the chief physician.

"In the direction of getting him up and about," said the Prince.

"Everything is being done that can properly be done," said the physician. "If your Royal Highness has not confidence in our knowledge and devotion—"

"Stow that," said the Prince. "Your devotion is all right; but your knowledge is bunk."

"Bunk!" exclaimed the chief physician, highly scandalized.

"Well, perhaps not all of it," said the Prince, feeling that he had gone a little too far; "but I cannot help knowing what everyone knows, and that is that according to your own best men nine-tenths of your official notions are fit only for the dustbin. I have a heap of letters, books, pamphlets, and magazines here which have been sent me; and they have disturbed me very much."

"I have not read these documents," said the physician. "If your Royal Highness can suggest any measure we have omitted, my opinion is at your service."

"Drugs, now?" said the Prince. "Drugs are bunk, are they not?"

"Undoubtedly, from a purely secular point of view, drugs are bunk," said the physician; "but in the case of a royal patient I could not possibly take the responsibility of withholding from His Majesty the official remedies from our *materia medica*."

"But," said the Prince, "there is a way of giving drugs in infinitesimal quantities to which all the latest discoveries and scientific speculations point as the right way."

"Infinitesimals," replied the physician, "are used only by homeopaths: that is, by empirics who, being ignorant of the nature of disease, merely treat its symptoms. If you bring a Chinese patient to a homeopath, he will treat him for yellow fever."

"Do you really know the nature of disease any more than a homeopath does?" said the Prince.

"Certainly," said the physician. "I have passed an examination in pathology, and written books about it. What a strange question!"

"What is the nature of my father's complaint?" said the Prince.

"It is what we call pleurisy," said the physician.

"I know that," said the Prince. "I know its name; and I know its symptoms. What is its nature?"

"If I knew that," said the physician, "perhaps I could cure it."

"Then pathology is bunk," said the Prince, who had picked up this expression from a famous motor-car manufacturer, who had applied it to History. "Let us call in a homeopath."

"Unfortunately," said the physician, "the only one in London whose reputation and success would satisfy public opinion has not been admitted to our communion; and if I discussed the case with him I should be excommunicated."

"Well," said the Prince, "they say a lot of trouble comes from spinal displacements. What about my father's spine?"

"It looks all right," said the physician.

"But there are chaps who are trained to feel whether it is all right or not," said the Prince. "There is a machine that will register on a galvanometer displacements that nobody can feel."

"I never heard of it," said the physician. "I can assure you that these people who feel spines are almost all ignorant Americans who have spent two years in mere manual training instead of in the study of pathology."

"All the same," said the Prince, "they bring off cures occasionally; so why not call one in?"

"I should be excommunicated if I were seen speaking to one," said the physician.

"Why not do it yourself?" said the Prince. "You are a surgeon."

"I have not had the two years' training," said the physician: "it is not part of our official surgery."

"Official surgery is a wash-out," said the Prince. "What about testing my father's blood for radiations? That can be done by a rheostat, can't it?

And there is some method of neutralizing the rays that sometimes cures, isn't there?''

''But it was discovered by an American,'' said the physician.

''I am prepared to overlook that if my father's health can be restored by his method,'' said the Prince.

''Impossible,'' said the physician. ''He was not only an American, but a Jew.''

''I understand he was a proper doctor all the same,'' persisted the Prince.

''No doubt,'' said the physician; ''but the treatment would involve attaching His Majesty to the electric light switch; and public opinion would never tolerate that.''

''Public opinion be blowed!'' said the Prince. ''Do you suppose I am going to let my father lose a chance because people are fools? Besides, we can use a private battery.''

''It may not be,'' said the physician. ''This discovery reached us only about a dozen years ago, and is not yet recognized by our Vatican. I dare not take the responsibility of experimenting on the King with a treatment that has not been proved by at least fifty years' experience.''

''Proved to do what?'' said the Prince. ''To cure the disease?''

''To have stood the test of being taught in our medical schools as the logical and appropriate treatment,'' said the physician.

''Do the patients recover under your logical and appropriate treatments?'' said the Prince.

''Sometimes,'' said the physician. ''Quite frequently.''

''They might do that if they had no treatment at all,'' said the Prince.

''That is true,'' said the physician. ''The recuperative power of the human organism is marvellous. Quacks take advantage of that, I am sorry to say.''

''I am not satisfied about all this,'' said the Prince. ''It seems to me that my father, just because he is a king, is cut off from the benefit of all the new discoveries and treatments that are available for the meanest of his subjects.''

''I exhort your Royal Highness to be patient,'' said the physician. ''Your royal father is in the hands of God.''

''You mean that we should call in a Christian Science practitioner?'' said the Prince.

''Most certainly not,'' said the physician. ''I and my colleagues would be obliged to withdraw at once if such a person were admitted to the palace.''

''Another wash-out,'' said the Prince.

''Not at all,'' said the physician. ''We should not object to a visit from

His Majesty's domestic chaplain; though of course we could not allow him to treat the case; and anything in the nature of a consultation would be out of the question."

"In short," said the Prince, "my poor father is in the hands of your confounded Vatican. However, I suppose we must make the best of it. I should like to call in your Pope for a consultation."

"We should have to tell him what to say beforehand," said the physician. "You see, he was qualified more than half a century ago, and may not be quite up to date."

"But I have looked him up in Who's Who," said the Prince; "and he has ninety distinctions and qualifications, entitling him to a dozen medical letters after his name. I attach great importance to a lot of letters because I have nothing else to go by."

"As I myself have only six, you naturally consider his opinion twice as valuable as mine," said the physician.

"Well, if the letters don't mean that, they don't mean anything," said the Prince.

"Precisely," said the physician.

"Then your Pope is another wash-out," said the Prince. "Are there any laymen on your Vatican council to represent my father and all the other patients?"

"A notorious enemy of our profession has succeeded, after years of agitation, in having one layman appointed," said the physician.

"Well, don't you agree with that?" said the Prince.

"Officially, no," said the physician.

"But unofficially—as between man and man?" pleaded the Prince.

"Since your Royal Highness is good enough to admit me to that footing," said the physician, "I am bound to say, as between man and man, that the exclusion of laymen from a body whose business it is to safeguard the general interests of the laity against the sectional interests of the medical profession is only one out of the many instances of the almost incredible incapacity of the Half Mad for taking care of themselves. In respect of the art of life, our people must be set aside as unqualified practitioners."

"This is a world of bunk," said the Prince; "and the boasted capacity of my father's subjects for self-government is the biggest bunk of the lot. But my father's life is in danger. I appeal to you to throw over your silly Vatican and be a friend to us in our need. If they give you the sack you shall have a dukedom and a pension of a hundred thousand a year. Tell me what is the most up-to-date scientific treatment for my father?"

"I have already ordered it," said the physician. "And you will be glad to hear that it will involve no conflict on my part with my colleagues."

"Splendid!" said the Prince. "I will never forget this proof of your sympathy and devotion. What is the treatment?"

"The seaside," said the physician.

"The seaside!" cried the Prince. "You call that the latest! Why, it is what my great-grandmother would have recommended."

"Yes," said the physician, "but not for the true scientific reason. She thought that the benefit arose from change of air."

"Then what does it arise from?" said the Prince.

"That," said the physician, "is a professional secret which I can impart to you only under a solemn pledge that it shall go no further."

"I give you my word of honor," said the Prince. "What will the seaside really do to cure my father?"

The physician stooped to the Prince's ear, and whispered: "It will get him away from the doctors."

Shortly afterwards, the King recovered.

GEORGE BERNARD SHAW
The Doctor's Dilemma

SIR PATRICK. What did you find out from Jane's case?

RIDGEON. I found out that the inoculation that ought to cure sometimes kills.

SIR PATRICK. I could have told you that. I've tried these modern inoculations a bit myself. I've killed people with them; and I've cured people with them; but I gave them up because I never could tell which I was going to do.

RIDGEON [*taking a pamphlet from a drawer in the writing-table and handing it to him*] Read that the next time you have an hour to spare; and you'll find out why.

SIR PATRICK [*grumbling and fumbling for his spectacles*] Oh, bother your pamphlets. Whats the practice of it? [*Looking at the pamphlet*] Opsonin? What the devil is opsonin?

RIDGEON. Opsonin is what you butter the disease germs with to make your white blood corpuscles eat them. [*He sits down again on the couch*].

SIR PATRICK. Thats not new. I've heard this notion that the white corpuscles—what is it that whats his name?—Metchinikoff—calls them?

RIDGEON. Phagocytes.

SIR PATRICK. Aye, phagocytes: yes, yes, yes. Well, I heard this theory that the phagocytes eat up the disease germs years ago: long before you came into fashion. Besides, they don't always eat them.

RIDGEON. They do when you butter them with opsonin.

SIR PATRICK. Gammon.

RIDGEON. No: it's not gammon. What it comes to in practice is this. The phagocytes won't eat the microbes unless the microbes are nicely buttered for them. Well, the patient manufactures the butter for himself all right; but my discovery is that the manufacture of that butter, which I call opsonin, goes on in the system by ups and downs—Nature being always rhythmical, you know—and that what the inoculation does is to stimulate the ups and downs, as the case may be. If we had inoculated Jane Marsh when her butter factory was on the up-grade, we should have cured her arm. But we got in on the down-grade and lost her arm for her. I call the up-grade the positive phase and the down-grade the negative phase. Everything depends on your inoculating at the right moment. Inoculate when the patient is in the negative phase and you kill: inoculate when the patient is in the positive phase and you cure.

SIR PATRICK. And pray how are you to know whether the patient is in the positive or the negative phase?

RIDGEON. Send a drop of the patient's blood to the laboratory at St. Anne's; and in fifteen minutes I'll give you his opsonin index in figures. If the figure is one, inoculate and cure: if it's under point eight, inoculate and kill. Thats my discovery: the most important that has been made since Harvey discovered the circulation of the blood. My tuberculosis patients don't die now.

SIR PATRICK. And mind do when my inoculation catches them in the negative phase, as you call it. Eh?

RIDGEON. Precisely. To inject a vaccine into a patient without first testing his opsonin is as near murder as a respectable practitioner can get. If I wanted to kill a man I should kill him that way.

EMMY [looking in] Will you see a lady that wants her husband's lungs cured?

RIDGEON [impatiently] No. Havn't I told you I will see nobody? [To Sir Patrick] I live in a stage of siege ever since it got about that I'm a magician who can cure consumption with a drop of serum. [To Emmy] Don't come to me again about people who have no appointments. I tell you I can see nobody.

EMMY. Well, I'll tell her to wait a bit.

RIDGEON [furious] You'll tell her I can't see her, and send her away: do you hear?

EMMY [unmoved] Well, will you see Mr. Cutler Walpole? He don't want a cure: he only wants to congratulate you.

RIDGEON. Of course. Shew him up. [She turns to go]. Stop. [To Sir Patrick] I want two minutes more with you between ourselves. [To Emmy] Emmy: ask Mr. Walpole to wait just two minutes, while I finish a consultation.

EMMY. Oh, He'll wait all right. He's talking to the poor lady. [She goes out].

SIR PATRICK. Well? what is it?

RIDGEON. Don't laugh at me. I want your advice.

SIR PATRICK. Professional advice?

RIDGEON. Yes. There's something the matter with me. I don't know what it is.

SIR PATRICK. Neither do I. I suppose you've been sounded.

RIDGEON. Yes, of course. There's nothing wrong with any of the organs:

nothing special, anyhow. But I have a curious aching: I don't know where: I can't localize it. Sometimes I think it's my heart: sometimes I suspect my spine. It doesn't exactly hurt me; but it unsettles me completely. I feel that something is going to happen. And there are other symptoms. Scraps of tunes come into my head that seem to me very pretty, though they're quite commonplace.

SIR PATRICK. Do you hear voices?

RIDGEON. No.

SIR PATRICK. I'm glad of that. When my patients tell me that they've made a greater discovery than Harvey, and that they hear voices, I lock them up.

RIDGEON. You think I'm mad! That's just the suspicion that has come across me once or twice. Tell me the truth: I can bear it.

SIR PATRICK. You're sure there are no voices?

RIDGEON. Quite sure.

SIR PATRICK. Then it's only foolishness.

RIDGEON. Have you ever met anything like it before in your practice?

SIR PATRICK. Oh, yes: often. It's very common between the ages of seventeen and twenty-two. It sometimes comes on again at forty or thereabouts. You're a bachelor you see. It's not serious—if you're careful.

RIDGEON. About my food?

SIR PATRICK. No: about your behavior. There's nothing wrong with your spine; and there's nothing wrong with your heart; but there's something wrong with your common sense. You're not going to die; but you may be going to make a fool of yourself. So be careful.

RIDGEON. I see you don't believe in my discovery. Well, sometimes I don't believe in it myself. Thank you all the same. Shall we have Walpole up?

SIR PATRICK. Oh, have him up. [*Ridgeon rings*]. He's a clever operator, is Walpole, though he's only one of your chloroform surgeons. In my early days, you made your man drunk; and the porters and students held him down; and you had to set your teeth and finish the job fast. Nowadays you work at your ease; and the pain doesn't come until afterwards, when you've taken your cheque and rolled up your bag and left the house. I tell you, Colly, chloroform has done a lot of mischief. It's enabled every fool to be a surgeon.

RIDGEON. [*to Emmy, who answers the bell*] Shew Mr. Walpole up.

EMMY. He's talking to the lady.

RIDGEON [*exasperated*] Did I not tell you—

Emmy goes out without heeding him. He gives it up, with a shrug, and plants himself with his back to the console, leaning resignedly against it.

SIR PATRICK. I know your Cutler Walpoles and their like. They've found out that a man's body's full of bits and scraps of old organs he has no mortal use for. Thanks to chloroform, you can cut half a dozen of them out without leaving him any the worse, except for the illness and the guineas it costs him. I knew the Walpoles well fifteen years ago. The father used to snip off the ends of people's uvulas for fifty guineas, and paint throats with caustic every day for a year at two guineas a time. His brother-in-law extirpated tonsils for two hundred guineas until he took up women's cases at double the fees. Cutler himself worked hard at anatomy to find something fresh to operate on; and at last he got hold of something he calls the nuciform sac, which he's made quite the fashion. People pay him five hundred guineas to cut it out. They might as well get their hair cut for all the difference it makes; but I suppose they feel important after it. You can't go out to dinner now without your neighbor bragging to you of some useless operation or other.

EMMY. [announcing] Mr. Cutler Walpole. [She goes out].

Cutler Walpole is an energetic, unhesitating man of forty, with a cleanly modelled face, very decisive and symmetrical about the shortish, salient, rather pretty nose, and the three trimly turned corners made by his chin and jaws. In comparison with Ridgeon's delicate broken lines, and Sir Patrick's softly rugged aged ones, his face looks machine-made and beeswaxed; but his scrutinizing, daring eyes give it life and force. He seems never at a loss, never in doubt: one feels that if he made a mistake he would make it thoroughly and firmly. He has neat, well-nourished hands, short arms, and is built for strength and compactness rather than for height. He is smartly dressed with a fancy waistcoat, a richly colored scarf secured by a handsome ring, ornaments on his watch chain, spats on his shoes, and a general air of the well-to-do sportsman about him. He goes straight across to Ridgeon and shakes hands with him.

WALPOLE. My dear Ridgeon, best wishes! heartiest congratulations! You deserve it.

RIDGEON. Thank you.

WALPOLE. As a man, mind you. You deserve it as a man. The opsonin is simple rot, as any capable surgeon can tell you; but we're all delighted to see your personal qualities officially recognized. Sir Patrick: how are you? I sent you a paper lately about a little thing I invented: a new saw. For shoulder blades.

SIR PATRICK [meditatively] Yes: I got it. It's a good saw: a useful, handy instrument.

WALPOLE. [confidently] I knew you'd see its points.

SIR PATRICK. Yes: I remember that saw sixty-five years ago.

WALPOLE. What!

SIR PATRICK. It was called a cabinetmaker's jimmy then.

WALPOLE. Get out! Nonsense! Cabinetmaker be—

RIDGEON. Never mind him, Walpole. He's jealous.

WALPOLE. By the way, I hope I'm not disturbing you two in anything private.

RIDGEON. No no. Sit down. I was only consulting him. I'm rather out of sorts. Overwork, I suppose.

WALPOLE. [*swiftly*] I know what's the matter with you. I can see it in your complexion. I can feel it in the grip of your hand.

RIDGEON. What is it?

WALPOLE. Blood-poisoning.

RIDGEON. Blood-poisoning! Impossible.

WALPOLE. I tell you, blood-poisoning. Ninety-five per cent of the human race suffer from chronic blood poisoning, and die of it. It's as simple as A.B.C. Your nuciform sac is full of decaying matter—undigested food and waste products—rank ptomaines. Now you take my advice, Ridgeon. Let me cut it out for you. You'll be another man afterwards.

SIR PATRICK. Don't you like him as he is?

WALPOLE. No I don't. I don't like any man who hasn't a healthy circulation. I tell you this: in an intelligently governed country people wouldn't be allowed to go about with nuciform sacs, making themselves centres of infection. The operation ought to be compulsory: it's ten times more important than vaccination.

SIR PATRICK. Have you had your own sac removed, may I ask?

WALPOLE. [*triumphantly*] I havn't got one. Look at me! I've no symptoms. I'm as sound as a bell. About five per cent of the population havn't got any; and I'm one of the five per cent. I'll give you an instance. You know Mrs. Jack Foljambe: the smart Mrs. Foljambe? I operated at Easter on her sister-in-law, Lady Gorran, and found she had the biggest sac I ever saw: it held about two ounces. Well, Mrs. Foljambe had the right spirit—the genuine hygienic instinct. She couldn't stand her sister-in-law being a clean, sound woman, and she simply a whited sepulchre. So she insisted on my operation on her, too. And by George, sir, she hadn't any sac at all. Not a trace! Not a rudiment!! I was so taken aback—so interested, that I forgot to take the sponges out, and was stitching them up inside her when the nurse missed them. Somehow, I'd made sure she'd have an exceptionally large one. [*He sits down on the couch, squaring his shoulders and shooting his hands out of his cuffs as he sets his knuckles akimbo.*]

EMMY [*looking in*] Sir Ralph Bloomfield Bonington.

A long and expectant pause follows this announcement. All look to the door; but there is no Sir Ralph.

RIDGEON [*at last*] Where is he?

EMMY [*looking back*] Drat him, I thought he was following me. He's stayed down to talk to that lady—

RIDGEON [*exploding*] I told you to tell that lady—[*Emmy vanishes*]

WALPOLE [*jumping up again*] Oh, by the way, Ridgeon, that reminds me. I've been talking to that poor girl. It's her husband; and she thinks it's a case of consumption: the usual wrong diagnosis: these damned general practitioners ought never to be allowed to touch a patient except under the orders of a consultant. She's been describing his symptoms to me; and the case is as plain as a pikestaff: bad blood-poisoning. Now she's poor. She can't afford to have him operated on. Well, you send him to me: I'll do it for nothing. There's room for him in my nursing home. I'll put him straight, and feed him up and make her happy. I like making people happy. [*He goes to the chair near the window*].

EMMY [*looking in*] Here he is.

Sir Ralph Bloomfield Bonington wafts himself into the room. He is a tall man, with a head like a tall and slender egg. He has been in his time a slender man; but now, in his sixth decade, his waistcoat has filled out somewhat. His fair eyebrows arch good-naturedly and uncritically. He has a most musical voice; his speech is a perpetual anthem; and he never tires of the sound of it. He radiates an enormous self-satisfaction, cheering, reassuring, healing by the mere incompatibility of disease or anxiety with his welcome presence. Even broken bones, it is said, have been known to unite at the sound of his voice: he is a born healer, as independent of mere treatment and skill as any Christian Scientist. When he expands into oratory or scientific exposition, he is as energetic as Walpole; but it is with a bland, voluminous, atmospheric energy, which envelops its subject and its audience, and makes interruption or inattention impossible, and imposes veneration and credulity on all but the strongest minds. He is known in the medical world as B. B.; and the envy roused by his success in practice is softened by the conviction that he is, scientifically considered, a colossal humbug: the fact being that, though he knows just as much (and just as little) as his contemporaries, the qualifications that pass muster in common men reveal their weakness when hung on his egregious personality.

B. B. Aha! Sir Colenso. Sir Colenso, eh? Welcome to the order of knighthood.

RIDGEON. [*shaking hands*] Thank you, B. B.

B. B. What! Sir Patrick! And how are we to-day? a little chilly? a little stiff? but hale and still the cleverest of us all [*Sir Patrick grunts*]. What! Walpole! the absent-minded beggar: eh?

WALPOLE. What does that mean?

B. B. Have you forgotten the lovely opera singer I sent you to have that growth taken off her vocal cords?

WALPOLE. [*springing to his feet*] Great heavens, man, you don't mean to say you sent her for a throat operation!

B. B. [*archly*] Aha! Ha ha! Aha! [*trilling like a lark as he shakes his finger at Walpole*] You removed her nuciform sac. Well, well! force of habit! force of habit! Never mind, ne-e-e-ver mind. She got back her voice after it, and thinks you the greatest surgeon alive; and so you are, so you are, so you are.

CLINICAL DESCRIPTIONS IN LITERATURE

Some of the most graphic accounts of illness available in print have appeared not in the medical journals but in novels. It is the writer's business to recognize dramatic situations—which abound in clinical medicine. And when the situation happens to the writer herself or himself, it is as difficult for the writer to avoid writing about it as it is for most patients to avoid talking about it. But the value to the medical profession of such reports or memoirs is that they provide an inner view of the perceptions and feelings that sometimes are no less pertinent than the diagnostic tests.

SAUL BELLOW
Mr. Sammler's Planet

SAUL BELLOW (1915-   ) is noted for his novels portraying the inner
feelings of characters placed in harried urban lifestyles. *Mr. Sammler's
Planet* uses the author's memories of his own parents' emigration from
Eastern Europe.

Sammler didn't at first understand what an aneurysm meant; he heard from
Angela that Gruner was in the hospital for throat surgery. The day after the
pickpocket had cornered him, he went to the East Side to visit Gruner. He
found him with a bandaged neck.

"Well, Uncle Sammler?"

"Elya—how are you? You look all right." And the old man, reaching
beneath himself with a long arm, smoothing the underside of the trench
coat, bending thin legs, sat down. Between the tips of cracked wrinkled
black shoes he set the tip of his umbrella and leaned with both palms on the
curved handle, stooping toward the bed with Polish-Oxonian politeness.
Meticulously, the sickroom caller. Finely, intricately wrinkled, the left side
of his face was like the contour map of difficult terrain.

Dr. Gruner sat straight, unsmiling. His expression after a lifetime of
good-humored appearance was still mainly pleasant. This was not pertinent
at present, merely habitual.

"I am in the middle of something."

"The surgery was successful?"

"There is a gimmick in my throat, Uncle."

"For what?"

"To regulate the flow of blood in the artery—the carotid."

"Is that so? Is it a valve or something?"

"More or less."

"It's supposed to reduce the pressure?"

"Yes, that's the idea."

"Yes. Well, it seems to be working. You look as usual. Normal, Elya."

Evidently there was something which Dr. Gruner had no intention of
letting out. His expression was neither dire nor grim. Instead of hardness
Mr. Sammler thought he could observe a curious kind of tight lightness.

The doctor in the hospital, in pajamas, was a good patient. He said to the nurses, "This is my uncle. Tell him what kind of patient I am."

"Oh, the doctor is a wonderful patient."

Gruner had always insisted on having affectionate endorsements, approbation, the good will of all who drew near.

"I am completely in the surgeon's hands. I do exactly as he says."

"He is a good doctor?"

"Oh, yes. He's a hillbilly. A Georgia red-neck. He was a football star in college. I remember reading about him in the papers. He played for Georgia Tech. But he's professionally very able; and I take orders from him, and I never discuss the case."

"So you're satisfied completely with him?"

"Yesterday the screw was too tight."

"What did that do?"

"Well, my speech got thick. I lost some coordination. You know the brain needs its blood supply. So they had to loosen me up again."

"But you are better today?"

"Oh, yes."

The mail was brought, and Dr. Gruner asked Uncle Sammler to read a few items from the Market Letter. Sammler lifted the paper to his right eye, concentrating window light upon it. "The U.S. Justice Department will file suit to force Ling-Temco-Vought to divest its holdings of Jones and Laughlin Steel. Moving against the huge conglomerate . . ."

"Those conglomerates are soaking up all the business in the country. One of them, I understand, has acquired all the funeral parlors in New York. I hear reports that Campbell, Riverside, have been bought by the same company that publishes *Mad* magazine."

"How curious."

"Youth is a big business. Schoolchildren spend fantastic amounts. If enough kids get radical, that's a new mass market, then it's a big operation."

"I have a general idea."

"Very little is holding still. First making money, then keeping your money from shrinking by inflation. How you invest it, whom you trust— you trust nobody—what you get with it, how you save it from those Federal taxation robbers, the gruesome Revenue Service. And how you leave it . . . wills! Those are the worst problems in life. Excruciating."

Uncle Sammler now understood fully how it was. His nephew Gruner had in his head a great blood vessel, defective from birth, worn thin and frayed with a lifetime of pulsation. A clot had formed from leakage. The whole jelly trembled. One was summoned to the brink of the black. Any beat of the heart might open the artery and spray the brain with blood. These facts shimmered their way into Sammler's mind. Was it the time? *The* time? How terrible! But yes! Elya would die of a hemorrhage. Did he know this? Of course he did. He was a physician, so he must know. But he was human, so he could arrange many things for himself. Both knowing and not knowing—one of the more frequent human arrangements. Then Sammler, making himself intensely observant, concluded after ten or twelve minutes that Gruner definitely knew. He believed that Gruner's moment of honor had come, that moment at which the individual could call upon his best qualities. Mr. Sammler had lived a long time and understood something about these cases of final gallantry. *If* there were time, occasionally good things were done. *If* one had a certain kind of luck.

"Uncle, try some of these fruit jellies. The lime and orange are the best. From Beersheba."

"Aren't you watching your weight, Elya?"

"No, I'm not. They're making terrific stuff in Israel these days." The doctor had been buying Israel bonds and real estate. In Westchester, he served Israeli wine and brandy. He gave away heavily embossed silver ball-point pens, made in Israel. You could sign checks with them. For ordinary purposes they were not useful. And on two occasions Dr. Gruner, as he was picking up his fedora, had said, "I believe I'll go to Jerusalem for a while."

"When are you leaving?"

"Now."

"Right away?"

"Certainly."

"Just as you are?"

"Just as I am. I can buy my toothbrush and razor when I land. I love it there."

He had his chauffeur drive him to Kennedy Airport.

"I'll cable you, Emil, when I'm coming back."

In Jerusalem were more old relatives like Sammler, and Gruner did genealogies with them, one of his favorite pastimes. More than a pastime. He had a passion for kinships. Sammler found this odd, especially in a physician. As one whose prosperity had been founded in the female generative slime, he might have had less specific sentiment about his own tribe. But now, seeing a fatal dryness in the circles under his eyes, Sammler better understood the reason for this. To each according to his intimations. Gruner had not worked in his profession for ten years. He had had a heart attack and retired on insurance. After a year or two of payments, the insurance company insisted that he was well enough to practice, and there had been a lawsuit. Then Dr. Gruner learned that insurance companies kept the finest legal talent in the city on retainer. The best lawyers were tied up, and the courts were deliberately choked with trivial suits by the companies, so that it was years before his case came to trial. But he won. Or was about to win. He had disliked his trade—the knife, blood. He had been conscientious. He had done his duty. But he hadn't liked his trade. He was still, however, fastidiously manicured like a practicing surgeon. Here in the hospital the manicurist was sent for, and during Sammler's visit Gruner's fingers were being soaked in a steel basin. The strange tinge of male fingers in the suds. The woman in her white smock, every single hair of the neckless head the same hue of dyed black, without variation, was gloomy, sloven-footed in orthopedic white shoes. Heavy-shouldered, she bent with instruments over his nails, concentrating on her work. She had quite a wide, tear-pregnant nose. Dr. Gruner had to woo reactions from her. Even from such a dismal creature.

As it might not be many times more (for Elya) the room was filled with sunny light. In which familiar human postures were struck. From which no great results had come in the past. From which little could be expected at this late hour. What if the manicurist were to take a liking to Dr. Gruner? What if she should requite his longing? What was his longing? Mr. Sammler had a thing about these unprofitable instants of clarity. Seeing the singular human creature demand more when the sum of human facts could not yield more. Sammler did not like such instants, but they came nevertheless.

The woman pushed back the cuticle. She would not be tempted up from her own underground galleries. Intimacy was refused.

"Uncle Artur, can you tell me anything about my grandmother's brother in the old country?"

"Who?"

"Hessid was the man's name."

"Hessid? Hessid? Yes, there was a Hessid family."

"He had a mill for cornmeal, and a shop near the Castle. Just a small place with a few barrels."

"You must be mistaken. I remember no one in the family who ground anything. However, you have an excellent memory. Better than mine."

"Hessid. A fine-looking old man with a broad white beard. He wore a derby, and a very fancy vest with watch and chain. Called up often to read from the Torah, though he couldn't have been a heavy contributor to the synagogue."

"Ah, the synagogue. Well, you see, Elya, I didn't have much to do with the synagogue. We were almost free-thinkers. Especially my mother. She had a Polish education. She gave me an emancipated name: Artur.''

Sammler regretted that he was so poor at family reminiscences. Contemporary contacts being somewhat unsatisfactory, he would gladly have helped Gruner to build up the past.

"I loved old Hessid. You know, I was a very affectionate child.''

"I'm sure you were,'' said Sammler. He could hardly remember Gruner as a boy. Standing, he said, "I won't tire you with a long visit.''

"Oh, you aren't tiring me. But you probably have things to do. At the public library. One thing, before you go, Uncle—you're in pretty good shape still. You took that last trip to Israel very well, and that was a tough one. Do you still like to run in Riverside Park, as you used to do?''

"Not lately. I feel too stiff for it.''

"I was going to say, it's not safe to run down there. I don't want you mugged. When you're winded from running, some crazy sonofabitch jumps out and cuts your throat! Anyway, if you are too stiff to run you're far from feeble. I know you're not a sickly type, apart from your nervous trouble. You still get that small payment from the West Germans? And the Social Security? Yes, I'm glad we had the lawyer set that up, about the Germans. And I don't want you to worry, Uncle Artur.''

"About what?''

"About anything at all. Security in old age. Being in a home. You stay with Margotte. She's a good woman. She'll look after you. I realize Shula is a little too nutty for you. She amuses other people but not her own father. I know how that can be.''

"Yes, Margotte is decent. You couldn't ask for better.''

"So, remember, Uncle, no worries.''

"Thank you, Elya.''

A confusing, frowning moment, and, getting into the breast, the head, and even down into the bowels and about the heart, and behind the eyes—something gripping, aching, smarting. The woman was buffing Gruner's nails, and he sat straight in the fully buttoned pajama coat; above it, the bandage hiding the throat with its screw. His large ruddy face was mainly unhandsome, his baldness, his big-eared plainness, the large tip of the nose; Gruner belonged to the common branch of the family. It was, however, a virile face, and, when superficial objections were removed, a kindly face. Sammler knew the defects of his man. Saw them as dust and pebbles, as rubble on a mosaic which might be swept away. Underneath, a fine, noble expression. A dependable man—a man who took thought for others.

"You've been good to Shula and me, Elya.''

Gruner neither acknowledged nor denied this. Perhaps by the rigidity of his posture he fended off gratitude he did not deserve in full.

In short, if the earth deserves to be abandoned, if we are not to be driven streaming into other worlds, starting with the moon, it is not because of the likes of you, Sammler would have said. He put it more briefly. "I'm grateful."

"You're a gentleman, Uncle Artur."

"I'll be in touch."

"Yes, come back. It does me good."

Sammler, outside the rubber-silenced door, put on his Augustus John hat. A hat from the Soho that was. He went down the corridor in his usual quick way, favoring the sightful side slightly, putting forward the right leg and the right shoulder. When he came to the anteroom, a sunny bay with soft plastic orange furniture, he found Wallace Gruner there with a doctor in a white coat. This was Elya's surgeon.

"My dad's uncle—Dr. Cosbie."

"How do you do, Dr. Cosbie." The conceivably wasted fragrance of Mr. Sammler's manners. Who was there now to be aware of such Old World stuff! Here and there perhaps a woman might appreciate his style of greeting. But not a Doctor Cosbie. The ex-football star, famous in Georgia, struck Sammler as a sort of human wall. High and flat. His face was mysteriously silent, and very white. The upper lip was steep and prominent. The mouth itself thin and straight. Somewhat unapproachable, he kept his hands behind his back. He had the air of a general whose mind is on battalions in a bloody struggle, just out of sight over a hill. To a civilian pest who came up to him at that moment he had nothing to say.

"How is Dr. Gruner?"

"Makin' good progress, suh. A very fine patient."

Dr. Gruner was being seen as he wished to be seen. Every occasion had its propaganda. Democracy was propaganda. From government, propaganda entered every aspect of life. You had a desire, a view, a line, and you disseminated it. It took, everyone spoke of the event in the appropriate way, under your influence. In this case Elya, a doctor, a patient, made it known that he was the patient of patients. An allowable foible; boyish, but what of it? It had a certain interest.

Faced with a doctor, Sammler had his own foible, for he often wanted to ask about his symptoms. This was repressed of course. But the impulse was there. He wanted to mention that he woke up with a noise inside his head, that his good eye built up a speck at the corner which he couldn't scratch out, it stuck in the fold, that his feet burned intolerably at night, that he suffered from *pruritis ani*. Doctors loathed laymen with medical phrases. All, naturally, was censored. The tachycardia last of all. Nothing was shown to Cosbie but a certain cool, elderly rosiness. A winter apple. A busy-minded old man. Colored specs. A wide wrinkled hat brim. An umbrella on a sunny day—inconsequent. Long narrow shoes, cracked but highly polished.

* * *

Elya was a physician and a businessman. With his own family, to his credit, he had not been businesslike. Nevertheless, he had the business outlook. And business, in business America, was also a training system for souls. The fear of being unbusinesslike was very great. As he was dying Elya might conceivably draw strength from doing business. He had in fact done that. He kept talking to Widick. And Sammler had nothing with a business flavor to offer him. But at the very end business would not do for Elya. Some, many, would go on with business to the last breath, but Elya was not like that, not so limited. Elya was not finally ruled by business considerations. He was not in that insect and mechanical state—such a surrender, such an insect disaster for human beings. Even now (now perhaps more than ever) Elya was accessible. In fact Sammler had not seen this in time. Yesterday, when Elya began to speak of Wallace, when he denounced Angela, he, Sammler, ought to have stayed with him. Any degree of frankness might have been possible. In the going phrase, a moment of truth. Meaning that most conversation was a compilation of lies, of course. But Elya's was not one of those sealed completed impenetrable systems, he was not one of your monstrous crystals or icicles.

* * *

Detesting *Kulturny* physicians who wanted to discuss Heidegger or Wittgenstein. Real doctors had no time for that phony stuff. He was a keen spotter of phonies. He could easily afford this car, but had none of the life that went with it. No Broadway musicals, no private jet. His one glamorous eccentricity was to fly to Israel on short notice and stroll into the King David Hotel without baggage, his hands in his pockets. That struck him as a sporting thing to do. Of course, thought Sammler, Elya was also peculiar; surgery was psychically peculiar. To enter an unconscious body with a knife? To take out organs, sew in the flesh, splash blood? Not everyone could do that. And perhaps he kept the car for Emil's sake. What would Emil do if there were no Rolls? Now there was the likeliest answer of all.

The protective instinct was strong in Elya. Undisclosed charities were his pleasure. He had many strategems of benevolence. I have reason to know. How very odd—astonishing, the desire to relieve and protect us. It was astonishing because Elya the surgeon also despised incompetence and weakness. Only great and powerful instincts worked so deeply and deviously, coming out on the side of things despised. But how could Elya afford to have rigid ideas of strength? He himself was a hooked man. Hilda had been far stronger than he. In the Mafioso swagger were pretensions of lawless liberty. But it was little Hilda with the rod-like legs and the bouffant hair and faultless hemlines and sweet refinements who was the real criminal. She had had her hook in Elya. And there had never been any help for Elya. Who was there to help him? He was the sort of individual from whom help emanated. There were no arrangements for return. However, it would soon be over. It was about to wash away.

*   *   *

The one-time football star in his white coat held his upper lip pressed by the nether one. The bloodless face and gas-blue eyes had been trained to transmit surgeons' messages. The message was plain. It was all over.

"When did he die?" said Sammler. "Just now?"

While I was stupidly urging Angela!

"A little while back. We had him down in the special unit, doin' the maximum possible."

"You couldn't do anything about a hemorrhage, I see, yes."

"You are his uncle. He asked me to say good-by to you."

"I wish I had been able to say it also to him. So it didn't happen in one rush?"

"He knew it was startin'. He was a doctor. He knew it. He asked me to take him from the room."

"He asked you to?"

"It was obvious he wanted to spare his daughter. So I said tests. It's Miss Angela?"

"Yes, Angela."

"He said he preferred downstairs. He knew I'd take him anyway."

"Of course. As a surgeon, Elya knew. He certainly knew the operation was futile, all that torture of putting a screw in his throat." Sammler removed his glasses. His eyes, one a sightless bubble, under the hair of overhanging brows, were level with Dr. Cosbie's. "Of course it was futile."

"The procedure was correct. He knew it was."

"My nephew wished always to agree. Of course he knew. It might have been kinder though not to make him go through it."

"I suppose you want to go in and tell Miss Angela?"

"Please tell Miss Angela yourself. What I want is to see my nephew. How do I get to him? Give me directions."

"You'll have to wait and see him at the chapel, sir. It's not allowed."

"Young man, it is important and you had better allow me. Take my word for it. I am determined. Let us not have a bad scene out here in the corridor. You would not want that, would you?"

"Would you make one?"

"I would."

"I'll send his nurse with you," said the doctor.

They went down in the elevator, the gray woman and Mr. Sammler, and through lower passages paved in speckled material, through tunnels, up and down ramps, past laboratories and supply rooms. Well, this famous truth for which he was so keen, he had it now, or it had him. He felt that he was being destroyed, what was left of him. He wept to himself. He walked at the habitual rapid sweeping pace, waiting at crossways for the escorting nurse. In stirring air flavored with body-things, sickness, drugs. He felt that he was breaking up, that irregular big fragments inside were melting, sparkling with pain, floating off. Well, Elya was gone. He was deprived of one more thing, stripped of one more creature. One more reason to live trickled out. He lost his breath. Then the woman came up. More hundreds of yards in this winding underground smelling of serum, of organic soap, of fungus, of cell brew. The nurse took Sammler's hat and said, "In there." The door sign read P.M. That would mean post-mortem. They were ready to do an autopsy as soon as Angela signed the papers. And of course she would sign. Let's find out what went wrong. And then cremation.

"To see Dr. Gruner. Where?" said Sammler.

The attendant pointed to the wheeled stretcher on which Elya lay. Sammler uncovered his face. The nostrils, the creases were very dark, the shut eyes pale and full, the bald head high-marked by gradients of wrinkles. In the lips bitterness and an expression of obedience were combined.

Sammler in a mental whisper said, "Well, Elya. Well, well, Elya." And then in the same way he said, "Remember, God, the soul of Elya Gruner, who, as willingly as possible and as well as he was able, and even to an intolerable point, and even in suffocation and even as death was coming was eager, even childishly perhaps (may I be forgiven for this), even with a certain servility, to do what was required of him. At his best this man was much kinder than at my very best I have ever been or could ever be. He was aware that he must meet, and he did meet—through all the confusion and degraded clowning of this life through which we are speeding—he did meet the terms of his contract. The terms which, in his inmost heart, each man knows. As I know mine. As all know. For that is the truth of it—that we all know, God, that we know, that we know, we know, we know.''

WILLIAM BLAKE
The Island in the Moon

————◦∞◦————

WILLIAM BLAKE (1757-1827) was a symbolic artist noted for his visionary poems and engravings. In this selection, *The Island in the Moon*, Blake satirizes one of his wealthy patrons, a surgeon.

"Ah!" said Sipsop, "I only wish Jack Tearguts had had the cutting of Plutarch. He understands Anatomy better than any of the Ancients. He'll plunge his knife up to the hilt in a single drive, and thrust his fist in, and all in the space of a Quarter of an hour. He does not mind their crying, tho' they cry ever so. He'll swear at them & keep them down with his fist, & tell them that he'll scrape their bones if they don't lay still & be quiet. What the devil should the people in the hospital that have it done for nothing make such a piece of work for?"

"Hang that," said Suction; "let us have a song."

Then the Cynic sang—

I.
"When old corruption first begun.
  "Adorn'd in yellow vest,
"He committed on flesh a whoredom—
  "O, what a wicked beast!

2.
"From then a callow babe did spring,
  "And old corruption smil'd
"To think his race should never end,
  "For now he had a child.

3.
"He call'd him surgery, & fed
  "The babe with his own milk,
"For flesh & he could ne'er agree,
  "She would not let him suck.

4.
"And this he always kept in mind,
  "And form'd a crooked knife,

195

''And ran about with bloody hands
''To seek his mother's life.

5.

''And as he ran to seek his mother
   ''He met with a dead woman,
''He fell in love & married her,
   ''A deed which is not common.

6.

''She soon grew pregnant & brought forth
   ''Scurvy & spott'd fever.
''The father grin'd & skipt about,
   ''And said, 'I'm made for ever!

7.

'' 'For now I have procur'd these imps
   '' 'I'll try experiments.'
''With that he tied poor scurvy down
   ''& stopt up all its vents.

8.

''And when the child began to swell,
   ''He shouted out aloud,
'' 'I've found the dropsy out, & soon
   '' 'Shall do the world more good.'

9.

''He took up fever by the neck
   ''And cut out all its spots,
''And thro' the holes which he had made
   ''He first discover'd guts.''

"Ah," said Sipsop, "you think we are rascals—& we think you are rascals. I do as I chuse. What is it to any body what I do? I am always unhappy too. When I think of Surgery—I don't know. I do it because I like it. My father does what he likes & so do I. I think, somehow, I'll leave it off. There was a woman having her cancer cut, & she shriek'd so that I was quite sick."

SIR ARTHUR CONAN DOYLE
The Curse of Eve

———◅∞▻———

SIR ARTHUR CONAN DOYLE (1859-1930) is famous for his creation of
the adventures of Sherlock Holmes, in which he, more than anyone
else, defined the modern detective story genre. What is little known
about Doyle is the fact that he practiced medicine for several years
before devoting himself fully to a successful writing career. Some of his
medical experiences are recounted here.

Robert Johnson was an essentially commonplace man, with no feature to
distinguish him from a million others. He was pale of face, ordinary in
looks, neutral in opinions, thirty years of age, and a married man. By trade
he was a gentlemen's outfitter in the New North Road, and the competition
of business squeezed out of him the little character that was left. In his hope
of conciliating customers he had become cringing and pliable, until working
ever in the same routine from day to day he seemed to have sunk into a
soulless machine rather than a man. No great question had ever stirred him.
At the end of this snug century, self-contained in his own narrow circle, it
seemed impossible that any of the mighty, primitive passions of mankind
could ever reach him. Yet birth, and lust, and illness, and death are
changeless things, and when one of these harsh facts springs out upon a
man at some sudden turn of the path of life, it dashes off for the moment his
mask of civilisation and gives a glimpse of the stranger and stronger face
below.

Johnson's wife was a quiet little woman, with brown hair and gentle
ways. His affection for her was the one positive trait in his character.
Together they would lay out the shop window every Monday morning, the
spotless shirts in their green cardboard boxes below, the neckties above
hung in rows over the brass rails, the cheap studs glistening from the white
cards at either side, while in the background were the rows of cloth caps
and the bank of boxes in which the more valuable hats were screened from
the sunlight. She kept the books and sent out the bills. No one but she knew
the joys and sorrows which crept into his small life. She had shared his
exultations when the gentleman who was going to India had bought ten
dozen shirts and an incredible number of collars, and she had been as

197

stricken as he when, after the goods had gone, the bill was returned from the hotel address with the intimation that no such person had lodged there. For five years they had worked, building up the business, thrown together all the more closely because their marriage had been a childless one. Now, however, there were signs that a change was at hand, and that speedily. She was unable to come downstairs, and her mother, Mrs. Peyton, came over from Camberwell to nurse her and to welcome her grandchild.

Little qualms of anxiety came over Johnson as his wife's time approached. However, after all, it was a natural process. Other men's wives went through it unharmed, and why should not his! He was himself one of a family of fourteen, and yet his mother was alive and hearty. It was quite the exception for anything to go wrong. And yet in spite of his reasonings the remembrance of his wife's condition was always like a sombre background to all his other thoughts.

Dr. Miles of Bridport Place, the best man in the neighbourhood, was retained five months in advance, and, as time stole on, many little packets of absurdly small white garments with frill work and ribbons began to arrive among the big consignments of male necessities. And then one evening, as Johnson was ticketing the scarfs in the shop, he heard a bustle upstairs, and Mrs. Peyton came running down to say that Lucy was bad and that she thought the doctor ought to be there without delay.

It was not Robert Johnson's nature to hurry. He was prim and staid and liked to do things in an orderly fashion. It was a quarter of a mile from the corner of the New North Road where his shop stood to the doctor's house in Bridport Place. There were no cabs in sight so he set off upon foot, leaving the lad to mind the shop. At Bridport Place he was told that the doctor had just gone to Harman Street to attend a man in a fit. Johnson started off for Harman Street, losing a little of his primness as he became more anxious. Two full cabs but no empty ones passed him on the way. At Harman Street he learned that the doctor had gone on to a case of measles, fortunately he had left the address—69 Dunstan Road, at the other side of the Regent's Canal. Robert's primness had vanished now as he thought of the women waiting at home, and he began to run as hard as he could down the Kingsland Road. Some way along he sprang into a cab which stood by the curb and drove to Dunstan Road. The doctor had just left, and Robert Johnson felt inclined to sit down upon the steps in despair.

Fortunately he had not sent the cab away, and he was soon back at Bridport Place. Dr. Miles had not returned yet, but they were expecting him every instant. Johnson waited, drumming his fingers on his knees, in a high, dim lit room, the air of which was charged with a faint, sickly smell of ether. The furniture was massive, and the books in the shelves were sombre, and a squat black clock ticked mournfully on the mantelpiece. It told him that it was half-past seven, and that he had been gone an hour and a quarter. Whatever would the women think of him! Every time that a distant door slammed he sprang from his chair in a quiver of eagerness.

His ears strained to catch the deep notes of the doctor's voice. And then, suddenly, with a gush of joy he heard a quick step outside, and the sharp click of the key in the lock. In an instant he was out in the hall, before the doctor's foot was over the threshold.

"If you please, doctor, I've come for you," he cried; "the wife was taken bad at six o'clock."

He hardly knew what he expected the doctor to do. Something very energetic, certainly—to seize some drugs, perhaps, and rush excitedly with him through the gaslit streets. Instead of that Dr. Miles threw his umbrella into the rack, jerked off his hat with a somewhat peevish gesture, and pushed Johnson back into the room.

"Let's see! You *did* engage me, didn't you?" he asked in no very cordial voice.

"Oh, yes, doctor, last November. Johnson the outfitter, you know, in the New North Road."

"Yes, yes. It's a bit overdue," said the doctor glancing at a list of names in a note-book with a very shiny cover. "Well, how is she?"

"I don't—"

"Ah, of course, it's your first. You'll know more about it next time."

"Mrs. Peyton said it was time you were there, sir."

"My dear sir, there can be no very pressing hurry in a first case. We shall have an all-night affair, I fancy. You can't get an engine to go without coals, Mr. Johnson, and I have had nothing but a light lunch."

"We could have something cooked for you—something hot and a cup of tea."

"Thank you, but I fancy my dinner is actually on the table. I can do no good in the earlier stages. Go home and say that I am coming, and I will be round immediately afterwards."

A sort of horror filled Robert Johnson as he gazed at this man who could think about his dinner at such a moment. He had not imagination enough to realise that the experience which seemed so appallingly important to him, was the merest everyday matter of business to the medical man who could not have lived for a year had he not, amid the rush of work, remembered what was due to his own health. To Johnson he seemed little better than a monster. His thoughts were bitter as he sped back to his shop.

"You've taken your time," said his mother-in-law reproachfully, look-ing down the stairs as he entered.

"I couldn't help it!" he gasped. "Is it over?"

"Over! She's got to be worse, poor dear, before she can be better. Where's Dr. Miles?"

"He's coming after he's had dinner."

The old woman was about to make some reply, when, from the half-opened door behind a high whinnying voice cried out for her. She ran back and closed the door, while Johnson, sick at heart, turned into the shop. There he sent the lad home and busied himself frantically in putting up shutters and turning out boxes. When all was closed and finished he seated himself in the parlour behind the shop. But he could not sit still. He rose incessantly to walk a few paces and then fell back into a chair once more. Suddenly the clatter of china fell upon his ear, and he saw the maid pass the door with a cup on a tray and a smoking teapot.

"Who is that for, Jane?" he asked.

"For the mistress, Mr. Johnson. She says she would fancy it."

There was immeasurable consolation to him in that homely cup of tea. It wasn't so very bad after all if his wife could think of such things. So light-hearted was he that he asked for a cup also. He had just finished it when the doctor arrived, with a small black leather bag in his hand.

"Well, how is she?" he asked genially.

"Oh, she's very much better," said Johnson, with enthusiasm.

"Dear me, that's bad!" said the doctor. "Perhaps it will do if I look in on my morning round!"

"No, no," cried Johnson, clutching at his thick frieze overcoat. "We are so glad that you have come. And, doctor, please come down soon and let me know what you think about it."

The doctor passed upstairs, his firm, heavy steps resounding through the house. Johnson could hear his boots creaking as he walked about the floor above him, and the sound was a consolation to him. It was crisp and decided, the tread of a man who had plenty of self-confidence. Presently, still straining his ears to catch what was going on, he heard the scraping of a chair as it was drawn along the floor, and a moment later he heard the door fly open and someone come rushing downstairs. Johnson sprang up with his hair bristling, thinking that some dreadful thing had occurred, but it was only his mother-in-law, incoherent with excitement and searching for scissors and some tape. She vanished again and Jane passed up the stairs with a pile of newly aired linen. Then, after an interval of silence, Johnson heard the heavy, creaking tread and the doctor came down into the parlour.

"That's better," said he, pausing with his hand upon the door. "You look pale, Mr. Johnson."

"Oh no, sir, not at all," he answered deprecatingly, mopping his brow with his handkerchief.

"There is no immediate cause for alarm," said Dr. Miles. "The case is not all that we could wish it. Still we will hope for the best."

"Is there danger sir?" gasped Johnson.

"Well, there is always danger, of course. It is not altogether a favourable case, but still it might be much worse. I have given her a draught. I saw as I passed that they have been doing a little building opposite to you. It's an improving quarter. The rents go higher and higher. You have a lease of your own little place, eh?"

"Yes, sir, yes!" cried Johnson, whose ears were straining for every sound from above, and who felt none the less that it was very soothing that the doctor should be able to chat so easily at such a time. "That's to say no, sir, I am a yearly tenant."

"Ah, I should get a lease if I were you. There's Marshall, the watchmaker, down the street. I attended his wife twice and saw him through the typhoid when they took up the drains in Prince Street. I assure you his landlord sprung his rent nearly forty a year and he had to pay or clear out."

"Did his wife get through it, doctor?"

"Oh yes, she did very well. Hullo! Hullo!"

He slanted his ear to the ceiling with a questioning face, and then darted swiftly from the room.

It was March and the evenings were chill, so Jane had lit the fire, but the wind drove the smoke downwards and the air was full of its acrid taint. Johnson felt chilled to the bone, though rather by his apprehensions than by the weather. He crouched over the fire with his thin white hands held out to the blaze. At ten o'clock Jane brought in the joint of cold meat and laid his place for supper, but he could not bring himself to touch it. He drank a glass of beer, however, and felt the better for it. The tension of his nerves seemed to have reacted upon his hearing, and he was able to follow the most trivial things in the room above. Once, when the beer was still heartening him, he nerved himself to creep on tiptoe up the stair and to listen to what was going on. The bedroom door was half an inch open, and through the slit he could catch a glimpse of the clean-shaven face of the doctor, looking wearier and more anxious than before. Then he rushed downstairs like a lunatic, and running to the door he tried to distract his thoughts by watching what was going on in the street. The shops were all shut, and some rollicking boon companions came shouting along from the public-house. He stayed at the door until the stragglers had thinned down, and then came back to his seat by the fire. In his dim brain he was asking himself questions which had never intruded themselves before. Where was the justice of it? What had his sweet, innocent little wife done that she should be used so? Why was nature so cruel? He was frightened at his own thoughts, and yet wondered that they had never occurred to him before.

As the early morning drew in, Johnson, sick at heart and shivering in every limb, sat with his great coat huddled round him, staring at the grey ashes and waiting hopelessly for some relief. His face was white and clammy, and his nerves had been numbed into a half conscious state by the long monotony of misery. But suddenly all his feelings leapt into keen life again as he heard the bedroom door open and the doctor's steps upon the stair. Robert Johnson was precise and unemotional in everyday life, but he almost shrieked now as he rushed forward to know if it were over.

One glance at the stern, drawn face which met him showed that it was no pleasant news which had sent the doctor downstairs. His appearance had altered as much as Johnson's during the last few hours. His hair was on end, his face flushed, his forehead dotted with beads of perspiration. There was a peculiar fierceness in his eye, and about the lines of his mouth, a fighting look as befitted a man who for hours on end had been striving with the hungriest of foes for the most precious of prizes. But there was a sadness too, as though his grim opponent had been overmastering him. He sat down and leaned his head upon his hand like a man who is fagged out.

"I thought it my duty to see you, Mr. Johnson, and to tell you that it is a very nasty case. You wife's heart is not strong, and she has some symptoms which I do not like. What I wanted to say is that if you would like to have a second opinion I shall be very glad to meet anyone whom you might suggest."

Johnson was so dazed by his want of sleep and the evil news that he could hardly grasp the doctor's meaning. The other, seeing him hesitate, thought that he was considering the expense.

"Smith or Hawley would come for two guineas," said he. "But I think Pritchard of the City Road is the best man."

"Oh, yes, bring the best man," cried Johnson.

"Pritchard would want three guineas. He is a senior man, you see."

"I'd give him all I have if he would pull her through. Shall I run for him?"

"Yes. Go to my house first and ask for the green baize bag. The assistant will give it to you. Tell him I want the A.C.E. mixture. Her heart is too weak for chloroform. Then go for Pritchard and bring him back with you."

It was heavenly for Johnson to have something to do and to feel that he was of some use to his wife. He ran swiftly to Bridport Place, his footfalls clattering through the silent streets and the big dark policemen turning their yellow funnels of light on him as he passed. Two tugs at the night-bell brought down a sleepy, half-clad assistant, who handed him a stoppered glass bottle and a cloth bag which contained something which clinked when you moved it. Johnson thrust the bottle into his pocket, seized the green bag, and pressing his hat firmly down ran as hard as he could set foot to ground until he was in the City Road and saw the name of Pritchard engraved in white upon a red ground. He bounded in triumph up the three steps which led to the door, and as he did so there was a crash behind him. His precious bottle was in fragments upon the pavement.

For a moment he felt as if it were his wife's body that was lying there. But the run had freshened his wits and he saw that the mischief might be repaired. He pulled vigorously at the night-bell.

"Well, what's the matter?" asked a gruff voice at his elbow. He started back and looked up at the windows, but there was no sign of life. He was approaching the bell again with the intention of pulling it, when a perfect roar burst from the wall.

"I can't stand shivering here all night," cried the voice. "Say who you are and what you want or I shut the tube."

Then for the first time Johnson saw that the end of a speaking-tube hung out of the wall just above the bell. He shouted up it,—

"I want you to come with me to meet Dr. Miles at a confinement at once."

"How far?" shrieked the irascible voice.

"The New North Road, Hoxton."

"My consultation fee is three guineas, payable at the time."

"All right," shouted Johnson. "You are to bring a bottle of A.C.E. mixture with you."

"All right! Wait a bit!"

Five minutes later an elderly, hard-faced man, with grizzled hair, flung open the door. As he emerged a voice from somewhere in the shadows cried,—

"Mind you take your cravat, John," and he impatiently growled something over his shoulder in reply.

The consultant was a man who had been hardened by a life of ceaseless labour, and who had been driven, as so many others have been, by the needs of his own increasing family to set the commercial before the philanthropic side of his profession. Yet beneath his rough crust he was a man with a kindly heart.

"We don't want to break a record," said he, pulling up and panting after attempting to keep up with Johnson for five minutes. "I would go quicker if I could, my dear sir, and I quite sympathise with your anxiety, but really I can't manage it."

So Johnson, on fire with impatience, had to slow down until they reached the New North Road, when he ran ahead and had the door open for the doctor when he came. He heard the two meet outside the bed-room, and caught scraps of their conversation. "Sorry to knock you up—nasty case—decent people." Then it sank into a mumble and the door closed behind them.

Johnson sat up in his chair now, listening keenly, for he knew that a crisis must be at hand. He heard the two doctors moving about, and was able to distinguish the step of Pritchard, which had a drag in it, from the clean, crisp sound of the other's footfall. There was silence for a few minutes and then a curious drunken, mumbling sing-song voice came quavering up, very unlike anything which he had heard hitherto. At the same time a sweetish, insidious scent, imperceptible perhaps to any nerves less strained than his, crept down the stairs and penetrated into the room. The voice dwindled into a mere drone and finally sank away into silence, and Johnson gave a long sigh of relief, for he knew that the drug had done its work and that, come what might, there should be no more pain for the sufferer.

But soon the silence became even more trying to him than the cries had been. He had no clue now as to what was going on, and his mind swarmed with horrible possibilities. He rose and went to the bottom of the stairs again. He heard the clink of metal against metal, and the subdued murmur of the doctors' voices. Then he heard Mrs. Peyton say something, in a tone as of fear or expostulation, and again the doctors murmured together. For twenty minutes he stood there leaning against the wall, listening to the occasional rumbles of talk without being able to catch a word of it. And then of a sudden there rose out of the silence the strangest little piping cry, and Mrs. Peyton screamed out in her delight and the man ran into the parlour and flung himself down upon the horse-hair sofa, drumming his heels on it in his ecstasy.

But often the great cat Fate lets us go only to clutch us again in a fiercer grip. As minute after minute passed and still no sound came from above save those thin, glutinous cries, Johnson cooled from his frenzy of joy, and lay breathless with his ears straining. They were moving slowly about. They were talking in subdued tones. Still minute after minute passing, and no word from the voice for which he listened. His nerves were dulled by his night of trouble, and he waited in limp wretchedness upon his sofa. There he still sat when the doctors came down to him—a bedraggled, miserable figure with his face grimy and his hair unkempt from his long vigil. He rose as they entered, bracing himself against the mantelpiece.

"Is she dead?" he asked.

"Doing well," answered the doctor.

And at the words that little conventional spirit which had never known until that night the capacity for fierce agony which lay within it, learned for the second time that there were springs of joy also which it had never tapped before. His impulse was to fall upon his knees, but he was shy before the doctors.

"Can I go up?"

"In a few minutes."

"I'm sure, doctor, I'm very—I'm very—" he grew inarticulate. "Here are your three guineas, Dr. Pritchard. I wish they were three hundred."

"So do I," said the senior man, and they laughed as they shook hands.

Johnson opened the shop door for them and heard their talk as they stood for an instant outside.

"Looked nasty at one time."

"Very glad to have your help."

"Delighted, I'm sure. Won't you step round and have a cup of coffee?"

"No, thanks. I'm expecting another case."

The firm step and the dragging one passed away to the right and the left. Johnson turned from the door still with that turmoil of joy in his heart. He seemed to be making a new start in life. He felt that he was a stronger and a deeper man. Perhaps all this suffering had an object then. It might prove to be a blessing both to his wife and to him. The very thought was one which he would have been incapable of conceiving twelve hours before. He was full of new emotions. If there had been a harrowing there had been a planting too.

"Can I come up?" he cried, and then, without waiting for an answer, he took the steps three at a time.

Mrs. Peyton was standing by a soapy bath with a bundle in her hands. From under the curve of a brown shawl there looked out at him the strangest little red face with crumpled features, moist, loose lips, and eyelids which quivered like a rabbit's nostrils. The weak neck had let the head topple over, and it rested upon the shoulder.

"Kiss it, Robert!" cried the grandmother. "Kiss your son!"

But he felt a resentment to the little, red, blinking creature. He could not forgive it yet for that long night of misery. He caught sight of a white face in the bed and he ran towards it with such love and pity as his speech could find no words for.

"Thank God it is over! Lucy, dear, it was dreadful!"

"But I'm so happy now. I never was so happy in my life."

Her eyes were fixed upon the brown bundle.

"You mustn't talk," said Mrs. Peyton.

"But don't leave me," whispered his wife.

So he sat in silence with his hand in hers. The lamp was burning dim and the first cold light of dawn was breaking through the window. The night had been long and dark but the day was the sweeter and the purer in consequence. London was waking up. The roar began to rise from the street. Lives had come and lives had gone, but the great machine was still working out its dim and tragic destiny.

DOCTORS
AND
STUDENTS

It would be possible to put together a small library consisting only of writings by physicians. The tradition of the physician-writer is a rich one in literature. Among the famous names represented would be Chekhov, Rabelais, Oliver Wendell Holmes, Arthur Conan Doyle, and William Carlos Williams. Somerset Maugham drew most of his material for *Of Human Bondage* and a number of short stories from experiences as a medical student and his work in hospitals. Among those who intended to be physicians but never completed their studies were John Keats and Gertrude Stein.

LOUIS-FERDINAND CÉLINE
Journey to the End of the Night

———❧———

LOUIS-FERDINAND CÉLINE (1894-1961) was wounded in the head
during World War I but survived to study medicine and become a
practicing physician. He became well known in the '30s and '40s for his
highly controversial writings. His *Journey to the End of the Night*,
although fictional, closely resembles his own life story.

Here in hospital, as in those nights in Flanders, death harried us—only that
here we were not so closely threatened by it, though it was just as
inexorable as it had been out there, once the vigilant care of the authorities
had aimed it at you.

We weren't yelled at here, it's true; we were even spoken to with
kindness; they spoke to us always on any subject except death—yet every
form we were asked to sign was our death warrant; we were sentenced in
every precaution they took on our behalf. Medals. . . . Identity disks. . . .
The least leave we were given, the smallest piece of advice. . . . We felt that
we were counted, supervised, numbered in the great reserve of those who
would be going off to-morrow. And so, naturally, all these civilians and
doctors who surrounded us seemed lighter-hearted than us by comparison.
The nurses, little bitches, did not share our destiny; their only thought was
to live long, and go on living and, of course, fall in love, and wander around,
and make love not once but again and again. Every one of these sweeties
nursed a little plan in her insides, like a convict,—a plan for later on, for
making love, when we should have died in the mud somewhere, God knows
how.

Then they would sigh for you with extra-special tenderness, which would
make them even more attractive than they were already, and in silence,
deeply moved, they would call to mind the tragic days of the war, the ghosts
of time gone by. . . . "Do you remember little Bardamu?" they would say,
thinking of me, as the evening shadows lengthened. "The boy who coughed
so, and we could never stop him coughing? Poor lad. I wonder what became
of him?"

A little sentimental regret at the right time and place becomes a woman as
well as wisps of fine-spun hair in the moonlight.

Behind everything they said, behind all their solicitude, what one had to be able to read was this: "You're going to die, soldier boy, you're going to die. There's a different life for each of us—a different part for each of us to play—a different death for each of us to face. We seem to be sharing the wretchedness of your lot—but death cannot be shared with any one. . . . Everything should be a matter of enjoyment for healthy souls and bodies, no more or less, and we are fine young women, beautiful, respected, healthy and well brought up. . . . For us everything becomes, by instinctive biological law, a joyous spectacle and a source of happiness! Our health demands that it should be so; we must not allow the ugliness of sorrow to encroach upon us. . . . What we need is something stimulating, nothing but stimulants. . . . We shall soon forget all about you, soldier boy. . . . Be kind, and hurry up and die . . . and let the war stop soon, and then we can marry one of your charming officers. A dark and handsome one, if possible. . . . Hurrah for our country, as Father always says! Mustn't love be wonderful when your beau comes back from the war! The man we shall marry will be a very distinguished soldier. . . . He'll have a lot of medals. . . . And you may polish his lovely boots on our happy wedding day, if you're still alive when that day comes, soldier boy. . . . Then won't you be glad to see us so happy, soldier boy?"

Every morning we saw our doctor, we kept on seeing him, with his nurses always in attendance. He was a very clever man, we were told. The old men from the almshouse near by used to come hobbling past our part of the building, unevenly and fatuously. They wandered from room to room, carrying with them their tainted breath and a store of wheezing, raggle-taggle gossip and jabbering, contemptible chitchat. Cloistered here in their official poverty, as in a moat of slime, these old workmen lived on the filth which accumulates about the human soul after long years of servitude—impotent hatreds rotted by the piddling idleness of communal living rooms. They devoted their last trembling energies to doing a bit of harm and destroying what little life and joy was left to them.

That was their supreme pleasure. There was no longer a single particle of their dried-up bodies that was not entirely cruel.

As soon as it was arranged that we soldiers should share the relative comforts of the bastion with these old men, they began to hate us in unison, though they gathered around all the same to beg through the windows for odds and ends of tobacco and bits of stale bread from under the benches. Their parchment faces were pressed at mealtimes against the panes of our refectory windows. They peered at us with screwed-up, bleary eyes, like greedy rats. One of these old wrecks seemed to be more cunning and quicker witted than the rest; he came and sang the popular ditties of his day to us for our amusement. Papa Birouette they called him. He was perfectly willing to do any mortal thing for you as long as you gave him tobacco—any mortal thing, that is, except walk past the morgue in the bastion, which was never empty. One of the usual jokes was to take him along in the direction of the morgue, as if for a stroll. "Won't you come on in?" you'd say to him just as you got level with the door. Then he'd rush away, wheezing, as fast and as far as his legs would carry him and you saw nothing more of Papa Birouette for a couple of days at least. He had caught sight of death.

For the purpose of putting some spirit into us, our medical officer, Doctor Bestombes, of the beautiful eyes, had had installed a lot of very complicated paraphernalia in the way of shining electrical apparatus with which he gave us shocks every so often. He claimed these currents had a tonic effect; one had to put up with them or be thrown out. It seems that he was a very rich man, Bestombes; he must have been, to be able to afford all these costly electrocuting gadgets. His father-in-law, a figure in the political world, had wangled things well in buying land for the Government and so could afford to allow him these extravagances.

One had to take advantage of it. Everything works out all right,—crimes and punishments. Such as he was, we did not hate him too much. He examined our nervous systems extraordinarily carefully and asked us questions with polite familiarity. This nicely regulated kindliness of his was the great delight of the nurses under him, who were all well-bred; dear little things, they looked forward each morning to the moment for enjoying his display of charming manners, like kiddies expecting a lump of candy. We were all acting in a play in which he, Bestombes, had chosen the part of the understanding philanthropist, the wise and kindly man of science. You had to know what you were at, then it was all right.

In this new hospital I shared a room with a Sergeant Branledore, who had served once and been called up again. Branledore was a hospital guest of long standing. For months and months he'd trailed his perforated guts from clinic to clinic, having run through four of them.

In the course of this progression he had learned how to attract and to hold the active sympathy of nurses. He brought up, and pissed, blood, and he bled internally pretty often, did Branledore, and he had very great difficulty in breathing; but these things would not have sufficed to win him the quite special good graces of the nursing staff, which had seen them frequently enough. So, if a doctor or a nurse was passing, between two fits of choking, Branledore would cry out, "Victory! Victory! It shall be ours!"—or he muttered it with as much or as little of the breath in his lungs as he could, according to the circumstances. Having fallen into line in this way with the right enthusiastically warlike ideals, thanks to an opportune piece of play-acting, he enjoyed the highest prestige. He'd got it taped all right.

The whole thing was pure theatre; you had to play a part, and Branledore was absolutely right. Nothing looks so silly and is more irritating, after all, than a dumb member of the audience who has strayed onto the stage by mistake. When you are there, dash it, you've got to enter into the spirit of the thing, you've got to wake up and act, make up your mind or clear out. The women, above all, wanted to see something going on and they were without pity for the amateur who dried up. There's no question about it, war goes straight to their tummies. They wanted heroes and those who weren't heroes either had to look as if they were or be prepared to undergo the utmost ignominy.

SIR ARTHUR CONAN DOYLE
A Medical Document

Medical men are, as a class, very much too busy to take stock of singular situations or dramatic events. Thus it happens that the ablest chronicler of their experiences in our literature was a lawyer. A life spent in watching over death-beds—or over birth-beds which are infinitely more trying—takes something from a man's sense of proportion, as constant strong waters might corrupt his palate. The overstimulated nerve ceases to respond. Ask the surgeon for his best experiences and he may reply that he has seen little that is remarkable, or break away into the technical. But catch him some night when the fire has spurted up and his pipe is reeking, with a few of his brother practitioners for company and an artful question or allusion to set him going. Then you will get some raw, green facts new plucked from the tree of life.

It is after one of the quarterly dinners of the Midland Branch of the British Medical Association. Twenty coffee cups, a dozen liqueur glasses, and a solid bank of blue smoke which swirls slowly along the high, gilded ceiling gives a hint of a successful gathering. But the members have shredded off to their homes. The line of heavy, bulge-pocketed overcoats and of stethoscope-bearing top hats is gone from the hotel corridor. Round the fire in the sitting-room three medicos are still lingering, however, all smoking and arguing, while a fourth, who is a mere layman and young at that, sits back at the table. Under cover of an open journal he is writing furiously with a stylographic pen, asking a question in an innocent voice from time to time and so flickering up the conversation whenever it shows a tendency to wane.

The three men are all of that staid middle age which begins early and lasts late in the profession. They are none of them famous, yet each is of good repute, and a fair type of his particular branch. The portly man with the authoritative manner and the white, vitriol splash upon his cheek is Charley Manson, chief of the Wormley Asylum, and author of the brilliant monograph—Obscure Nervous Lesions in the Unmarried. He always wears his collar high like that, since the half-successful attempt of a student of Revelations to cut his throat with a splinter of glass. The second, with the ruddy face and the merry brown eyes, is a general practitioner, a man of vast experience, who, with his three assistants and his five horses, takes twenty-five hundred a year in half-crown visits and shilling consultations out of the poorest quarter of a great city. That cheery face of Theodore Foster is seen at the side of a hundred sick-beds a day, and if he has one-third more names on his visiting list than in his cash book he always promises himself that he will get level some day when a millionaire with a chronic complaint—the ideal combination—shall seek his services. The third, sitting on the right with his dress shoes shining on the top of the fender, is Hargrave, the rising surgeon. His face has none of the broad humanity of Theodore Foster's, the eye is stern and critical, the mouth straight and severe, but there is strength and decision in every line of it, and it is nerve rather than sympathy which the patient demands when he is bad enough to come to Hargrave's door. He calls himself a jawman ''a mere jawman'' as he modestly puts it, but in point of fact he is too young and too poor to confine himself to a specialty, and there is nothing surgical which Hargrave has not the skill and the audacity to do.

''Before, after, and during,'' murmurs the general practitioner in answer to some interpolation of the outsider's. ''I assure you, Manson, one sees all sorts of evanescent forms of madness.''

''Ah, puerperal!'' throws in the other, knocking the curved grey ash from his cigar. ''But you had some case in your mind, Foster.''

''Well, there was only one last week which was new to me. I had been engaged by some people of the name of Silcoe. When the trouble came round I went myself, for they would not hear of an assistant. The husband who was a policeman, was sitting at the head of the bed on the further side. 'This won't do,' said I. 'Oh yes, doctor, it must do,' said she. 'It's quite irregular and he must go,' said I. 'It's that or nothing,' said she. 'I won't open my mouth or stir a finger the whole night,' said he. So it ended by my allowing him to remain, and there he sat for eight hours on end. She was very good over the matter, but every now and again *he* would fetch a hollow groan, and I noticed that he held his right hand just under the sheet all the time, where I had no doubt that it was clasped by her left. When it was all happily over, I looked at him and his face was the colour of this cigar ash, and his head had dropped on to the edge of the pillow. Of course I thought he had fainted with emotion, and I was just telling myself what I thought of myself for having been such a fool as to let him stay there, when suddenly I saw that the sheet over his hand was all soaked with blood; I whisked it down, and there was the fellow's wrist half cut through. The woman had one bracelet of a policeman's handcuff over her left wrist and the other round his right one. When she had been in pain she had twisted with all her strength and the iron had fairly eaten into the bone of the man's arm. 'Aye, doctor,' said she, when she saw I had noticed it. 'He's got to take his share as well as me. Turn and turn,' said she.''

"Don't you find it a very wearing branch of the profession?'' asks Foster after a pause.

"My dear fellow, it was the fear of it that drove me into lunacy work.''

"Aye, and it has driven men into asylums who never found their way on to the medical staff. I was a very shy fellow myself as a student, and I know what it means.''

"No joke that in general practice,'' says the alienist.

"Well, you hear men talk about it as though it were, but I tell you it's much nearer tragedy. Take some poor, raw, young fellow who has just put up his plate in a strange town. He has found it a trial all his life, perhaps, to talk to a woman about lawn tennis and church services. When a young man *is* shy he is shyer than any girl. Then down comes an anxious mother and consults him upon the most intimate family matters. 'I shall never go to that doctor again,' says she afterwards. 'His manner is so stiff and unsympathetic.' Unsympathetic! Why, the poor lad was struck dumb and paralysed. I have known general practitioners who were so shy that they could not bring themselves to ask the way in the street. Fancy what sensitive men like that must endure before they get broken in to medical practice. And then they know that nothing is so catching as shyness, and that if they do not keep a face of stone, their patient will be covered with confusion. And so they keep their face of stone, and earn the reputation perhaps of having a heart to correspond. I suppose nothing would shake *your* nerve, Manson.''

"Well, when a man lives year in and year out among a thousand lunatics, with a fair sprinkling of homicidals among them, one's nerves either get set or shattered. Mine are all right so far.''

"I was frightened once,'' says the surgeon. "It was when I was doing dispensary work. One night I had a call from some very poor people, and gathered from the few words they said that their child was ill. When I entered the room I saw a small cradle in the corner. Raising the lamp I walked over and putting back the curtains I looked down at the baby. I tell you it was sheer Providence that I didn't drop that lamp and set the whole place alight. The head on the pillow turned and I saw a face looking up at me which seemed to me to have more malignancy and wickedness than ever I had dreamed of in a nightmare. It was the flush of red over the cheekbones, and the brooding eyes full of loathing of me, and of everything else, that impressed me. I'll never forget my start as, instead of the chubby face of an infant, my eyes fell upon this creature. I took the mother into the next room. 'What is it?' I asked. 'A girl of sixteen,' said she, and then throwing up her arms, 'Oh, pray God she may be taken!' The poor thing, though she spent her life in this little cradle, had great, long, thin limbs which she curled up under her. I lost sight of the case and don't know what became of it, but I'll never forget the look in her eyes.''

''That's creepy,'' says Dr. Foster. ''But I think one of my experiences would run it close. Shortly after I put up my plate I had a visit from a little hunch-backed woman who wished me to come and attend to her sister in her trouble. When I reached the house, which was a very poor one, I found two other little hunched-backed women, exactly like the first, waiting for me in the sitting-room. Not one of them said a word, but my companion took the lamp and walked upstairs with her two sisters behind her, and me bringing up the rear. I can see those three queer shadows cast by the lamp upon the wall as clearly as I can see that tobacco pouch. In the room above was the fourth sister, a remarkably beautiful girl in evident need of my assistance. There was no wedding ring upon her finger. The three deformed sisters seated themselves round the room, like so many graven images, and all night not one of them opened her mouth. I'm not romancing, Hargrave; this is absolute fact. In the early morning a fearful thunderstorm broke out, one of the most violent I have ever known. The little garret burned blue with the lightning, and thunder roared and rattled as if it were on the very roof of the house. It wasn't much of a lamp I had, and it was a queer thing when a spurt of lightning came to see those three twisted figures sitting round the walls, or to have the voice of my patient drowned by the booming of the thunder. By Jove! I don't mind telling you that there was a time when I nearly bolted from the room. All came right in the end, but I never heard the true story of the unfortunate beauty and her three crippled sisters.''

''That's the worst of these medical stories,'' sighs the outsider. ''They never seem to have an end.''

''When a man is up to his neck in practice, my boy, he has no time to gratify his private curiosity. Things shoot across him and he gets a glimpse of them, only to recall them, perhaps, at some quiet moment like this. But I've always felt, Manson, that your line had as much of the terrible in it as any other.''

''More,'' groans the alienist. ''A disease of the body is bad enough, but this seems to be a disease of the soul. Is it not a shocking thing—a thing to drive a reasoning man into absolute Materialism—to think that you may have a fine, noble fellow with every divine instinct and that some little vascular change, the dropping, we will say, of a minute spicule of bone from the inner table of his skull on to the surface of his brain may have the effect of changing him to a filthy and pitiable creature with every low and debasing tendency? What a satire an asylum is upon the majesty of man, and no less upon the ethereal nature of the soul.''

"Faith and hope," murmurs the general practitioner.

"I have no faith, not much hope, and all the charity I can afford," says the surgeon. "When theology squares itself with the facts of life I'll read it up."

"You were talking about cases," says the outsider, jerking the ink down into his stylographic pen.

"Well, take a common complaint which kills many thousands every year, like G.P. for instance."

"What's G.P.?"

"General practitioner." suggests the surgeon with a grin.

"The British public will have to know what G.P. is," says the alienist gravely. "It's increasing by leaps and bounds, and it has the distinction of being absolutely incurable. General paralysis is its full title, and I tell you it promises to be a perfect scourge. Here's a fairly typical case now which I saw last Monday week. A young farmer, a splendid fellow, surprised his fellows by taking a very rosy view of things at a time when the whole country-side was grumbling. He was going to give up wheat, give up arable land, too, if it didn't pay, plant two thousand acres of rhododendrons and get a monopoly of the supply for Covent Garden—there was no end to his schemes, all sane enough but just a bit inflated. I called at the farm, not to see him, but on an altogether different matter. Something about the man's way of talking struck me and I watched him narrowly. His lip had a trick of quivering, his words slurred themselves together, and so did his handwriting when he had occasion to draw up a small agreement. A closer inspection showed me that one of his pupils was ever so little larger than the other. As I left the house his wife came after me. 'Isn't it splendid to see Job looking so well, doctor,' said she; 'he's that full of energy he can hardly keep himself quiet.' I did not say anything, for I had not the heart, but I knew that the fellow was as much as condemned to death as though he were lying in the cell at Newgate. It was a characteristic case of incipient G.P.''

"Good heavens!" cries the outsider. My own lips tremble. I often slur my words. I believe I've got it myself!''

Three little chuckles come from the front of the fire.

"There's the danger of a little medical knowledge to the layman."

"A great authority has said that every first year's student is suffering in silent agony from four diseases," remarks the surgeon. "One is heart disease, of course; another is cancer of the parotid. I forget the two other."

"Where does the parotid come in?"

"Oh, it's the last wisdom tooth coming through!"

"And what would be the end of that young farmer?" asks the outsider.

"Paresis of all the muscles, ending in fits, coma, and death. It may be a few months, it may be a year or two. He was a very strong young man and would take some killing."

"By-the-way," says the alienist, "did I ever tell you about the first certificate I signed? I came as near ruin then as a man could go."

"What was it, then?"

"I was in practice at the time. One morning a Mrs. Cooper called upon me and informed me that her husband had shown signs of delusions lately. They took the form of imagining that he had been in the army and had distinguished himself very much. As a matter of fact he was a lawyer and had never been out of England. Mrs. Cooper was of opinion that if I were to call it might alarm him, so it was agreed between us that she should send him up in the evening on some pretext to my consulting-room, which would give me the opportunity of having a chat with him and, if I were convinced of his insanity, of signing his certificate. Another doctor had already signed, so that it only needed my concurrence to have him placed under treatment. Well, Mr. Cooper arrived in the evening about half an hour before I had expected him, and consulted me as to some malarious symptoms from which he said that he suffered. According to his account he had just returned from the Abyssinian Campaign, and had been one of the first of the British forces to enter Magdala. No delusion could possibly be more marked, for he would talk of little else, so I filled in the papers without the slightest hesitation. When his wife arrived, after he had left, I put some questions to her to complete the form. 'What is his age?' I asked. 'Fifty,' said she. 'Fifty!' I cried. 'Why, the man I examined could not have been more than thirty!' And so it came out that the real Mr. Cooper had never called upon me at all, but that by one of those coincidences which take a man's breath away another Cooper, who really was a very distinguished young officer of artillery, had come in to consult me. My pen was wet to sign the paper when I discovered it," says Dr. Manson, mopping his forehead.

"We were talking about nerve just now," observes the surgeon. "Just after my qualifying I served in the Navy for a time, as I think you know. I was on the flag-ship on the West African Station, and I remember a singular example of nerve which came to my notice at that time. One of our small gunboats had gone up the Calabar river, and while there the surgeon died of coast fever. On the same day a man's leg was broken by a spar falling upon it, and it became quite obvious that it must be taken off above the knee if his life was to be saved. The young lieutenant who was in charge of the craft searched among the dead doctor's effects and laid his hands upon some chloroform, a hip-joint knife, and a volume of Gray's Anatomy. He had the man laid by the steward upon the cabin table, and with a picture of a cross section of the thigh in front of him he began to take off the limb. Every now and then, referring to the diagram, he would say: 'Stand by with the lashings, steward. There's blood on the chart about here.' Then he would jab with his knife until he cut the artery, and he and his assistant would tie it up before they went any further. In this way they gradually whittled the leg off, and upon my word they made a very excellent job of it. The man is hopping about the Portsmouth Hard at this day."

"It's no joke when the doctor of one of these isolated gunboats himself falls ill," continues the surgeon after a pause. "You might think it easy for him to prescribe for himself, but this fever knocks you down like a club, and you haven't strength left to brush a mosquito off your face. I had a touch of it at Lagos, and I know what I am telling you. But there was a chum of mine who really had a curious experience. The whole crew gave him up, and, as they had never had a funeral aboard the ship, they began rehearsing the forms so as to be ready. They thought that he was unconscious, but he swears he could hear every word that passed. 'Corpse comin' up the 'atchway!' cried the Cockney sergeant of Marines. 'Present harms!' He was so amused, and so indignant too, that he just made up his mind that he wouldn't be carried through that hatchway, and he wasn't, either."

"There's no need for fiction in medicine," remarks Foster, "for the facts will always beat anything you can fancy. But it has seemed to me sometimes that a curious paper might be read at some of these meetings about the uses of medicine in popular fiction."

"How?"

"Well, of what the folk die of, and what diseases are made most use of in novels. Some are worn to pieces, and others, which are equally common in real life, are never mentioned. Typhoid is fairly frequent, but scarlet fever is unknown. Heart disease is common, but then heart disease, as we know it, is usually the sequel of some foregoing disease, of which we never hear anything in the romance. Then there is the mysterious malady called brain fever, which always attacks the heroine after a crisis, but which is unknown under that name to the text books. People when they are over-excited in novels fall down in a fit. In a fairly large experience I have never known anyone to do so in real life. The small complaints simply don't exist. Nobody ever gets shingles or quinsy, or mumps in a novel. All the diseases, too, belong to the upper part of the body: The novelist never strikes below the belt.''

''I'll tell you what, Foster,'' says the alienist, ''there is a side of life which is too medical for the general public and too romantic for the professional journals, but which contains some of the richest human materials that a man could study. It's not a pleasant side, I am afraid, but if it is good enough for Providence to create, it is good enough for us to try and understand. It would deal with strange outbursts of savagery and vice in the lives of the best men, curious momentary weaknesses in the record of the sweetest women, known but to one or two, and inconceivable to the world around. It would deal, too, with the singular phenomena of waxing and of waning manhood, and would throw a light upon those actions which have cut short many an honoured career and sent a man to a prison when he should have been hurried to a consulting-room. Of all evils that may come upon the sons of men, God shield us principally from that one!''

''I had a case some little time ago which was out of the ordinary,'' says the surgeon. ''There's a famous beauty in London society—I mention no names—who used to be remarkable a few seasons ago for the very low dresses which she would wear. She had the whitest of skins and most beautiful of shoulders, so it was no wonder. Then gradually the frilling at her neck lapped upwards and upwards, until last year she astonished everyone by wearing quite a high collar at a time when it was completely out of fashion. Well, one day this very woman was shown into my consulting-room. When the footman was gone she suddenly tore off the upper part of her dress. 'For God's sake do something for me!' she cried. Then I saw what the trouble was. A rodent ulcer was eating its way upwards, coiling on in its serpiginous fashion until the end of it was flush with her collar. The red streak of its trail was lost below the line of her bust. Year by year it had ascended and she had heightened her dress to hide it, until now it was about to invade her face. She had been too proud to confess her trouble, even to a medical man.''

''And did you stop it?''

''Well, with zinc chloride I did what I could. But it may break out again. She was one of those beautiful white-and-pink creatures who are rotten with struma. You may patch but you can't mend.''

''Dear! dear! dear!'' cries the general practitioner, with that kindly softening of the eyes which had endeared him to so many thousands. ''I suppose we mustn't think ourselves wiser than Providence, but there are times when one feels that something is wrong in the scheme of things. I've seen some sad things in my life. Did I ever tell you that case where Nature divorced a most loving couple? He was a fine young fellow, an athlete and a gentleman, but he overdid athletics. You know how the force that controls us gives us a little tweak to remind us when we get off the beaten track. It may be a pinch on the great toe if we drink too much and work too little. Or it may be a tug on our nerves if we dissipate energy too much. With the athlete, of course, it's the heart or the lungs. He had bad phthisis and was sent to Davos. Well, as luck would have it, she developed rheumatic fever, which left her heart very much affected. Now, do you see the dreadful dilemma in which those poor people found themselves? When he came below four thousand feet or so, his symptoms became terrible. She could come up about twenty-five hundred and then her heart reached its limit. They had several interviews half way down the valley, which left them nearly dead, and at last, the doctors had to absolutely forbid it. And so for four years they lived within three miles of each other and never met. Every morning he would go to a place which overlooked the chalet in which she lived and would wave a great white cloth and she answer from below. They could see each other quite plainly with their field glasses, and they might have been in different planets for all their chance of meeting.''

"And one at last died,'' says the outsider.

"No, sir. I'm sorry not to be able to clinch the story, but the man recovered and is now a successful stockbroker in Drapers Gardens. The woman, too, is the mother of a considerable family. But what are you doing there?''

"Only taking a note or two of your talk.''

The three medical men laugh as they walk towards their overcoats.

"Why, we've done nothing but talk shop,'' says the general practitioner. "What possible interest can the public take in that?''

JOHANN WOLFGANG VON GOETHE
Faust

SCHOLAR
Excuse me, sir, if still I trouble you:
There's just one other favour I would win—
To hear a trenchant word or two
Touching the art of medicine.
Three years, Heaven knows, are quickly gone,
One has so large a field to work upon:
Had I some hint, some sign before me,
I soon should see my way more plain!

MEPHISTOPHELES *(aside)*
This sober style begins to bore me;
'Tis time I played the Devil himself again.
(Aloud)
The spirit of medicine is grasped with ease:
First try to know both worlds, the large and small,
And at the end let things befall
As God may please.
The search for truth is but a wild-goose chase,
For each will only master what he can:
But he who grasps the moments in their race,
He is the real man.
A decent figure you can boast,
And are as bold, no doubt, as most;
And trust in self once fairly gained,
Your neighbour's trust is soon attained.
With women chiefly you must learn to deal:
Their everlasting sighs and groans,
Their thousand moans,
And if you show but passable decorum,
You soon enough will lord it o'er 'em.
A sounding title first declares
Your wondrous skill, and leaves 'em much impressed:
By way of greeting, then, you'll handle all those wares,

Which others have for years but touched at best.
Next press her pulse (a safe advance!)
And then with sly and fiery glance
You'll catch her round her slender waist,
To see how tightly she is laced.

SCHOLAR
Ah! that sounds better far! one sees the why and how!

MEPHISTOPHELES
Grey, worthy friend, is all philosophy,
And green and fresh life's golden tree.

SCHOLAR
To me 'tis all a dream, I vow:
But may I wait upon you in due course
And drink your wisdom at the source?

MEPHISTOPHELES
Whate'er I can, I'll gladly give you!

SCHOLAR
I cannot bring myself to leave you!
Here is my album—may I first secure
The honour of your signature?

MEPHISTOPHELES
With pleasure. *(Writes and returns it.)*

SCHOLAR *(reads)*
Eritis sicut Dei, scientes bonum et malum.
(Bows respectfully and withdraws.)

OLIVER WENDELL HOLMES
Elsie Venner

---◆◇◆---

OLIVER WENDELL HOLMES (1809-1894), Boston Brahmin, father of the
Associate Justice of the United States Supreme Court, was a practicing
physician, professor of anatomy, and Dean of the Harvard Medical
School, who would have been flattered if someone had referred to him
primarily as a poet and philosopher. He infused both poetry and
philosophy into his education of medical students, as this talk may
indicate.

THE DOCTOR CALLS ON ELSIE VENNER.

If that primitive physician, CHIRON, M. D., appears as a Centaur, as we
look at him through the lapse of thirty centuries, the modern country-
doctor, if he could be seen about thirty miles off, could not be distinguished
from a wheel-animalcule. He *inhabits* a wheel-carriage. He thinks of
stationary dwellings as Long Tom Coffin did of land in general; a house may
be well enough for incidental purposes, but for a "stiddy" residence give
him a "kerridge." If he is classified in the Linnæan scale, he must be set
down thus: Genus *Homo*; Species *Rotifer infusorius,*—the wheel-animal of
infusions.

The Dudley mansion was not a mile from the Doctor's; but it never
occurred to him to think of walking to see any of his patients' families, if he
had any professional object in his visit. Whenever the narrow sulky turned
in at a gate, the rustic who was digging potatoes, or hoeing corn, or *swishing*
through the grass with his scythe, in wave-like crescents, or stepping short
behind a loaded wheelbarrow, or trudging lazily by the side of the swinging,
loose-throated, short-legged oxen, rocking along the road as if they had just
been landed after a three-months' voyage,—the toiling native, whatever he
was doing, stopped and looked up at the house the Doctor was visiting.

"Somebody sick over there t' Haynes's. Guess th' old man's ailin' ag'in.
Winder's haäf-way open in the chamber,—should n' wonder 'f he was dead
and laid aout. Docterin' a'n't no use, when y' see th' winders open like that.
Wahl, money a'n't much to speak of to th' old man naow! He don' want but
tew cents,—'n' old Widah Peake, she knows what he wants them for!"

224

Or again,—

"Measles raound pooty thick. Briggs's folks buried two children with 'em laäs' week. Th' ol' Doctor, he 'd h' ker'd 'em threugh. Struck in 'n' p'dooced mo't'f'cation,—so they say."

This is only meant as a sample of the kind of way they used to think or talk, when the narrow sulky turned in at the gate of some house where there was a visit to be made.

Oh, that narrow sulky! What hopes, what fears, what comfort, what anguish, what despair, in the roll of its coming or its parting wheels! In the spring, when the old people get the coughs which give them a few shakes and their lives drop in pieces like the ashes of a burned thread which have kept the thread-like shape until they were stirred,—in the hot summer noons, when the strong man comes in from the fields, like the son of the Shunamite, crying, "My head, my head,"—in the dying autumn days, when youth and maiden lie fever-stricken in many a household, still-faced, dull-eyed, dark-flushed, dry-lipped, low-muttering in their daylight dreams, their fingers moving singly like those of slumbering harpers,—in the dead winter, when the white plague of the North has caged its wasted victims, shuddering as they think of the frozen soil which must be quarried like rock to receive them, if their perpetual convalescence should happen to be interfered with by any untoward accident,—at every season, the narrow sulky rolled round freighted with unmeasured burdens of joy and woe.

*   *   *

WHY DOCTORS DIFFER.

The two Doctors had taken two arm-chairs and sat squared off against each other. Their conversation is perhaps as well worth reporting as that of the rest of the company, and, as it was carried on in a louder tone, was of course more easy to gather and put on record.

It was a curious sight enough to see those two representatives of two great professions brought face to face to talk over the subjects they had been looking at all their lives from such different points of view. Both were old; old enough to have been moulded by their habits of thought and life; old enough to have all their beliefs "fretted in," as vintners say,—thoroughly worked up with their characters. Each of them looked his calling. The Reverend Doctor had lived a good deal among books in his study; the Doctor, as we will call the medical gentleman, had been riding about the country for between thirty and forty years. His face looked tough and weather-worn; while the Reverend Doctor's, hearty as it appeared, was of finer texture.

*   *   *

"*Ubi tres medici, duo athei,* you know, Doctor. Your profession has always had the credit of being lax in doctrine,—though pretty stringent in *practice,* ha! ha!"

"Some priest said that," the Doctor answered, dryly. "They always talked Latin when they had a bigger lie than common to get rid of."

"Good!" said the Reverend Doctor; "I'm afraid they would lie a little sometimes. But isn't there some truth in it, Doctor? Don't you think your profession is apt to see 'Nature' in the place of the God of Nature,—to lose sight of the great First Cause in their daily study of secondary causes?"

"I've thought about that," the Doctor answered, "and I've talked about it and read about it, and I've come to the conclusion that nobody believes in God and trusts in God quite so much as the doctors; only it isn't just the sort of Deity that some of your profession have wanted them to take up with. There was a student of mine wrote a dissertation on the Natural Theology of Health and Disease, and took that old lying proverb for his motto. He knew a good deal more about books than ever I did, and had studied in other countries. I'll tell you what he said about it. He said the old Heathen Doctor, Galen, praised God for his handiwork in the human body, just as if he had been a Christian, or the Psalmist himself. He said they had this sentence set up in large letters in the great lecture-room in Paris where he attended: *I dressed his wound and God healed him.* That was an old surgeon's saying. And he gave a long list of doctors who were not only Christians, but famous ones. I grant you, though, ministers and doctors are very apt to see differently in spiritual matters."

"That's it," said the Reverend Doctor; "you are apt to see 'Nature' where we see God, and appeal to 'Science' where we are contented with Revelation."

"We don't separate God and Nature, perhaps, as you do," the Doctor answered. "When we say that God is omnipresent and omnipotent and omniscient, we are a little more apt to mean it than your folks are. We think, when a wound heals, that God's *presence* and *power* and *knowledge* are there, healing it, just as that old surgeon did. We think a good many theologians, working among their books, don't see the facts of the world they live in. When we tell 'em of these facts, they are apt to call us materialists and atheists and infidels, and all that. We can't help seeing the facts, and we don't think it's wicked to mention 'em."

"Do tell me," the Reverend Doctor said, "some of these facts we are in the habit of overlooking, and which your profession thinks it can see and understand."

"That's very easy," the Doctor replied. "For instance: you don't understand or don't allow for idiosyncrasies as we learn to. We know that food and physic act differently with different people; but you think the same kind of truth is going to suit, or ought to suit, all minds. We don't fight with a patient because he can't take magnesia or opium; but you are all the time quarrelling over your beliefs, as if belief did not depend very much on race and constitution, to say nothing of early training."

"Do you mean to say that every man is not absolutely free to choose his beliefs?"

"The men you write about in your studies are, but not the men we see in the real world. There is some apparently congenital defect in the Indians, for instance, that keeps them from choosing civilization and Christianity. So with the Gypsies, very likely. Everybody knows that Catholicism or Protestantism is a good deal a matter of race. Constitution has more to do with belief than people think for. I went to a Universalist church, when I was in the city one day, to hear a famous man whom all the world knows, and I never saw such pews-full of broad shoulders and florid faces, and substantial, wholesome-looking persons, male and female, in all my life. Why, it was astonishing. Either their creed made them healthy, or they chose it because they were healthy. Your folks have never got the hang of human nature."

"I am afraid this would be considered a degrading and dangerous view of human beliefs and responsibility for them," the Reverend Doctor replied. "Prove to a man that his will is governed by something outside of himself, and you have lost all hold on his moral and religious nature. There is nothing bad men want to believe so much as that they are governed by necessity. Now that which is at once degrading and dangerous cannot be true."

"No doubt," the Doctor replied, "all large views of mankind limit our estimate of the absolute freedom of the will. But I don't think it degrades or endangers us, for this reason, that, while it makes us charitable to the rest of mankind, our own sense of freedom, whatever it is, is never affected by argument. *Conscience won't be reasoned with.* We feel that *we* can practically do this or that, and if we choose the wrong, we know we are responsible; but observation teaches us that this or that other race or individual has not the same practical freedom of choice. I don't see how we can avoid this conclusion in the instance of the American Indians. The science of Ethnology has upset a good many theoretical notions about human nature.''

"Science!" said the Reverend Doctor, "science! that was a word the Apostle Paul did not seem to think much of, if we may judge by the Epistle to Timothy: 'Oppositions of science falsely so called.' I own that I am jealous of that word and the pretensions that go with it. Science has seemed to me to be very often only the handmaid of skepticism.''

"Doctor!" the physician said, emphatically, "science is knowledge. Nothing that is not *known* properly belongs to science. Whenever knowledge obliges us to doubt, we are always safe in doubting. Astronomers foretell eclipses, say how long comets are to stay with us, point out where a new planet is to be found. We see they *know* what they assert, and the poor old Roman Catholic Church has at last to knock under. So Geology *proves* a certain succession of events, and the best Christian in the world must make the earth's history square with it. Besides, I don't think you remember what great revelations of himself the Creator has made in the minds of the men who have built up science. You seem to me to hold his human masterpieces very cheap. Don't you think the 'inspiration of the Almighty' gave Newton and Curvier 'understanding'?''

The Reverend Doctor was not arguing for victory. In fact, what he wanted was to call out the opinions of the old physician by a show of opposition, being already predisposed to agree with many of them. He was rather trying the common arguments, as one tries tricks of fence merely to learn the way of parrying. But just here he saw a tempting opening, and could not resist giving a home-thrust.

"Yes; but you surely would not consider it inspiration of the same kind as that of the writers of the Old Testament?''

That cornered the Doctor, and he paused a moment before he replied. Then he raised his head, so as to command the Reverend Doctor's face through his spectacles, and said,—

"I did not say that. You are clear, I suppose, that the Omniscient spoke through Solomon, but that Shakespeare wrote without his help?''

*   *   *

"No," she said, "there is nothing wrong, such as you are thinking of; I am not dying. You may send for the Doctor; perhaps he can take the pain from my head. That is all I want him to do. There is no use in the pain, that I know of; if he can stop it, let him.''

So they sent for the old Doctor. It was not long before the solid trot of

Caustic, the old bay horse, and the crashing of the gravel under the wheels, gave notice that the physician was driving up the avenue.

The old Doctor was a model for visiting practitioners. He always came into the sick-room with a quiet, cheerful look, as if he had a consciousness that he was bringing some sure relief with him. The way a patient snatches his first look at his doctor's face, to see whether he is doomed, whether he is reprieved, whether he is unconditionally pardoned, has really something terrible about it. It is only to be met by an imperturbable mask of serenity, proof against anything and everything in a patient's aspect. The physician whose face reflects his patient's condition like a mirror may do well enough to examine people for a life-insurance office, but does not belong to the sickroom. The old Doctor did not keep people waiting in dread suspense, while he stayed talking about the case,—the patient all the time thinking that he and his friends are discussing some alarming symptom or formidable operation which he himself is by-and-by to hear of.

He was in Elsie's room almost before she knew he was in the house. He came to her bedside in such a natural, quiet way, that it seemed as if he were only a friend who had dropped in for a moment to say a pleasant word. Yet he was very uneasy about Elsie until he had seen her; he never knew what might happen to her or those about her, and came prepared for the worst.

"Sick, my child?" he said, in a very soft, low voice.

Elsie nodded, without speaking.

The Doctor took her hand,—whether with professional views, or only in a friendly way, it would have been hard to tell. So he sat a few minutes, looking at her all the time with a kind of fatherly interest, but with it all noting how she lay, how she breathed, her color, her expression, all that teaches the practised eye so much without a single question being asked. He saw she was in suffering, and said presently,—

"You have pain somewhere; where is it?"

She put her hand to her head.

As she was not disposed to talk, he watched her for a while, questioned Old Sophy shrewdly a few minutes, and so made up his mind as to the probable cause of disturbance and the proper remedies to be used.

Some very silly people thought the old Doctor did not believe in medicine, because he gave less than certain poor half-taught creatures in the smaller neighboring towns, who took advantage of people's sickness to disgust and disturb them with all manner of ill-smelling and ill-behaving drugs. In truth, he hated to give anything noxious or loathsome to those who were uncomfortable enough already, unless he was very sure it would do good,—in which case, he never played with drugs, but gave good, honest, efficient doses. Sometimes he lost a family of the more boorish sort, because they did not think they got their money's worth out of him, unless they had something more than a taste of everything he carried in his saddle-bags.

He ordered some remedies which he thought would relieve Elsie, and left her, saying he would call the next day, hoping to find her better. But the next day came, and the next, and still Elsie was on her bed,—feverish, restless, wakeful, silent. At night she tossed about and wandered, and it became at length apparent that there was a settled attack, something like what they called, formerly, a "nervous fever."

On the fourth day she was more restless than common. One of the women of the house came in to help take care of her; but she showed an aversion to her presence.

"Send me Helen Darley," she said, at last.

The old Doctor told them, that, if possible, they must indulge this fancy of hers. The caprices of sick people were never to be despised, least of all of such persons as Elsie, when rendered irritable and exacting by pain and weakness.

SINCLAIR LEWIS
Arrowsmith

———◆◇◆———

SINCLAIR LEWIS (1885-1951) was the son of a physician and drew heavily on his observations for one of his major novels, *Arrowsmith*, from which this selection is drawn. He was the first American to win the Nobel Prize for literature. His novels satirized middle-class life in the American heartland. He was heralded as one of America's three or four greatest writers by the literary critics of his time, but his reputation has not been sustained in recent years. It is felt that his writing lacked grace and genuine literary distinction. Even so, he both reflected and portrayed an era in American life.

Professor Gottlieb was the mystery of the University. It was known that he was a Jew, born and educated in Germany, and that his work on immunology had given him fame in the East and in Europe. He rarely left his small brown weedy house except to return to his laboratory, and few students outside of his classes had ever identified him, but everyone had heard of his tall, lean, dark aloofness. A thousand fables fluttered about him. It was believed that he was the son of a German prince, that he had immense wealth, that he lived as sparsely as the other professors only because he was doing terrifying and costly experiments which probably had something to do with human sacrifice. It was said that he could create life in the laboratory, that he could talk to the monkeys which he inoculated, that he had been driven out of Germany as a devil-worshiper or an anarchist, and that he secretly drank real champagne every evening at dinner.

It was the tradition that faculty-members did not discuss their colleagues with students, but Max Gottlieb could not be regarded as anybody's colleague. He was impersonal as the chill northeast wind. Dr. Brumfit rattled:

"I'm sufficiently liberal, I should assume, toward the claims of science, but with a man like Gottlieb—I'm prepared to believe that he knows all about material forces, but what astounds me is that such a man can be blind to the vital force that creates all others. He says that knowledge is worthless unless it is proven by rows of figures. Well, when one of you scientific sharks can take the genius of a Ben Jonson and measure it with a yardstick, then I'll admit that we literary chaps, with our doubtless absurd belief in beauty and loyalty and the world o' dreams, are off on the wrong track!''

Martin Arrowsmith was not exactly certain what this meant and he enthusiastically did not care. He was relieved when Professor Edwards from the midst of his beardedness and smokiness made a sound curiously like ''Oh, hell!'' and took the conversation away from Brumfit. Ordinarily Encore would have suggested, with amiable malice, that Gottlieb was a ''crapehanger'' who wasted time destroying the theories of other men instead of making new ones of his own. But tonight, in detestation of such literary playboys as Brumfit, he exalted Gottlieb's long, lonely, failure-burdened effort to synthesize antitoxin, and his diabolic pleasure in disproving his own contentions as he would those of Ehrlich or Sir Almroth Wright. He spoke of Gottlieb's great book, ''Immunology,'' which had been read by seven-ninths of all the men in the world who could possibly understand it—the number of these being nine.

*   *   *

On his first day in medical school, Martin Arrowsmith was in a high state of superiority. As a medic he was more picturesque than other students, for medics are reputed to know secrets, horrors, exhilarating wickednesses. Men from the other departments go to their rooms to peer into their books. But also as an academic graduate, with a training in the basic sciences, he felt superior to his fellow medics, most of whom had but a high-school diploma, with perhaps one year in a ten-room Lutheran college among the cornfields.

For all his pride, Martin was nervous. He thought of operating, of making a murderous wrong incision; and with a more immediate, macabre fear, he thought of the dissecting-room and the stony, steely Anatomy Building. He had heard older medics mutter of its horrors: of corpses hanging by hooks, like rows of ghastly fruit, in an abominable tank of brine in the dark basement; of Henry the janitor, who was said to haul the cadavers out of the brine, to inject red lead into their veins, and to scold them as he stuffed them on the dumb-waiter.

There was prairie freshness in the autumn day but Martin did not heed. He hurried into the slate-colored hall of the Main Medical, up the wide stairs to the office of Max Gottlieb. He did not look at passing students, and when he bumped into them he grunted in confused apology. It was a portentous hour. He was going to specialize in bacteriology; he was going to discover enchanting new germs; Professor Gottlieb was going to recognize him as a genius, make him an assistant, predict for him—He halted in Gottlieb's private laboratory, a small, tidy apartment with racks of cotton-corked test-tubes on the bench, a place unimpressive and unmagical save for the constant-temperature bath with its tricky thermometer and electric bulbs. He waited till another student, a stuttering gawk of a student, had finished talking to Gottlieb, dark, lean, impassive at his desk in a cubbyhole of an office, then he plunged.

If in the misty April night Gottlieb had been romantic as a cloaked horseman, he was now testy and middle-aged. Near at hand, Martin could see wrinkles beside the hawk eyes. Gottlieb had turned back to his desk, which was heaped with shabby note-books, sheets of calculations, and a marvelously precise chart with red and green curves descending to vanish at zero. The calculations were delicate, minute, exquisitely clear; and delicate were the scientist's thin hands among the papers. He looked up, spoke with a hint of German accent. His words were not so much mispronounced as colored with a warm unfamiliar tint.

"Vell? Yes?"

"Oh, Professor Gottlieb, my name is Arrowsmith. I'm a medic freshman, Winnemac B.A. I'd like awfully to take bacteriology this fall instead of next year. I've had a lot of chemistry—"

"No. It is not time for you."

"Honest, I know I could do it now."

"There are two kinds of students the gods give me. One kind they dump on me like a bushel of potatoes. I do not like potatoes, and the potatoes they do not ever seem to have great affection for me, but I take them and teach them to kill patients. The other kind—they are very few!—they seem for some reason that is not at all clear to me to wish a liddle bit to become scientists, to work with bugs and make mistakes. Those, ah, those, I seize them, I denounce them, I teach them right away the ultimate lesson of science, which is to wait and doubt. Of the potatoes, I demand nothing; of the foolish ones like you, who think I could teach them something, I demand everything. No. You are too young. Come back next year."

"But honestly, with my chemistry—"

"Have you taken physical chemistry?"

"No, sir, but I did pretty well in organic."

"Organic chemistry! Puzzle chemistry! Stink chemistry! Drugstore chemistry! Physical chemistry is power, it is exactness, it is life. But organic chemistry—that is a trade for pot-washers. No. You are too young. Come back in a year."

Gottlieb was absolute. His talon fingers waved Martin to the door, and the boy hastened out, not daring to argue. He slunk off in misery. On the campus he met that jovial historian of chemistry, Encore Edwards, and begged, "Say, Professor, tell me, is there any value for a doctor in organic chemistry?"

"Value? Why, it seeks the drugs that allay pain! It produces the paint that slicks up your house, it dyes your sweetheart's dress—and maybe, in these degenerate days, her cherry lips! Who the dickens has been talking scandal about my organic chemistry?"

"Nobody. I was just wondering," Martin complained, and he drifted to the College Inn where, in an injured and melancholy manner, he devoured an enormous banana-split and a bar of almond chocolate, as he meditated:

"I want to take bacteriology. I want to get down to the bottom of this disease stuff. I'll learn some physical chemistry. I'll show old Gottlieb, damn him! Some day I'll discover the germ of cancer or something, and then he'll look foolish in the face! . . Oh, Lord, I hope I won't take sick, first time I go into the dissecting-room. . . . I want to take bacteriology— now!"

He recalled Gottlieb's sardonic face; he felt and feared his quality of dynamic hatred. Then he remembered the wrinkles, and he saw Max Gottlieb not as a genius but as a man who had headaches, who became agonizingly tired, who could be loved.

"I wonder if Encore Edwards knows as much as I thought he did? What *is* Truth?" he puzzled.

*   *   *

Martin was jumpy on his first day of dissecting. He could not look at the inhumanly stiff faces of the starveling gray men lying on the wooden tables. But they were so impersonal, these lost old men, that in two days he was, like the other medics, calling them "Billy" and "Ike" and "the Parson," and regarding them as he had regarded animals in biology. The dissecting-room itself was impersonal: hard cement floor, walls of hard plaster between wire-glass windows. Martin detested the reek of formaldehyde; that and some dreadful subtle other odor seemed to cling about him outside the dissecting-room; but he smoked cigarettes to forget it, and in a week he was exploring arteries with youthful and altogether unholy joy.

His dissecting partner was the Reverend Ira Hinkley, known to the class by a similar but different name.

Ira was going to be a medical missionary. He was a man of twenty-nine, a graduate of Pottsburg Christian College and of the Sanctification Bible and Missions School. He had played football; he was as strong and nearly as large as a steer, and no steer ever bellowed more enormously. He was a bright and happy Christian, a romping optimist who laughed away sin and doubt, a joyful Puritan who with annoying virility preached the doctrine of his tiny sect, the Sanctification Brotherhood, that to have a beautiful church was almost as damnable as the debaucheries of card-playing.

Martin found himself viewing "Billy," their cadaver—an undersized, blotchy old man with a horrible little red beard on his petrified, vealy face—as a machine, fascinating, complex, beautiful, but a machine. It damaged his already feeble belief in man's divinity and immortality. He might have kept his doubts to himself, revolving them slowly as he dissected out the nerves of the mangled upper arm, but Ira Hinkley would not let him alone. Ira believed that he could bring even medical students to bliss, which, to Ira, meant singing extraordinarily long and unlovely hymns in a chapel of the Sanctification Brotherhood.

"Mart, my son," he roared, "do you realize that in this, what some might call a sordid task, we are learning things that will enable us to heal the bodies and comfort the souls of countless lost unhappy folks?"

"Huh! Souls. I haven't found one yet in old Billy. Honest, do you believe that junk?"

Ira clenched his fist and scowled, then belched with laughter, slapped Martin distressingly on the back, and clamored, "Brother, you've got to do better than that to get Ira's goat! You think you've got a lot of these fancy Modern Doubts. You haven't—you've only got indigestion. What you need is exercise and faith. Come on over to the Y.M.C.A. and I'll take you for a swim and pray with you. Why, you poor skinny little agnostic, here you have a chance to see the Almighty's handiwork, and all you grab out of it is a feeling that you're real smart. Buck up, young Arrowsmith. You don't know how funny you are, to a fellow that's got a serene faith!"

To the delight of Clif Clawson, the class jester, who worked at the next table, Ira chucked Martin in the ribs, patted him, very painfully, upon the head, and amiably resumed work, while Martin danced with irritation.

*   *   *

In his second year of internship, when the thrills of fires and floods and murder became as obvious a routine as bookkeeping, when he had seen the strangely few ways in which mankind can contrive to injure themselves and slaughter one another, when it was merely wearing to have to live up to the pretentiousness of being The Doctor, Martin tired to satisfy and perhaps kill his guilty scientific lust by voluntary scrabbling about the hospital laboratory, correlating the blood counts in pernicious anemia. His trifling with the drugs of research was risky. Amid the bustle of operations he began to picture the rapt quietude of the laboratory. "I better cut this out," he said to Leora, "if I'm going to settle down in Wheatsylvania and 'tend to business and make a living—and I by golly am!"

Dean Silva often came to the hospital on consultations. He passed through the lobby one evening when Leora, returned from the office where she was a stenographer, was meeting Martin for dinner. Martin introduced them, and the little man held her hand, purred at her, and squeaked, "Will you children give me the pleasure of taking you to dinner? My wife has deserted me. I am a lone and misanthropic man."

He trotted between them, round and happy. Martin and he were not student and teacher, but two doctors together, for Dean Silva was one pedagogue who could still be interested in a man who no longer sat at his feet. He led the two starvelings to a chop-house and in a settle-walled booth he craftily stuffed them with roast goose and mugs of ale.

He concentrated on Leora, but his talk was of Martin:

"Your husband must be an Artist Healer, not a picker of trifles like these laboratory men."

"But Gottlieb's no picker of trifles," insisted Martin.

"No-o. But with him—It's a difference of one's gods. Gottlieb's gods are the cynics, the destroyers—crapehangers, the vulgar call 'em: Diderot and Voltaire and Elser; great men, wonder-workers, yet men that had more fun destroying other people's theories than creating their own. But my gods now, they're the men who took the discoveries of Gottlieb's gods and turned them to the use of human beings—made them come alive!

"All credit to the men who invented paint and canvas, but there's more credit, eh? to the Raphaels and Holbeins who used those discoveries! Laënnec and Osler, those are the men! It's all very fine, this business of pure research: seeking the truth, unhampered by commercialism or fame-chasing. Getting to the bottom. Ignoring consequences and practical uses. But do you realize if you carry that idea far enough, a man could justify himself for doing nothing but count the cobblestones on Warehouse Avenue—yes, and justify himself for torturing people just to see how they screamed—and then sneer at a man who was making millions of people well and happy!

"No, no! Mrs. Arrowsmith, this lad Martin is a passionate fellow, not a drudge. He must be passionate on behalf of mankind. He's chosen the highest calling in the world, but he's a feckless, experimental devil. You must keep at it my dear, and not let the world lose the benefit of his passion.

After this solemnity Dad Silva took them to a musical comedy and sat between them, patting Martin's shoulder, patting Leora's arm, choking with delight when the comedian stepped into the pail of whitewash. In midnight volubility Martin and Leora sputtered their affection for him, and saw their Wheatsylvania venture as glory and salvation.

But a few days before the end of Martin's internship and their migration to North Dakota, they met Max Gottlieb on the street.

Martin had not seen him for more than a year; Leora never. He looked worried and ill. While Martin was agonizing as to whether to pass with a bow, Gottlieb stopped.

"How is everything, Martin?" he said cordially. But his eyes said, "Why have you never come back to me?"

The boy stammered something, nothing, and when Gottlieb had gone by, stooped and moving as in pain, he longed to run after him.

Leora was demanding, "Is that the Professor Gottlieb you're always talking about?"

"Yes. Say! How does he strike you?"

"I don't—Sandy, he's the greatest man I've ever seen! I don't know how I know, but he is! Dr. Silva is a darling, but that was a *great* man! I wish—I wish we were going to see him again. There's the first man I ever laid eyes on that I'd leave you for, if he wanted me. He's so—oh, he's like a sword—no, he's like a brain walking. Oh, Sandy, he looked so wretched. I wanted to cry. I'd black his shoes!"

"God! So would I!"

But in the bustle of leaving Zenith, the excitement of the journey to Wheatsylvania, the scramble of his state examinations, the dignity of being a Practicing Physician, he forgot Gottlieb, and on that Dakota prairie radiant in early June, with meadow larks on every fence post, he began his work.

W. SOMERSET MAUGHAM
from The Summing Up

—⋘—

WILLIAM SOMERSET MAUGHAM (1874-1965) qualified as a surgeon at St. Thomas's Hospital, spent a year in practice in the slums of London, then, except for World War I Red Cross service, gave up medicine to become a playwright and novelist. His life's travels lent verisimilitude to best-selling novels set in Tahiti, the Middle East, and the United States, as well as in London and the south of France, where he lived for many years. He is as well known for his sparse, tightly drawn short stories. In his autobiography, *The Summing Up,* Maugham notes that authors are well aware of the mind-body connection. He points out that Flaubert suffered from the symptoms of arsenic poisoning while writing of Madame Bovary's suicide. Every novelist, he says, goes through similar experiences.

I do not know a better training for a writer than to spend some years in the medical profession. I suppose that you can learn a good deal about human nature in a solicitor's office; but there on the whole you have to deal with men in full control of themselves. They lie perhaps as much as they lie to the doctor, but they lie more consistently, and it may be that for the solicitor it is not so necessary to know the truth. The interests he deals with, besides, are usually material. He sees human nature from a specialized standpoint. But the doctor, especially the hospital doctor, sees it bare. Reticences can generally be undermined; very often there are none. Fear for the most part will shatter every defence; even vanity is unnerved by it. Most people have a furious itch to talk about themselves and are restrained only by the disinclination of others to listen. Reserve is an artificial quality that is developed in most of us but as the result of innumerable rebuffs. The doctor is discreet. It is his business to listen and no details are too intimate for his ears.

But of course human nature may be displayed before you and if you have not the eyes to see you will learn nothing. If you are hidebound with prejudice, if your temper is sentimental, you can go through the wards of a hospital and be as ignorant of man at the end as you were at the beginning. If you want to get any benefit from such an experience you must have an open mind and an interest in human beings. I look upon myself as very fortunate in that though I have never much liked men I have found them so interesting that I am almost incapable of being bored by them. I do not particularly want to talk and I am very willing to listen. I do not care if people are interested in me or not. I have no desire to impart any knowledge I have to others nor do I feel the need to correct them if they are wrong. You can get a great deal of entertainment out of tedious people if you keep your head. I remember being taken for a drive in a foreign country by a kind lady who wanted to show me round. Her conversation was composed entirely of truisms and she had so large a vocabulary of hackneyed phrases that I despaired of remembering them. But one remark she made has stuck in my memory as have few witticisms; we passed a row of little houses by the sea and she said to me: 'Those are week-end bungalows, if you understand what I mean; in other words they're bungalows that people go to on Saturdays and leave on Mondays.' I should have been sorry to miss that.

I do not want to spend too long a time with boring people, but then I do not want to spend too long a time with amusing ones. I find social intercourse fatiguing. Most persons, I think, are both exhilarated and rested by conversation; to me it has always been an effort. When I was young and stammered, to talk for long singularly exhausted me, and even now that I have to some extent cured myself, it is a strain. It is a relief to me when I can get away and read a book.

*　　*　　*

I would not claim for a moment that those years I spent at St. Thomas's Hospital gave me a complete knowledge of human nature. I do not suppose anyone can hope to have that. I have been studying it, consciously and subconsciously, for forty years and I still find men unaccountable; people I know intimately can surprise me by some action of which I never thought them capable or by the discovery of some trait exhibit a side of themselves that I never even suspected. It is possible that my training gave me a warped view, for at St. Thomas's the persons I came in contact with were for the most part sick and poor and ill-educated. I have tried to guard against this. I have tried also to guard against my own prepossessions. I have no natural trust in others. I am more inclined to expect them to do ill than to do good. This is the price one has to pay for having a sense of humour. A sense of humour leads you to take pleasure in the discrepancies of human nature; it leads you to mistrust great professions and look for the unworthy motive that they conceal; the disparity between appearance and reality diverts you and you are apt when you cannot find it to create it. You tend to close your eyes to truth, beauty and goodness because they give no scope to your sense of the ridiculous. The humorist has a quick eye for the humbug; he does not always recognize the saint. But if to see men one-sidedly is a heavy price to pay for a sense of humour there is a compensation that has a value too. You are not angry with people when you laugh at them. Humour teaches tolerance, and the humorist, with a smile and perhaps a sigh, is more likely to shrug his shoulders than to condemn. He does not moralize, he is content to understand; and it is true that to understand is to pity and forgive.

But I must admit that, with these reservations that I have tried always to remember, the experience of all the years that have followed has only confirmed the observations on human nature that I made, not deliberately, for I was too young, but unconsciously, in the out-patients' departments and in the wards of St. Thomas's Hospital. I have seen men since as I saw them then, and thus have I drawn them. It may not be a true picture and I know that many have thought it an unpleasant one. It is doubtless partial, for naturally I have seen men through my own idiosyncrasies. A buoyant, optimistic, healthy and sentimental person would have seen the same people quite differently. I can only claim to have seen them coherently. Many writers seem to me not to observe at all, but to create their characters in stock sizes from images in their own fancy. They are like draughtsmen who draw their figures from recollections of the antique and have never attempted to draw from the living model. At their best they can only give living shape to the fantasies of their own minds. If their minds are noble they can give you noble figures and perhaps it does not matter if they lack the infinite complication of common life.

I have always worked from the living model. I remember that once in the dissecting room when I was going over my 'part' with the demonstrator, he asked me what some nerve was and I did not know. He told me; whereupon I remonstrated, for it was in the wrong place. Nevertheless he insisted that it was the nerve I had been in vain looking for. I complained of the abnormality and he, smiling, said that in anatomy it was the normal that was uncommon. I was only annoyed at the time, but the remark sank into my mind and since then it has been forced upon me that it was true of man as well as of anatomy. The normal is what you find but rarely. The normal is an ideal. It is a picture that one fabricates of the average characteristics of men, and to find them all in a single man is hardly to be expected. It is this false picture that the writers I have spoke of take as their model and it is because they describe what is so exceptional that they seldom achieve the effect of life. Selfishness and kindliness, idealism and sensuality, vanity, shyness, disinterestedness, courage, laziness, nervousness, obstinacy, and diffidence, they can all exist in a single person and form a plausible harmony. It has taken a long time to persuade readers of the truth of this.

I do not suppose men in past centuries were any different from the men we know, but they must surely have appeared to their contemporaries more of a piece than they do to us now, or writers would not have thus represented them. It seemed reasonable to describe every man in his humour. The miser was nothing but miserly, the fop foppish, and the glutton gluttonous. It never occurred to anyone that the miser might be foppish and gluttonous; and yet we see constantly people who are; still less, that he might be an honest and upright man with a disinterested zeal for public service and a genuine passion for art. When novelists began to disclose the diversity that they had found in themselves or seen in others they were accused of maligning the human race. So far as I know the first novelist who did this with deliberate intention was Stendhal in *Le Rouge et le Noir*. Contemporary criticism was outraged. Even Sainte-Beuve, who needed only to look into his own heart to discover what contrary qualities could exist side by side in some kind of harmony, took him to task. Julien Sorel is one of the most interesting characters that a novelist has ever created. I do not think that Stendhal has succeeded in making him entirely plausible, but that, I believe, is due to causes that I shall mention in another part of this book. For the first three quarters of the novel he is perfectly consistent. Sometimes he fills you with horror; sometimes he is entirely sympathetic; but he has an inner coherence, so that though you often shudder you accept.

But it was long before Stendhal's example bore fruit. Balzac, with all his genius, drew his characters after the old models. He gave them his own immense vitality so that you accept them as real; but in fact they are humours as definitely as are the characters of old comedy. His people are unforgettable, but they are seen from the standpoint of the ruling passion that affected those with whom they were brought in contact. I suppose it is a natural prepossession of mankind to take people as though they were homogeneous. It is evidently less trouble to make up one's mind about a man one way or the other and dismiss suspense with the phrase, he's one of the best or he's a dirty dog. It is disconcerting to find that the saviour of his country may be stingy or that the poet who has opened new horizons to our consciousness may be a snob. Our natural egoism leads us to judge people by their relations to ourselves. We want them to be certain things to us, and for us that is what they are; because the rest of them is no good to us, we ignore it.

These reasons perhaps explain why there is so great a disinclination to accept the attempts to portray man with his incongruous and diverse qualities and why people turn away with dismay when candid biographers reveal the truth about famous persons. It is distressing to think that the composer of the quintet in the *Meistersinger* was dishonest in money matters and treacherous to those who had benefited him. But it may be that he could not have had great qualities if he had not also had great failings. I do not believe they are right who say that the defects of famous men should be ignored; I think it is better that we should know them. Then, though we are conscious of having faults as glaring as theirs, we can believe that that is no hindrance to our achieving also something of their virtues.

*   *   *

Besides teaching me something about human nature my training in a medical school furnished me with an elementary knowledge of science and scientific method. Till then I had been concerned only with art and literature. It was a very limited knowledge, for the demands of the curriculum at that time were small, but at all events it showed me the road that led to a region of which I was completely ignorant. I grew familiar with certain principles. The scientific world of which I thus obtained a cursory glimpse was rigidly materialistic and because its conceptions coincided with my own prepossessions I embraced them with alacrity; 'For men,' as Pope observed, 'let them say what they will, never approve any other's sense, but as it squares with their own.' I was glad to learn that the mind of man (himself the product of natural causes) was a function of the brain subject like the rest of his body to the laws of cause and effect and that these laws were the same as those that governed the movements of star and atom. I exulted at the thought that the universe was no more than a vast machine in which every event was determined by a preceding event so that nothing could be other than it was. These conceptions not only appealed to my dramatic instinct; they filled me besides with a very delectable sense of liberation. With the ferocity of youth I welcomed the hypothesis of the Survival of the Fittest. It gave me much satisfaction to learn that the earth was a speck of mud whirling round a second-rate star which was gradually cooling; and that evolution, which had produced man, would by forcing him to adapt himself to his environment deprive him of all the qualities he had acquired but those that were necessary to enable him to combat the increasing cold till at last the planet, an icy cinder, would no longer support even a vestige of life. I believed that we were wretched puppets at the mercy of a ruthless fate; and that, bound by the inexorable laws of nature, we were doomed to take part in the ceaseless struggle for existence with nothing to look forward to but inevitable defeat. I learnt that men were moved by a savage egoism, that love was only the dirty trick nature played on us to achieve the continuation of the species, and I decided that, whatever aims men set themselves, they were deluded, for it was impossible for them to aim at anything but their own selfish pleasures. When once I happened to do a friend a good turn (for what reasons, since I knew that all our actions were purely selfish, I did not stop to think) and wanting to show his gratitude (which of course he had no business to feel, for my apparent kindness was rigidly determined) he asked me what I would like as a present, I answered without hesitation Herbert Spencer's *First Principles*. I read it with complacency. But I was impatient of Spencer's maudlin belief in progress: the world I knew was going from bad to worse and I was as pleased as Punch at the thought of my remote descendants, having long forgotten art and science and handicraft, cowering skin-clad in caverns as they watched the approach of the cold and eternal night. I was violently pessimistic. All the same, having abundant vitality, I was getting on the whole a lot of fun out of life. I was ambitious to make a name for myself as a writer. I exposed myself to every vicissitude that seemed to offer a chance of gaining the greater experience that I wanted and I read everything I could lay my hands on.

ARTHUR SCHNITZLER
My Youth in Vienna

———⦅∞⦆———

ARTHUR SCHNITZLER (1862-1931) is well known as a playwright and novelist. His Viennese playboy lifestyle is reflected in witty, erotic dramas also noteworthy for their psychological insight. His early days as a student of medicine and psychiatry are drawn upon in detail in the autobiography, *My Youth in Vienna*.

Due to the fact that I had attended to medicine from the start in a highly desultory fashion, my interest could not be seriously or lastingly aroused, even where my predispositions—if they had been correctly channeled—would have found quite a few points of contact. My moods, to say nothing of my viewpoint, were soon influenced by the atmosphere of the halls in which the daily life of a medical student, even a not very industrious one, was played out. Before I entered the dissecting room for the first time, I had never seen a human corpse, but like all my colleagues I soon found out that the human body dead, if the observer is not moved by any personal relationship to the soul which has fled that body and especially when it is being demonstrated to a crowd of students in a sober hall of learning, solely as object, soon loses the dark, sinister character it seems to preserve for the sentimental layman (the layman as such is always sentimental). Yes, like my colleagues I too tended to exaggerate to some extent my indifference to the human creature become thing, as if in defense against just such lay sentimentality. But I never went so far in my cynicism as those who considered it something to be proud of when they munched roasted chestnuts with relish at the dissecting table, so to speak under the very nose of the corpse, a cynicism which may also spring from subconsciously logical considerations. At the head of the bed on which the dead man lies, even if the man who just breathed his last is unknown to you, stands Death, still a grandiose ghostly apparition. In the morgue he stalks like a pedantic schoolmaster whom the *baccalaureus* thinks he can deride. And only in infrequent moments, when the corpse apes the living man he once was in some grotesque motion or under a sudden light effect, does the composed, even the frivolous man involuntarily experience a feeling of embarrassment or fear.

The anatomical laboratory lay beside the dissecting room, and the relationship of the two to each other could be compared to that of church and sacristy, especially when the priestly eminent professor or one of his assistants stepped out of the room assigned to him, into the generally accessible ones, to mingle with the working or chattering students. By far the most interesting one of these assistants was Emil Zuckerkandl, a pale young man with a dark Van Dyke beard and black eyes, who in his robes looked exactly like one of the anatomists as depicted by Rembrandt. The almost legendary aura of his lively drink- and duel-happy fraternity days still wafted about him. He still enjoyed the reputation of being able to go straight from some night club or other, even from the arms of a beautiful woman, to his serious day's work, teaching and learning with incredible application until late in the evening. However, instead of letting him set me an example or at least taking advantage of his highly praised talents as an instructor by regularly attending his lectures, I preferred to let his romantically twilit figure, seen superficially from afar, inspire me to write a rather feeble poem which I called "Prosector." At about the same time I wrote a somewhat flat fantasy, *Spring Night in the Dissecting Room* (*Frühlingsnacht im Seziersaal*), which I never completed, and if I want to add the fragment, *Sebaldus,* already mentioned, then I have described everything for which the poet in me has the enigmatic, bleak impressions of anatomy to thank.

The atmosphere of the medical profession with which I was surrounded made impressions on me in other ways as well. I began to suffer from hypochondria, especially after I started to attend the clinical lecture halls and visit the hospital wards; and my awareness of this reaction probably played its part in alienating me from the areas that did most toward arousing it. Still, from time to time I could feel an honest professional interest struggling to life within me. Although I was disposed to classify my occasional hypochondriac emotions as "specific third-year manifestations," I already looked ahead with some apprehension to my maturer years, and wondered if I would ever have the strength to preserve my *joie de vivre* with a constantly more concentrated miasma of possible ailments all around me, which however did not prevent me from considering the publication of a book on natural philosophy in my fiftieth year.

It goes without saying that my father watched my activities and even more sharply the things I failed to do, with increasing displeasure. When I told him, in December, during my first university year, that I had passed my preliminary examination in mineralogy, with honors, a fact of which I informed him as we were passing the Stadttheater to which we were going together that evening, he cried out overjoyed, "What I would really like to do now is give you a kiss!" words that deeply touched me and my companion, Jacques Pichler. But from then on my father was to have only rare occasions for such expressions of fatherly satisfaction, although some of his reproaches were not entirely justified and a few of the vexations he suffered through me were all too exaggeratedly taken. It was quite impossible, for instance, to consider me a spendthrift, which was what he liked to call me, because I couldn't make do with my five gulden a week pocket money. When he insisted on reproaching me for coming home so late at night, with the declaration that he felt ashamed of my behavior in front of the caretaker, then he was only betraying again, as was his wont in pedagogic concerns, that he considered outer manifestations—what people might say—of disproportionate importance. Still I could understand, even if I objected to it, the displeasure, yes, even the anxiety of a man who had started at the bottom, and with only his own resources had risen to a status of esteem and prominence in his field, and to a satisfactory social position, and now saw the son he loved and considered talented showing signs of wavering at the outset of a career that had been prescribed and made easy for him, threatening to stray from it, even to losing his way, instead of moving steadily forward with at least some display of seriousness.

As an example of how I idled away my days, the description of one, told in my customary fashion, may serve as an example of many others: "13.2.80. Got up fairly late, as usual, and couldn't start anything much before nine, which was when my anatomy lecture began. After listening rather attentively to Langer's lecture on the larynx, I went over to the chemistry lab where I spent more time chatting with Richard Kohn than working. Then home, where I spent a quarter of an hour on zoology after which I worked on *Aegidius,* finally accompanied my brother on the piano. A Mozart sonata. After dinner, played the Wagner Faust overture with Mama, then off with Eugene to the Café Central where we played three games of chess. (I won the first, he won the second, the third was a draw.) Dillmann joined us just as I had to leave for the Maria-Theresienstrasse, the usual trysting spot. She came, we went to the Quai Park; spring heralded its arrival in our delightful chatter. Both of us were in a wonderful mood. She took my arm, it got darker and darker, and we frequently interrupted our conversation in the sweetest fashion with tender kisses. Then I met Kohn, spoke to Jacques, also to Eugene. Home again, I read Max Waldau's *According to Nature (Nach der Natur),* improvised on the piano and played cards and chess with my brother after a futile attempt to hypnotize him.''

Sometimes I wrote in my diary in sentimental, humorous, blank verse. For instance, on June 27, 1880, the following lines:

Life looks at me, although still young in years,
With pale expression, and I fail to see
What is intended to bring joy unto my soul,
What still might come to lavish on my heart
The jubilation of a lovelier life.
In order not to pine away with boredom,
I have decided to recount my day,
(It was so cool, and so banal,) and tell
The hollow tale, and so be rid of it.
This evening I went walking in the gardens,
Where people go for pleasure or for pain.
A young girl, sitting on a bench, Fännchen her name,
Her loving parents seated at her side.
(They were the ones who did create the maid.)
Words were exchanged, passed back and forth,
But for the two of us there was a diff'rent feeling.
Shyly, out of the corners of our eyes,
Presentiments and recollections darted
Forth from the faint glow of our furtive glances,
To, fro, and daring not to linger,
The all of me no longer rooted there
But long since gone toward the Langegasse,
Toward Vienna's Zuckerkandl-Kneipe.
Forward—my coat slung o'er my shoulders,
I strode, with one last lingering look
At my girl flower and the flower she wore,
A gift to signify my love and my devotion.
Eugene, Jacques, Rudolf, all went with me;
Soon we were lost in jollity and noise, in wildest drinking,
Babel of voices, clapping hands and raucous singing,
Which on the student ladder quickly rises
To utter drunkenness. Weaved back and forth
And swam in the most welcome pool. And yet
One leaves such waters but to find oneself with simple cold,
Which one then calls, with sheepish grin,
A *Katzenjammer,* for e'en a cat
On finding one in such condition

Would have to groan and moan.
I left. Tavern and witching-hour were over.
Alone and lonely I wandered off to rouse myself
Out of my semi-stupor, at a coffee-house.
Chattered a while with some loose women, drank black coffee,
Blew smoke into the sin-filled air.
Told curious tales of curious journeys,
Of how once shipwrecked, then again
Roaming through jungles to New York,
Lied my way thus through yet another hour
Until at last, with hat perched rakishly on head,
I hurried home. And since the night is gone,
I sit here now, again faced with my papers,
And write, lamenting. For lamentable 'tis
To have on this earth naught of which it may be said,
"This thing is mine. This thing I do delights me."

And continued in the same vein on the following day:

In the fresh air, in kindly Nature,
But in the company of those who neither
Free nor kindly were—although beloved,
I spent my yesterday. The Brühl,
So beautiful, encircled us within
The shadows of its woods, and with
The sensuous scent of its wild flowers.
I strolled through the green meadows,
Holding a book which does divide all life
In no time into cells. Its name is Botany.
And all things blossoming around me
Suddenly were naught but albumen, but wretched protoplasm.
Then cosily I ate my cheese and butter
And ham—the best—also salami,
Must not forget to mention milk,
Mixed with my coffee's pleasant black,
Let it flow thoughtfully between my lips.
Three pretty girls passed back and forth,
And some prim misses, charming figures,
Their pretty faces graced the terrace.

WILLIAM CARLOS WILLIAMS
Autobiography

———❧———

WILLIAM CARLOS WILLIAMS (1883-1963) is one of a small number of physicians who have successfully combined medical and literary careers. He practiced medicine in New Jersey and wrote novels and poetry based on everyday urban life. His autobiography is a paean to the examined life of a doctor.

THE CITY OF THE HOSPITAL

The city of the hospital is my final home. You bring into it what you are, what your forebears were before you, first-generation Americans in many cases, who bring Europe with them also, peasant Europe with all its kindness, greed, cupidity and its despair.

There are good doctors and bad doctors; you can't tell them by their names; thieves, even murderers, with the most respectable names. On the other hand there are the most painstaking and humane priests of healing whose names show their origin to have been the ghettos of Poland or Sicily's stricken villages. There are financial geniuses whose parents not so many years back started operations at some corner fruit stand, men who could well give our Morgans and Rockefellers points on how to improve the complexion of a nickel. They are just what you might expect from their heritage, those who prey on others of their own kind. But there are also men and women who pain over every dollar they charge the sick for their cure and live virtually poverty-stricken lives of devoted service to mankind—which doesn't on the other hand make them the best doctors by any means.

It's a strange thing how many phases go into the making of a good, serviceable physician. Some have hands, just good surgeon's hands, and if by luck they have a head and a heart to go with them, they can reach the heights. Others are a menace to the community they inhabit. How are you going to tell them apart? Most of their fellows know them. But the human animal is an untrustworthy self-seeker, and the worst doctors know how to make themselves attractive. They are usually popular.

Who, when he has to pay the rent or his office nurse's salary, would hesitate to take out a pair of tonsils if he is offered the opportunity to do so?

No matter what the contours of the pharynx will look like afterward, he's licensed to do it and he'll go ahead. He doesn't even know the significance of the anatomical picture, much less care about the end results.

My own conception of the job has been to consider myself a man in the front line, in the trenches. It's the only way I can respect myself and go on treating what comes to me, men, women and children. I don't know everything about medicine and surgery but I *must* know well what I do know, besides which I must be thoroughly aware of what I do not know. I can't handle everything but I must never miss anything. I must play the game to win every time, often by referring a case with the greatest possible speed to someone else, get for the patient the finest service I can find in my region, at the least possible cost consistent with his ability to pay.

By and large we couldn't live in the world today, were it not for the medical profession, and I mean just that. We'd plain die, masses of us, tomorrow, if medical techniques were not kept up no matter what our fractional beliefs might be. On the other hand we may be populating the world with idiots. No one knows the answer.

I am grateful at least that I studied medicine (which is an idea: to study medicine but not to practice it) that I might know what goes on in myself as well as others. Gertrude Stein spoke of this clearly in her own life. She took it from the top down. She began with the psychic factors under William James and was, according to his testimony, a brilliant student. Then finding she did not want to limit herself to the abstractions but preferred rather the study of the whole man, went to Johns Hopkins for the somatic factor, the study of the physical body to make her knowledge whole. For the practice of letters concerns the whole man no matter what the stylistic variants may be. What better then than to know your subject thoroughly in all its aspects before beginning to exploit it? That was, at least, Gertrude Stein's conception of the advantages of knowing medicine if you wish to be a writer.

Obviously enough, the entire world today is a hospital so that, one thing canceling the other, that makes the hospital a very normal environment. It is only incidentally concerned with illness: quite casually, to itself, it measures, with some indifference, the decay of flesh, its excreta, bad odors and even its ecstasies of birth and cure. Cure to a physician is a pure accident, to the pathologist in his laboratory almost a disappointment. The real thing is the excitement of the chase, the opportunity for exercise of precise talents, the occasion for batting down a rival to supersede him, to strut, to boast and get on with one's fellows. Discovery is the great goal—and the accumulation of wealth.

Today the hospital is part of the fairgrounds for the commercial racket carried on by the big pharmaceutical houses. Almost every day there are exhibits of the latest drugs put on by the sales force of this or that manufacturer in the doctor's waiting room. It is a place as busy as the city editor's desk of a big newspaper, for the latest cures are front-page stuff today. If the physician does not hand out the latest variant of the popular cure-all, he will fast lose his practice. Rightly so. The practice of medicine and surgery is close to the realm of necromancy today; miracles are being looked for and performed; knowledge *has* increased at such a rate that one should be ashamed to die of anything short of decapitation over the edge of a windshield.

Then we have the managerial staff, and after them the nursing staff—which has many occupations apart from techniques. They are women, they are young women, they are for the most part intelligent young women and frequently, in their crisp and becoming uniforms, they appear as beautiful young women with whom the distresses of mankind have little to do directly. It is their own backgrounds out of which the "call" comes to serve humanity that determine their lives. Fine eyes, velvet skin (or coarse), arms built for love, breasts casqued in starched linen, never to be pictured or kissed.

What shall they do? The discipline is rigid. I have long listened to their stories.

"She has decided to stay there."

"Where?"

"Where she is now, at Grasslands."

"The insane?"

"Yes, she loves it. The only one in her class. They get two hundred and fifty a month. Of course thirty-five dollars of it is taken out for meals."

"You mean little Audrey?"

"She has signed up to go on from two to eleven."

"They get a day off?"

"Two days, up there. But she doesn't want the women. She only wants to take care of the men. She can't stand the women."

"Good for her."

"Do you know Nellie De Graff is up there?"

"You mean . . . ?"

"Yes. She is in a private cottage."

"I did hear that she's been hitting the bottle recently."

"A hopeless case. Her children signed her in. I'm sorry for her husband. Three to five hundred a week, the poor man, he can't stand it."

* * *

One New Year's morning I wasn't too steady myself when a little redhead came up to me.

"What time is it?"

"11:15."

"O God, if I can only hold out till noon."

"What's the matter with your eye?"

"Fell downstairs this morning—at four A.M."

This was the same one whom her friends had dragged in soused to the gills through the dormitory window while they were serving their time at the Contagious Hospital in Newark. They undressed her, pushed her under the shower to get her on duty at seven.

Some of them (one is all I remember) are so well-made they can land a job, let's say, as "hostess" at some night club. But that's not the only type. There are the ones with powerful legs, hair to entice a Botticelli or a Modigliani to draw them. They are lost or almost lost in most cases.

These are the necessities that drive them to decide on their choice of service.

And what becomes of them? Some stay on, think of Alaska or Korea, but never get there. A few with wit or the intelligence or the stomachs to do it, marry the medical men, still unattached, who serve as interns in the places. Good marriages. But most marry men, good fellows who cannot hope to afford their wives the sorts of associations they have grown used to in their three years of hospital service, in the private rooms and among the older men on the attending staff. These are individuals of far greater culture in many cases than the girls have been used to, far greater wealth and talent also than is usually available to them. The girls are tempted. The prospect is at times a glittering one. They are deeply affected. Shall they deny themselves this last chance at distinction before the plunge into mediocrity and the raising of a family?

And the older men? Here is often charm, loyalty, devotion to very love itself—shown in a roseate cloud—offered not crudely if hesitatingly, but even courageously. The opportunities are manifold, the late time of duty, the freedom from restraint at strange hours, the very intimate character of the occupation with the human carcass, at times under great stress, the complete (but not complete) knowledge of its processes. The girls have to witness everything there is to see and to know. Surgery is complete knowledge, and witnessing births gives detailed plans of what they themselves are built for.

The only thing the girls lack is the practice of the physiology of love. Its knowledge is old-hat to them before they have been two years out of high school, and they themselves are ripe, in fact, sadly enough, overripe. That intensifies the loss: the knowledge, the opportunities denied, the constant attack they are under from all sides leave them worn out often before they have started. They have caught a glimpse of love, have been offered endless opportunities for its physical fulfillment but, in the end, come away, ignorant, their fine bodies wasted and their minds unsatisfied. Not that all of them have minds or even sensibilities, but at least the hospital has swallowed them.

One day I was coming out of the cloakroom when I ran into a young surgeon whom I very much like, a really good guy. I greeted him affectionately and received a gruff reply. This was unlike the man.

"Hey," I said, grabbing him by the shoulder as he was passing me, "what's the idea?"

"Oh, nothing," he said.

But I kept hold of him and continued. "Don't give me that stuff," I said. "What's biting you? Come on, give."

"You wanna know?"

"Sure, that's why I asked you." We were standing in the passage to the lobby.

"I was over at the other hospital this morning. I had an operation scheduled since yesterday. But when I got there at eight o'clock, somebody else had the place sewed up."

"And . . .?"

"I went to the scrub room to find what was up. There he was, the whole place was crowded with them." He paused a moment and I waited.

"So, I said to him, 'What have you got this morning, a gall bladder?' "

" 'No, just an appendix,' he told me. That made me mad. You know him."

"Yes, I know him," I said.

"Well, I stood there a minute, the whole room was listening. Then I said to him, 'You know, I got an idea: The next man that comes into your office, when you look at him and decide you want to take out his gall bladder, you have a little gun in the top drawer of your desk and point it at his belly and you say to him, "For two hundred and fifty dollars I won't take out your gall bladder." He looks at you and he sees you mean business'—they were all scrubbing up and all listening to me. 'Then he gives you the money.' "

"Did you really say that to him?" I asked, fascinated and gleefully chuckling to myself, thinking of this cocky little chap standing behind the first, twice his size, who had stopped scrubbing as had all the others to listen.

" 'In that way,' " went on my friend, " 'you accomplish three things: first, you get the money; two, you save a lot of time for everyone: and third, your patient escapes a needless operation.' "

*   *   *

Men at operating tables drop dead, sometimes, at their tasks. The young are always pushing their elders, as in all corporate work. Brilliant work gets done and is often never acclaimed. There is much genius among physicians, as in any occupation to which a man or woman can devote himself, great work done casually in the course of duty for which no praise is asked and none given other than a nurse's smile or a friend's nod of the head, superb accomplishments. For what? For a few bucks? But that, the crown of the physician, is not today the thing most recognized.

An old friend of my father's once said to me when I was one day raving against a flagrant miscarriage of justice in our local courts, "Willie, what do you think you can get in a court of law?"

"Why the least you can ask for," I said, "is common justice."

"Oh, no," he replied, "you won't get justice, that's impossible. All you'll get is the best that is available in your locality."

It's no different with medicine, a rat race, if there ever was one, in which the ones most devoted to humanity often come in second best. But it can't be helped. If a man brings me his son, saying to me that the boy has "an appendix" which the father wants out and I tell him the boy is perfectly well and shouldn't be touched, what does the father do? He goes to the next man down the block who takes on the job without even looking. Who's the sucker? Why, I am, of course. Multiply that by a thousand times and add to it the fact that in the end all cases are lost, while the postponement of the evil is all we hope for, and you'll grasp at once the money that's in the racket.

The doctor is admitted to all houses. Often a man will say, "I'm leaving the front door open, Doc, you'll find her in bed. Go ahead in. She's looking for you." It's a great ticket of admission to a lot of things.

When the girls come up for their nurse's graduation and stand on the platform in their starched uniforms to receive their diplomas, some of them will appear to the onlookers as the most beautiful women in the world, which they are.

And then the grinning head of the Board of Governors will stand at the front, as I have often seen it done, with a list in his hand and call the girls up one by one, each to receive her scroll. He may start in, "Miss Adams"—

but then, as he goes on, he will begin to arrive at a sticker (the fool could have studied the name previously), he hesitates: "Miss—tch"—he laughs, the audience is howling and the girl, recognizing what he is trying to say, comes red-faced to the front. That's the mark of her condition. She is embarrassed by the offensive snobbery of the man.

*   *   *

FRENCH HOSPITAL

But innocence is hard to beat. Even the building of the old French Hospital itself is gone now—it stood opposite what is now the exit of the Lincoln Tunnel on West Thirty-fourth Street—completely vanished. It seems impossible that it was there I met the big Greek on the medical ward, stark naked as he was, and wrestled with him.

The big Greek had pneumonia and lay in the far bed to the left coming from the corridor. Miss McGrath, by no means "*petite*," was giving him a bath behind the usual screen when, as I learned later, the man hit her suddenly between the eyes with his clenched fist. She fell backward carrying the screen, covered with a sheet, over with her. As she scrambled up he was after her, naked, a big guy muscled like a wrestler. When I got there he was standing in the middle of the floor struggling to possess the clay water pitcher we always had on a table in the center of the ward, which a little guy, convalescent from typhoid, was hanging onto with all his might. The Sister in charge with McGrath was standing barring his exit and the other girls, back of her, fascinated, were watching the show.

As I came in, the man let go of the pitcher and came for me. All I could do was grab him. Luckily for me, he'd been ill, had a high fever at the moment, perhaps 106° or more. I got him around the neck and tried to throw him, but he sank his teeth into my shoulder. I got one foot back of him and down we went to the floor together, I, fortunately, on top. All the fight suddenly went out of him. I let him stand, then, and led him back to his bed. But at that moment it became startlingly apparent that he was naked! The girls scattered, Gaskins, one of the interns, grinning like a fool, a sheet held between his hands, came behind us sashaying like a dancer from side to side. What a clown.

*   *   *

I remember Eugene Pool accosted me when my time in the French was finally up and asked me what I was going to do. It was he who had given me the name "the boy surgeon" when he had come upon me one day while I was trying to dissect out a Bartholin cyst abscess.

"One thing I'm not going to do," I told him, "and that's surgery."

"Why not?"

"I don't fancy a life spent dabbling in people's guts."

He laughed. "I think you're wise at that," he said. "There are plenty of young men, your age, with three times the surgery you've had, who are having a hard time getting on here in the city."

"I'm going to the suburbs," I said, "but not yet. I think I'll take another internship in obstetrics and diseases of children, then go in for general practice."

"Good boy," he said. "If you stay in the city it will take you twenty years (it's always twenty years that has to elapse between desire and achievement) then, just as you're on your feet, making a name for yourself, you're an old fogey." I knew at the time that Pool himself had married the daughter of one of the directors of the New York Hospital—crazy like a fox, I thought, and thanked him. Of course, he had money; I had no money and had no idea of ever getting any.

Once they brought in a French fisherman who had been lost for two weeks on the Grand Banks in an open boat, with only a sip of fresh water a day and a few biscuits to stead him. He had been a powerful man, but starvation had reduced him to skin and bones. And once we took care of a big Frenchman, with thick brown beard, from Valencia, Spain, exiled from France because of his Royalist inclinations, and performances too, I can well imagine. We had case after case of malaria and typhoid among the sailors. Once a drunk swallowed a basinful of a 1/10,000 corrosive sublimate solution. He clamped his teeth, refusing to let us use a stomach tube on him. Sure, he'd let me give him a shot in the arm. Why not? But he didn't know it was apomorphine. The change in the expression of his face when the uncontrollable vomiting started was belly-shaking to behold. I once took a knife from under a sailor's pillow. The nurses were kind—but wanted marriage.

*   *   *

At the French Hospital, I was lying on my back naked one summer's day, resting before returning to my duties in the operating room. It was a brute of a day and I was tired. How old was I? Twenty-three or -four before I became fully aware of what had been a mystery theretofore called "love." No wonder I thought to myself when I remembered Doc Martin's lecture on the subject, "Everyone in this class has committed masturbation including

your present instructor—don't let's be overimpressed by its importance."
I hadn't known what he meant.

The French Sisters who did most of the ordinary work about the premises were always friendly to me, largely because I spoke French. They were of all ages and conditions, from the fat Sister Pelagia—who could hardly get out of her own way and whom the patients hated because of her indifferent clumsiness—to little wide-eyed Elizabeth, a pure peasant who was shocked when she found I, who could be so nice, was not a Catholic. Bless her sweet heart—a baby robin or a kitten was what she represented to me.

But Sister Julianna, the Sister Superior, an older black-eyed woman with a whiplike intelligence, was something else again. She was boss and no prude. We respected her. One day an old gal, one of our "chronics" hopped a window from the fifth floor going clean down into the concrete areaway in front of the building. The alarm was sounded. I jumped bare-legged into white pants and lit out for the elevator. Sister J. made the same car I did. We were laughing, merely doing our duty, no one was very excited.

"Look what I've got on," I said to her.

"Well, look what I've got on," said she, pulling her nun's habit above her naked knee. I loved her, a marvelous woman. I needed to love her and she me, for more than once it was her intercession alone that kept me in the place.

There were five of us interns if you count Krumwiede—what a name for the French hospital! We called him "The Wrath of God" from the way he looked at breakfast every morning. Smith, who fell on his back beside a recently operated-on and beautiful girl patient—he had been trying to do a handstand on the bar at the foot of her bed—his feet hit her pillow! Maloney, who was unjustly dismissed over a complaint he made to the newspapers about the way we were fed, and Gaskins, my immediate pal—one of the most hilarious, comical men I've ever met and the best pal in the world. Eberhard came after Maloney had been fired. He was a fat guy from Brooklyn.

Charles Krumwiede, the pathologist, would get up late mornings after reading until two or three A.M. at his 20-volume *System of Abnormal Anatomy*. We all respected him, but we'd be sore because we'd have to make a seven or eight o'clock schedule and it didn't go so well with us to have him lazing in to a leisurely breakfast just as we were swallowing our last sip of weak coffee preparatory to going on duty. Krumwiede particularly liked me because of his piano. Playing the scores of various of the operas, I'd dub in the voice with my fiddle as he'd play the orchestra parts. We'd have grand times together.

Once we four interns had a maid, if you could call her that, a rough-and-ready dish smasher who at least did bring our food in to us and inhabited a skin as tightly packed with goodies as a young intern could desire to pinch. She was Irish and she was quick, strong and ready. Eberhard caught her off balance one day and took her in his arms, but she came back swinging and broke away. He followed. As she ran through the glass-paneled pantry door, he no more than a whisker behind her, she swung the door back so that his powerful right paw went through the glass—without really hurting him. I never saw four men disappear so suddenly. I never did discover how they did it.

I was Senior at the time. With the crash of the glass, or so it seemed, Sister Superior was in the room. I hadn't moved.

"What's going on in here?" she shouted.

"Nothing very serious, Sister," I told her. "We'll pay for the glass."

She stood there looking at me a moment and then smiled.

"Tell me what happened."

I told her.

"Well," she said, "as long as it's you, we'll say nothing more about it."

"Thank you, Sister."

"But don't let it happen again."

"No, Sister."

One night I came in with a bad cold. I was hardly able to talk. Sister Julianna happened to meet me in the lobby and took me by the shoulder.

"Come with me," she said. "You young men!"

We went into the Sisters' dining room, it was late, the room was empty. There she made me sit at one of the little tables. She brought out a saucer and placed a teacup on it. She got the sugar bowl filled with lump sugar, then she dug out a bottle of brandy and began her operations.

First she put three lumps, square lumps of sugar, in the bottom of the cup. On top of them she placed two lumps and finally one lump to complete the pyramid. I watched her intently. Next she filled the cup with brandy, and I mean filled it.

"Hey, wait a minute," I said.

"You wait a minute," she said. "*I'm* doing this."

At that she struck a match and lit the top lump of brandied sugar. Together we watched the blue flame while she lectured me on my behavior and gave many such admonishments. The brandy burned and burned—it took several minutes finally to flicker and die out. At that moment, the sugar dissolved, the solution heated from the burning, much of the alcohol gone, she pointed to the cup and said to me, "Drink it!"

I drank it down in one sweep.

"Now go to bed and behave yourself."

Perhaps it was the next evening I was passing Saks's window at the corner of Thirty-fourth Street and Sixth Avenue. I came on an incident that really startled me.

It was cold, wet and gusty with hardly anyone out. There was a cab at the gutter and standing, her back against the shop window, was a young woman. It was a spot much frequented by the prostitutes of the quarter. In front of her was a priest facing her and arguing with her intently. I could see from her looks what was going on. I'd seen it for half a block before I actually came up to them: he was talking to her earnestly, trying to get her to go straight. She was looking down, turned slightly away from him, refusing to listen—when just as I passed, I saw the cab driver come up behind him. The priest didn't see the man until he tapped him on the shoulder from behind. The priest turned. The man smiled inviting him and the girl to take advantage of his cab and go off together. I had just time to witness the outraged fury of the holy man and the girl's guilty smile.

This was the French quarter where Mouquin had his celebrated restaurant of iron grilles and outdoor stairs leading up to the ornate second floor.

Poor priests, I heard enough of priests, for the most part Paulist Fathers, and their unhappiness, in that hospital to last me a lifetime. I washed out their stomachs, comforted them as best I could and saw them die too, more than once. I pitied them. One told me that he blamed his bad stomach on the life he led somewhere in one of the far western parishes where he would have to go fifteen to twenty miles horseback between churches, sometimes, to say Mass, but could not eat a bite until the last was over. They found me patient. The one I am thinking of would let no one else pass the stomach tube. God rest his soul.

But we had all sorts. A poor whore came in one morning in an awful state. I hardly knew women and felt tender to them all, especially, like any man, if they retained some vestige of beauty. This woman was young and full-breasted. She had been cruelly beaten. Her eyes were closed, her lips bloody where her teeth had cut them and her arms bruised and bleeding. But the thing that knocked me over was that her breasts were especially lacerated and on one could be seen the deeply imbedded marks of teeth, as if some animal had attempted to tear the tissues away.

*   *   *

The old hospital, on Thirty-fourth between Ninth and Tenth Avenues, was one short block away from the excavation then being made for the new Pennsylvania Station. We had sandblast victims in the clinic every day. But one day they brought in, unconscious, a big lump of a man in dirty overalls. He'd been dumping broken stone from a wheelbarrow off the end of a trestle to the pile below when for some reason he'd fallen, barrow and all, onto the heap twenty feet down. When we saw him he was messed up generally, bleeding from the mouth and nose and, as I say, unconscious. I looked at him, smelled whisky and told the girls to undress him. I wasn't sure whether he had a fracture of the skull or was malingering. It isn't always easy to make a snap diagnosis in such a case.

I went back to sit in the chair at the chart desk but almost at once heard the girls cry out and come piling from behind the screen.

"What's up?"

"Come see."

I went and was not a little astonished at what they had discovered. The man was a big guy, a plump specimen in bloody clothes, but when they had begun to remove the outer clothing, they found he had on a woman's silk chemise with little ribbons at his nipples; that his chest and finally his legs were shaved; that he wore women's panties and long silk stockings.

The girls wouldn't have anything more to do with him. I called the orderly, and that was that! He was still unconscious and obviously in bad shape. His wife was notified of the accident and when told of her man's unusual dress, said merely that he liked that sort of thing, that he was a good husband and that she had no complaint of him. She was genuinely broken up by his critical condition and went away weeping.

The next morning—the man still being unconscious with an obvious skull fracture—a magnificent open car of the 1907 breed, something of unusual luxuriousness, pulled up in front of the hospital and out of it stepped a figure which cannot be forgotten. He was over six feet tall, erect and so dressed that everyone about him looked like a lackey. He inquired for his friend, the injured workman. I saw and spoke to him in the lobby. His hair, pure white, was worn in tight curls covering his really fine head. He was quiet but insistent. I reported the condition to his friend and told him how the cards lay.

"Have him moved to a private room. Give him the best there is." No, he didn't want to see him. "Send all the bills to me." He gave me his name—which was one of the most prominent in the state—and came every day thereafter to inquire about the man's condition. When the man died, the body was returned to the wife for a decent funeral.

*   *   *

It was sometime after this that Maloney left. He was forced out. We'd had an emergency case one night. I took care of it, though I didn't see the first part of the show. A cab had driven in to the ambulance entrance. Before we could identify anyone, a young guy was pushed out and his friends had gone. So we looked him over and found a stab wound in the chest, not too bad. But in those days, any wound of the chest was bad, and we admitted him—just a kid in his teens.

But next day, the reporters were on our necks getting past the Sister at the window, coming up the elevators unannounced, trying to pick up a story. There was no story to amount to anything, just a stabbing. So one of the brighties of the press began snooping around for something to send to the city desk. I don't know how he hit on it, but he got hold of Maloney and perhaps by chance asked how the food was in the place. As it happened, the grub was rotten at that moment, as it often is in certain hospitals, and we had more than once kicked about it. For instance, they had served us for dinner a brain of some animal, perhaps a sheep or calf or pig for all we knew; there it lay ungarnished on the platter looking as if had come from some autopsy table. We damned near threw it out the window.

So poor Maloney let go on all our gripes, and the reporter made a hit story of it. If I recall the time correctly, there had been similar incidents in other hospitals of the city, so that we merely confirmed such findings. Maloney was hauled before the Board of Governors and out he went. I was moved up six months and so instead of serving two years in the hospital, served only eighteen months before going over to the Nursery and Child's. It certainly altered my life.

HANS ZINSSER
As I Remember Him

———◆◇◆———

Dr. Kerr is now dead. He is probably forgotten by all but a few old farmers' wives. He had neither fame nor more than a frugal living. He was probably unhappy, while he lived, not for the reasons mentioned, but because he never could do for his people as much as he wanted to do. He practised in St. Lawrence County, near Chippewa Bay. His office was a little surgery extension of a small village house. He was tall, thin, and very dark, with hairy wrists, a big nose, a busy moustache, and kind, tired brown eyes. I was camping on my island in the bay and was known to the grocer in the village as a young doctor from New York. One day at about 4 A.M. a motorboat approaching my island aroused me and the grocer's son shouted through the fog and drizzle that Dr. Kerr needed my help in a difficult case. He landed while I dressed, and we were off four miles to the village. There Dr. Kerr was waiting for me with his buggy. I had never seen him before and he impressed me, in my young self-confidence, as probably a poor country bonesetter whom I would have to show how a case should be handled. This, however, lasted only until we were bumping along a muddy country lane and he had begun to tell me about the patient.

It was a woman, a farm hand's wife, who was having her first baby. She had developed eclampsia seven months along, and the child had died. She was having convulsions. The problem was to deliver the dead baby from a uterus with an undistended cervix, and the mother dangerously toxic. At this point, I was thoroughly scared. I had had training at the Sloane Maternity, but this was a "high forceps" under difficulties, a case for Professor Cragin in a well-equipped operating room, with an assistant and two or three nurses.

We drove about four miles into the river flats. I could see the little unpainted cottage next to a haystack a mile away. I offered no suggestion while I was trying to recover my old ambulance courage. He didn't ask me any questions.

The place was a picture of abject poverty. The husband, a pathetic little bandy-legged, redheaded fellow in torn overalls, was waiting at the door, anxious and silent. The kitchen was a mess from his efforts at housekeeping. In the next room the woman, half-conscious, her bloated face twitching, lay on a dirty double bed, on a mattress without sheets under an old quilt half kicked off, leaving her almost naked.

While I stood looking at her with frightened sympathy, Dr. Kerr unpacked his bag. Without asking me to do anything, he filled a wash boiler with hot water from a kettle, added a little lysol, and put on his forceps to boil. Then he took of his coat, rolled up his sleeves, filled a basin, and began to soap and lysol his hands. Not until he was doing this did he speak.

Then he began to give me directions. In a few minutes I was cleaning up the patient, spreading clean towels under her, preparing a chloroform cone and jumping at his words as though in Dr. Cragin's clinic. With no essential help from me, he performed as neat a cervix dilation and forceps delivery as I had ever seen. When, after the long and arduous task, with everything complete as possible, he began to clean up, he didn't even thank me. He took it for granted that, being a doctor and being in the neighborhood, I was on call. It was his only compliment, except for a friendly smile.

He asked me to stay there the rest of the day while he made his rounds, gave me a few directions, and left a sedative. Then he went out, patted the husband on the back, and drove away. The woman recovered. Dr. Kerr, I heard later, spent the first two nights after this on a rocking chair, drinking cider with the husband, and napping when he could. His fee, I also heard, accepted to please the husband, was a peck of potatoes.

Some time later, I had occasion to ask him to open a boil on my neck. He sat me down in a chair, wiped my neck with alcohol, took a knife out of a little leather case, wiped that with alcohol, and let me have it. I made no suggestion whatever. I saw him often after that, and I sincerely hope—even now—that he liked me.

One of Dr. Kerr's colleagues from up near Ogdensburg, whom I had met at this time, did a most extraordinary thing. I met him on the river one day when we were both fishing off the head of Watch Island. Just as I came in sight of him as I rounded the point, he pulled out a magnificent pickerel.

"Good for you, doctor!" I shouted to him.

"What d'ye think, young feller?" he called back. "I caught that fish with a nice fat appendix I took out this mornin'."

*　　*　　*

Young Americans who entered medicine at the time that R. S. did were more fortunate than they knew, for they were destined to participate in a professional evolution that has few parallels. The development of modern medicine in our country is a thrilling chapter in its intellectual history, and illustrates, more than is generally recognized, the magnificent self-corrective vitality of this profession. At the present time, there is a strong popular movement for the socialization of medical practice, and an effort, essentially praiseworthy, to bring the benefits of discovery and of improved care within the reach of the population as a whole, irrespective of ability to pay. This is as it should be, and there is little question of the fact that the old system of charity clinics and hospitals no longer meets modern requirements. Moreover, it is morally sound to postulate that all discovered means of alleviating suffering and sorrow, maintaining health and preventing death, should be freely available to all that need them—without reference to social, racial, or economic condition. This will demand a complete reorganization of practice, in which the medical profession must, and should, play the leading role; and undoubtedly it will—though there has been a tendency on the part of reformers, sociologists, government agencies, and professors of the teachers' union type to assume that reluctance to accept any and all proposals indicates a conservatism of self-preservation based on purely venal motives. Let it not be forgotten that the situation as it now exists is entirely the consequence of the progress made in medical discovery by the profession itself; that the enhanced power for good which is now claimed as the latest of the inalienable rights of man is the result of the labors of medical investigators and practitioners, and that public-health organization, social service, group practice, and all other advances which have revolutionized the relationship of medical knowledge to the population—even housing, nutrition, and the sociological conditions that influence health, such as wage scales, public parks, industrial hygiene, etc., etc.—were given their basis of factual observation and their early organization for practical application by the insight of medical men.

There is in the practice of medicine a unique quality that is a source both of inspiration and of terror to the conscientious young physician. Dealing as it does with matters of life and death, any lack of knowledge or of skill becomes a positive fault of omission and even guilt. If a patient dies or is incapacitated—with all the heartbreak and suffering that this implies— because the attending practitioner was ignorant of measures that are available and that might have brought another outcome in more skillful hands, he is as responsible as though he had committed a willful injury. This is true not only of surgical procedures, but equally—perhaps more frequently so—in infectious diseases, where speed and precision of diagnosis by well-known methods and vigorous intelligent treatment may decide the issue within a few hours, one way or the other. It is this consideration, more than any other, which—with the growing accumulation of knowledge that no one man can hope to master completely—has automatically led to the organization of group medicine, the increasing coöperation of city and state health departments, and the more generalized utilization of hospital facilities. And since it is essential that all effective knowledge must be applied to rich and poor alike, unless our profession is to lose the fine, ancient traditions of its history, a considerable readjustment of its activities is inevitable. These simple considerations are at the bottom of all the agitation for the so-called "socialization" of medicine on which great volumes of reports have already been issued. It should not be forgotten, however, by the ardent lay reformers that evolution in these directions has long been going on within the profession itself, and, within a single span of professional life, enormous progress—almost entirely originated by public-spirited doctors—has been achieved. Controversies have turned not at all on the objectives to be attained, but rather upon the manner in which the reorganization is to be carried out.

Now it is always relatively easy to conceive an ideal scheme of organization which shall represent the perfect mechanism for social reform. But such conceptions are likely to neglect certain imponderable human values without which the machinery of service cannot run smoothly. In medicine, the problem is to find a solution which shall meet the requirements of effective scientific care of all those who require it, and retain at the same time that sense of personal responsibility, compassion, and judgment without which the physician becomes a mere technician. It is this consideration which has given the impression of exaggerated conservatism in many actually progressive physicians. We realize—more acutely than most of the lay reformers—the obligations of greater precision of practice and wider and cheaper application of the benefits of progress. But we are reluctant to lose our "horse and buggy" doctors, or to deprive the suffering patient of that solace and support which only the close personal relationship with a wise and compassionate physician can give.

During little more than the space of the professional lives of R. S.'s generation, American medicine developed from a relatively primitive dependence upon European thought to its present magnificent vigor. How this came about is a unique illustration of coöperative effort, wise benevolence, and healthy self-criticism. To understand it wholly, we must sketch the dependence of modern medical development upon that of the basic sciences, its emergence—in Europe—from mediaevalism, and the manner in which these influences were transported to the new continent.

Since the Renaissance there have been no complete breaks in the continuity of the sciences comparable to those sterile periods which have, from time to time, interrupted the progress of the arts. There has been an alternation of slowing down and acceleration, but the progress has been a reasonably steady one, the intervals between great advances being occupied with the organization of strong points within the conquered territory. The preparatory accumulation of minor discoveries and of accurately observed details by conscientious drones is, in scientific pursuits, almost as important for the mobilization of great forward drives as the periodic correlation of these disconnected observations into principles and laws by the vision of genius. In this, the lesser men of science are happier than the minor poets or painters. Thus the roots of modern medicine trace back deeply into the seventeenth and eighteenth centuries.

The earliest of the great Baconians, Harvey, not only clarified the facts concerning the circulation of man, but carried his observations into the animal world and, in his *De Generatione Animalium,* into the field of exact study of embryological development. If any single individual can be named as the first to introduce, into medical thought, exact methods of observation and experiment for the correlation of structure and function, this credit belongs to William Harvey. Moreover, it is probably not unreasonable to appraise him as the most important individual force in the transition from mediaeval into modern medicine, in the sense that there could be no rational physiology until Harvey had refuted the old doctrine of Galen that there were two kinds of blood—the venous and the arterial—serving different functions respectively.

The period in which Harvey lived was the most momentous in the history of science. Harvey was born in 1578. Between 1564 and 1596 were born Galileo, Kepler, and Descartes. Pascal was born in 1623, and Newton nineteen years later. Between 1623 and 1630, when Kepler died, all these men except Newton were alive. Even when compared with the flowering period of biology which laid the foundations of modern medicine in the nineteenth century, this golden age of physics and mathematics represents the most powerful foward surge of the human intellect, equaled in the history of art only by the miracles of Homer, or Leonardo, of Shakespeare, of Bach and a very few others. And it is quite clear that in the logical continuity of scientific evolution, this development of physics must have preceded any possible advances in chemistry and biology and—therefore—in medicine.

Apart from Malpighi, the first great histologist, and Mayow, who anticipated—within the limitations of available chemistry—Lavoisier's discoveries on the physiology of breathing, Harvey had no contemporary peers. The nature of medical practice was, in that age, discouraging to scientific inquiry.

In Bacon's words, "the physician . . . hath no particular acts demonstrative of his ability . . . for who can tell if a patient die or recover . . . whether it be art or accident? And, therefore, many times the impostor is prized and the man of virtue taxed. Nay, we see the weakness and credulity of men is such, as they will often prefer a mountebank [Montabank] or witch before a learned physician. And, therefore, the poets were clear-sighted in discerning this extreme folly, when they made Aesculapius and Cierce brother and sister, both children of the Sun. . . . And what followeth? Even this, that physicians say to themselves, as Solomon expresseth it upon a higher occasion: If it befall me as it befalleth to the fool, why should I labour to be more wise?"

That a competition of physicians with superstition and gullibility, if not with witchcraft, still persists is attested by the power of Christian Science, osteopathy, chiropractice, and the mass of purely meretricious advertising. There have lately also been lapses into a sort of rationalized mysticism on the part of individuals—sometimes eminent scientists—which are dangerous only when they are combined with skill in popular exposition, as in the case of Dr. Carrel, to whom we shall refer presently. That the fight is practically won, however, is apparent from the fact that, except among the lowest classes of intelligence, "cults" such as those mentioned are themselves attempting to find justification in scientific reasoning, and are slipping into legitimate medicine by the back door.

From Harvey's time on, there was a consistent effort on the part of leading physicians to emancipate the profession from superstition and tradition, and to evolve a science of medicine. Anatomy—and with it the beginnings of physiology—was considerably enriched by Meckel, Morgagni, Boerhaave, Haller, and their followers. In clinical medicine, Sydenham, John Hunter, Auenbrugger,—the inventor of percussion,—Benjamin Bell, and a host of others were applying principles of exact observation to case studies, and thinking in terms of the primitive physiology at their disposal; progressive schools of surgery appeared in England and on the Continent.

Early eighteenth-century medicine made its chief advances in practical directions. Physics and mathematics were not ready for any kind of immediate influence upon medical theory or methodology; the intermediary—that is, chemistry—was still too primitive in technique and conception to bring the two together. It was the century of philosophy, and the reaction of all human thought against theological domination had a considerable indirect influence upon medicine as well. Helvetius, Maupertuis, and above all Voltaire,—who, with the aid of the *éducation de l'oreiller* from the learned Marquise du Châtelet, brought the Newtonian

physics to France,—these, with Diderot, d'Alembert, and others, revolutionized the attitude of all educated men toward the observation of
nature. La Mettrie, who anticipated Schopenhauer in his postulation of
egoism as the basis of morals, was a military surgeon. Cabanis was a
medical man. Buffon had timid suspicions of the common origin of animals.
Linnaeus classified men with the apes. The Abbé Spallanzani was leading
up to Pasteur's refutation of the spontaneous generation of life. Stahl, to be
sure, put a handful of sand into the scientific gears with his conceptions of
"Vitalism"; but Boerhaave of Leyden and his pupil Haller were beginning
to teach medicine on the basis of what was known of physiology and of
microscopic anatomy, and trained some of the most eminent physicians of
the next generation. It was a period of preparation for the true beginning of
sound medical theory, which started gradually toward the end of the
century with the chemistry of Priestley, Boyle, and above all Lavoisier.

American medicine, quite naturally, was during this century under the
influence of the British school, and the most eminent physicians of
Revolutionary times were pupils of such great clinicians as John Fothergill,
Huxham, John Hunter, and others. Progress, however, was largely along
purely empirical, clinical directions. Surgery advanced remarkably, considering the lack of anaesthetics. But, though there were men of unusual
wisdom and skill, no fundamental advances were made—except in the
discovery of Jennerian vaccination, which, against considerable opposition, was established in America, with the aid of Thomas Jefferson, by Dr.
Waterhouse of Boston. The history of these times would reveal an
interesting collection of strong personalities, wise and alert, but would be
found, with a few exceptions like that of Jenner, to be largely a period of
groping, without any notable advances in the discovery of fundamental
fact. It was a time of theorizing and of "systems." John Brown of
Edinburgh founded a school which explained all disease as fluctuations in
the "irritability" of the nervous system to external and internal stimuli. It is
not worthwhile to detail his views, since it is all clever nonsense; but
"Brownianism" developed a considerable vogue in other European countries. Then there was "Vitalism," founded by Sauvages, Bordeu, and
Barthez, at Montpellier. As in the "Animism" of Stahl, the "life principle"
or "soul" was, for the Vitalists, the seat of all morbid processes; and the
vital principle resided in the central nervous system, in which all disturbances from the normal originated. It was a primitive neurology, based on
speculation without structural investigation, and it became curiously
involved with the observations, by Galvani, of the stimulation of muscle
contractions by electrical currents. Galvani observed, too, that a muscle
contracted when it and its nerve were placed in contact with two dissimilar

metals. He postulated the existence of "animal electricity," and thus it was a short cry from Vitalism to elaborate theories of electrical "fluids" as governors of all life processes. And, even the soul acquired a galvanometrically measurable quality.

An interesting offshoot of this was "Mesmerism," a movement which had much similarity to the sort of thing that survives in the best modern medical circles. The first thought that comes to one on reading Dr. Carrel's book is that there is nothing new under the sun. The same sort of thing that seems to be happening to our distinguished friend happened to many medical men in the days during and following the cult of Mesmerism.

Franz Anton Mesmer studied medicine in Vienna, where—thanks to a rich wife—he became a successful general practitioner. There he developed theories of therapeutics dependent on the influence of magnetism upon the human nervous system. Out of this there rapidly grew a school of treatment in which a sort of "chiropractic" massage at the hands of a strongly "psychic" physician (as he would now be called) claimed a considerable number of extraordinary cures. The medical profession, skeptical then as now, was not at first persuaded; but Mesmer appeared before various academies and found enthusiastic disciples in Paris, in spite of the unfavorable report of a commission—one of whose members was Lavoisier. By Parisian followers, the theory of "Animal Magnetism" was then expanded into what was called "Magnetic Somnambulism" and, by the influence of the Marquis de Puységur, it became a theory of clairvoyance. Thus Mesmer said that "living creatures, which are in contact (by magnetic waves) with all of nature, are capable of feeling (or perceiving) other distant living bodies and events. From this, it is easy to understand that the will of one person can be communicated—by an inner sense—to the will of another."

The thing spread far and wide, as this sort of business does to-day, was taken up by imaginative writers like the physician-poet Justinus Kerner, who projected the mesmeric communication into the spirit world, into ghosts and creatures like "Margery's" brother, the brakeman. Finally, in 1815, in the hands of German professors, the movement developed into a "Christian Science," and Ennemoser, Windisschman, and others declared that all disease originated in sin, and what was needed was a *Christliche Heilkunde*. The French shook it off at this point, but in England a great physician of St. Thomas's Hospital and the physiologist Herbert Mayo swallowed it hook, bait, and sinker, until—as in some more recent cases—it was discovered that these learned gentlemen had had their legs pulled. It is almost a modern story.

It is not to be supposed that medicine stood still or receded during these years of speculation. Much practical progress was made. There were notable advances in obstetrical and surgical technique; there was sound progress in the botany of drugs; and, above all, the development of general anatomy was clearing the ground for pathology and physiology. Much exact anatomical observation had resulted from the studies of the Vitalists of Montpellier. A great deal had been added by others, notably by Galvani and the Italian school. Chemistry began to assume physiological significance through Lavoisier. Buffon and Linné had developed logical systems of nature.

Strangely enough, it was Bichat, pupil of Montpellier and convinced Vitalist, who was so far able to separate his theoretical prejudices from his observational precision that he became the actual founder of the modern conceptions of structure as the basis of function and thus, in his *Anatomie Générale,* made possible the immediate development of rational pathology and physiology. Bichat may be regarded as the most powerful single influence in the rise of the French school of clinicians which, by the middle of the nineteenth century, had become the most effective and intelligent medical group in the world.

THE
PRACTICE

Of the varieties of human experience, none are more compelling and vivid than those observed and described by physicians in the course of their everyday work. The doctor sees life at its extremes—not just in birth and death but in the heightened human interest it produces along the way.

Any branch of knowledge, in order to qualify as a science, must be able to discern its own errors. It is doubtful whether any science has recognized its errors more consistently than has medicine. Approaches, methods, and practices constantly change. It was only sixty years ago that key discoveries were made about insulin; only fifty years ago that sulfonamide drugs were introduced; only forty years ago that penicillin was used medically; only thirty years ago that psychotropic drugs altered the treatment of mental illness; only twenty-five years ago that polio vaccine began to save countless lives. And so it goes. But all these advances in the science of medicine serve mainly to dramatize the fact that the art of medicine remains essentially the same. The physician who has the confidence of the patient is not at a disadvantage alongside the physician who stays close to his science and maintains a discreet distance from patients.

LOUIS-FERDINAND CÉLINE
Journey to the End of the Night

⎯⎯⎯⎯⎯❦⎯⎯⎯⎯⎯

Molly had been right. I was beginning to understand what she meant. Studies change you, they make a man proud. Before, one was only hovering around life. You think you are a free man, but you get nowhere. Too much of your time's spent dreaming. You slither along on words. That's not the real thing at all. Only intentions and appearances. You need something else. With my medicine, though I wasn't very good at it, I had come into closer contact with men, beasts and creation. Now it was a question of pushing right ahead, foursquare, into the heart of things. Death comes chasing along after you, you've got to get a move on, and you have to find something to eat too, while you're searching, and dodge war as well. That makes an awful lot of things to do. It isn't easy.

*   *   *

They often kill guys around here, don't they?'' Bébert remarked. I crossed his puddle of dust but the municipal sweeper rumbled past at that moment and a great typhoon swirled up from the gutters, filling the whole street with even thicker and more peppery clouds of dust. You couldn't see a thing. Bébert skipped about with joy, sneezing and yelping. His haggard little face, his mop of greasy hair, his legs like an emaciated monkey's, all bobbed about convulsively at the end of his broom.

Bébert's aunt came back from shopping. She'd already had her little tot of something and she smelt slightly too of ether; that was a habit she'd picked up once when she worked for a doctor and had had such aches in her wisdom-teeth. She only had two teeth left in the front of her mouth but these she brushed assiduously. ''When you have worked for a doctor, like I have, you know what hygiene means.'' She gave medical consultations in the neighbourhood, and further afield, as far as Bezons.

I should have liked to know whether Bébert's aunt ever thought about anything. No, she didn't think at all. She talked a hell of a lot without thinking at all. When we were alone, with no possible eavesdroppers about, she would try to get free medical advice out of me. It was flattering, in a sort of way.

273

"Bébert, Doctor—I can tell you because you're a medical man—is a nasty, dirty little boy! He abuses himself. I've noticed it going on for two months now and I can't think who can have taught him such a loathsome habit. I've always brought him up well. . . . I tell him he mustn't. But he won't listen to me."

"Tell him he'll go mad," I said: classical advice.

Bébert, who was listening, wasn't a bit pleased. "I don't; it's not true. It was the Gagat kid who suggested I—"

"There you are, you see; I thought so," said his aunt. "You know the Gagats, the people on the fifth floor? They are a vicious family. It seems that the grandfather used to go in for flagellation. . . . Ugh, I ask you, flagellation! Look, Doctor, while we're on the subject, couldn't you make him out a syrup of some kind that would stop him playing with himself?"

I followed her into the lodge to prescribe an anti-vice tonic for little Bébert. Of course, I was too kind to every one, I realize that. No one ever paid me. I gave consultations on sight, chiefly out of curiosity. It's a mistake. People revenge themselves for the kindnesses you do them. Bébert's aunt, like all the rest, took advantage of my being so disinterested and proud, the most unfair advantage. I did nothing about it. I let myself be fooled. These sick people had me in their power, they snivelled more and more each day, they led me by the nose. And at the same time they showed me, one after another, all the horrible deformities hidden away in their hearts which they revealed to no one but me. Such hideousness cannot be adequately paid for. It slips through your fingers like a slimy snake.

I'll spill it all one day, if I can live long enough to tell everything. "Listen, you swine! Let me be nice to you for a few more years; don't kill me yet. Just look humble and helpless and I'll tell you everything. I promise you that. And you'll suddenly turn tail like those sticky caterpillars that used to crawl around my hut in Africa, and I will make you more cunningly cowardly and obscene than ever, so much so that at the last maybe you'll die of it."

"Is it sweet?" asked Bébert, meaning the syrup.

"For heaven's sake, don't make it sweet," the aunt said: "dirty little beast! He doesn't deserve it should be sweet, and anyway, he steals enough sugar from me as it is. He is thoroughly naughty, thoroughly depraved! He'll end up by murdering his mother!"

"I haven't got a mother," Bébert flatly retorted, knowing exactly what he was about.

"Hell!" said his aunt. "I'll lay across you with the broom handle, if you answer me back." She went and seized the broom, but Bébert had slipped out into the street. "You vicious old thing!" he shouted at her from the doorway. His aunt blushed and came back into the lodge. There was a silence. We changed the conversation.

"Doctor, perhaps you ought to go and see the lady at Number 4, Rue des Mineures. The husband used to work at the notary's office; he's been told about you. I said you were the kindest doctor in the world with ill people."

I knew at once that Bébert's aunt was going to lie to me. Frolichon is her favourite doctor. She always recommends him when she can, and me she invariably runs down if she gets the chance. My humanitarianism makes her hate me in a thoroughly animal way. After all, she is an animal; one mustn't forget that. Only Frolichon, whom she admires, makes her pay on the nail, so she consults me on the quiet. It must be an absolutely gratuitous visit for her to have recommended me, or else some extremely shady affair. But as I left, I remembered Bébert.

"You ought to take him for walks," I said; "the kid doesn't get out enough."

"Where could the two of us go? I can't stray far from my lodge."

"Well, take him to the Park on Sundays then."

"But the Park's even more full of people and dust than this place is! You're all on top of one another."

She's quite right in what she says. I think of somewhere else to suggest.

Timidly, I suggest the cemetery. The cemetery at Garenne-Rancy is the only place of any size in the whole neighbourhood where there are a few trees.

"Why, that's true, I hadn't thought of that; we could go there, of course!" At that moment Bébert reappeared.

So they left her to look after herself for a while in her hut. All the same, they insisted on showing me the old lady, by hook or by crook; that's what I had come for, and all sorts of subterfuges were necessary before she'd receive us. But I couldn't really make out what was wanted of me. Bébert's aunt, the concierge, had told them I was a nice doctor, a very kind and easy-going man. . . . They wanted to know if I could make the old woman keep quiet just by giving her some medicines to take. . . . But what they really wanted more, at bottom (particularly the daughter-in-law) was that I should get her shut up for them once and for all. . . .After we had knocked at her door for a good half hour, she finally flung it open suddenly, and popped out there in front of me, with her watery red eyes. . . . But a bright expression danced in them above her flaccid, grey cheeks, a lively glance which you noticed at once and which made you forget all the rest, because it was light and youthful and gave you a feeling of pleasure, in spite of yourself, and instinctively you found yourself trying to remember and retain something of it afterwards.

This gay glance of hers enlivened everything in the shadows round with something young and blithe about it, a minute but sparkling enthusiasm of a kind we no longer possess. Her voice, which was hoarse when she shouted, sounded sprightly and charming when she talked normally; then she made her words and her sentences frisk about and skip and come bouncing merrily back, as people could with their voices and everything in the days when not to be able to tell a story well or sing a song when necessary was considered feeble, deplorable and stupid.

Age had covered her, like an old, swaying tree, with jaunty branches.

She was a gay old Henrouille; discontented and grimy, yet gay. The bleakness she had lived in for more than twenty years had affected her spirit not at all. On the contrary, it was from the outside world that she had shrunk in self-defence, as if the growing cold and all the frightfulness and death itself were to come to her from there, not from inside. From inside herself she seemed to fear nothing. She seemed certain of her own head as of something definite and solid and understood, understood once and for all.

And there was I, always chasing after mine, chasing it all over the world.

Mad, they said she was, "mad"; it's easily said. She hadn't come out of her burrow more than three times in twelve years, that's all it was! Maybe she had her own reasons. . . . She didn't want to lose anything. . . . She wasn't going to tell *us* though, who wouldn't have been wise enough to understand her, anyway.

Her daughter harked back to her scheme of getting the old lady shut up. "Don't you think that she is mad, Doctor? We can't get her to go out. . . . And yet that would do her good occasionally. . . . Yes, Grandma, it would do you good, really it would. . . . Don't say that it wouldn't! I assure you it would do you good." The old woman shook her head, firmly, obstinately, angrily, when she was spoken to like that.

"She won't let us look after her properly. . . . The shed's in a filthy mess. It's cold in there and she hasn't a fire . . . Really, we can't have her going on living like that. We can't, can we, Doctor?"

I pretended not to understand. As for Henrouille, he had stayed behind by the stove; he preferred not to know exactly what we were all up to, his wife, his mother and me.

Then the old lady became angry again.

"Give me back all my belongings and I tell you I'll go away from here! I have enough to live on! You need never hear of me again! And we'll have done with all this once and for all."

"Enough to live on? But, Grandma, you'd never be able to get along on your three thousand francs a year, Grandma! Living has become much more expensive since the last time you went out. Wouldn't it be ever so much better, Doctor, if she were to go and live with the Sisters, as we tell her she should? The Sisters would look after her well. . . . They're so sweet and good.''

But the prospect of St. Vincent's horrified her.

''Me go to the Sisters? The Sisters?'' she rejoined at once. ''I've never been to them yet. . . . Why shouldn't I go to the curé while you're about it? Eh? If I haven't enough money, as you say, well then, I'll go to work again!''

''Work? Why, Grandmamma! Where will you work? Ah, Doctor, just listen to that! Work—at her age! When she's nearly eighty! That's madness, Doctor. Who would dream of taking her? You're mad, Grandma!''

''Mad! Nonsense! Not at all! But *you're* certainly wrong somewhere, you dirty little beast!''

''Listen to her, Doctor—raving and insulting me! How do you expect us to keep her here?''

Then the old lady turned to me, against me, her new danger.

''How does that man know whether I am mad or not? Is *he* inside my head? Or inside yours? Would he have to be to know? Clear out, both of you! Go away, leave my house! You are wickeder than a hell full of devils, the way you bully me! Why don't you go and see my son, instead of standing here, jabbering drivel among the weeds. . . . He needs a doctor far more than I do. He hasn't any teeth left, that son of mine, and he used to have such beautiful teeth when I looked after him. Go on, go on, get out, I tell you, the two of you!'' And she banged the door in our faces.

She peered out at us from behind her lamp, watching us go away up the court. When we had crossed it, when we were far enough away, she began to laugh. She had defended herself well.

On our return from this unpleasant expedition, Henrouille was still standing by the stove with his back turned to us. But his wife went on harrying me with questions, all of them with a single meaning. . . . She had a little round, dark head. She kept her elbows glued to her sides while she talked, making no gestures of any sort. But she was very keen that this visit of the doctor's should not be wasted, that it should serve some purpose. . . . The cost of living was going up every day. . . . The mother-in-law's contribution was no longer enough. . . . After all, they too were growing old. . . . They could not always live in fear of the old lady dying without proper care, as they had in the past. . . . Of her setting fire to the place, for example. . . . Of her dying amid fleas and filth like that. Instead of going to a nice, proper asylum, where they would look after her well. . . .

As I looked as if I agreed with them, they became even more amiable, both of them. . . . They promised to say a lot of nice things about me in the neighbourhood. . . . If I would only help them, take pity on them. Rid them of the old woman. . . . She must be so unhappy herself in the surroundings she so obstinately insisted on living in.

"And we might be able to let her cottage," the husband suggested, suddenly waking up. . . . A *faux pas,* talking like that in front of me. His wife trod on his foot under the table. He couldn't understand why.

While they wrangled, I thought of the thousand franc note I could so easily pocket just by signing that certificate of madness for them. They seemed to want it frightfully badly. . . . Bébert's aunt had probably told them all about me and explained that there wasn't another doctor in all Rancy in such miserable straits. . . . That I could be had for the asking. . . . Frolichon they wouldn't have offered a job like that to. Frolichon was straight, a virtuous man.

I was quite absorbed in these reflections when the old woman burst into the room where we sat plotting. You'd have said she had guessed as much. What a surprise! She had caught up her full skirts against her stomach and here she was, like that, suddenly letting fly at us and at me in particular. She had come from the bottom of her courtyard just for this.

"Blackguard!" she yelled straight at me. "You can go now, I've told you so already—get out! There's no point in your staying here. I'm not going to any madhouse, I tell you, and I won't go to the convent either! You can talk and lie as much as you like—you won't get *me,* you rascal! These rogues will go before me, these fleecers of an old woman! And you too, you scum, you'll go to gaol, let me tell you, and pretty damn quick!"

I was out of luck all right. Just when there was a thousand francs going begging at one fell swoop! I left at once.

When I was back in the street she leaned out over a little balcony to shout after me, far in the darkness that was hiding me. "You cad! You swine!" she yelled. The echoes rang with it. Damn the rain. I ran from one lamp-post to the next as far as the public convenience on the Place des Fêtes—the first shelter there was.

ANTON CHEKHOV
Letters

————✠————

ANTON CHEKHOV (1860-1904), Russia's best-loved dramatist, was a practicing physician who wrote stories and plays for both love and money. Many of his characters dream of a privileged past. They are frustrated in their inability to communicate with one another. This non-fiction selection, from his *Letters*, evokes the pathos of Siberian exile seen by Chekhov on a trip to a penal colony for a public health survey.

TO A. S. SUVORIN

Moscow, March 9, 1890
(The Feast of Forty Martyrs and of
Ten Thousand Larks)

Both of us are mistaken about Sakhalin, but you probably more than I. I am going there fully convinced that my trip will not result in any valuable contribution to either literature or science: I lack the knowledge, the time, and the pretensions for that. My plans are not those of a Humboldt or a Kennan,[1] I want to write one hundred to two hundred pages and thereby pay off some of my debt to medicine, toward which, as you know, I have behaved like a pig. Perhaps I shall not be able to write anything; nevertheless the journey does not lose its attraction for me: by reading, looking around and listening, I shall get to know and to learn a great deal. I haven't left yet, but thanks to the books that I have been obliged to read, I have learned much of what everyone should know under penalty of forty lashes, and of which I was formerly ignorant. Besides, I believe that the trip will mean six months of incessant work, physical and mental, and this I need, for I am a Khokhol[2] and have already begun to be lazy. One must keep in training. My trip may be a trifle, the result of obstinacy, a whim, but

[1] At the invitation of the Czar, Alexander von Humboldt explored Siberia in 1829; in the 1880s George E. Kennan made a thorough study of the Siberian penal system for *Century* magazine.
[2] Having been born in Taganrog, which lies on the border of Ukrainian territory, Chekhov sometimes called himself a Khokhol to account for his laziness, allegedly a southern characteristic. As a matter of fact, both his parents were of Great Russian stock.

279

consider and tell me what I lose by going. Time? Money? Shall I be undergoing privations? My time is worth nothing, money I never have anyway, as for privations. I shall travel by carriage not more than twenty-five to thirty days—and all the rest of the time I shall be sitting on the deck of a steamer or in a room and constantly bombarding you with letters.

Suppose the trip gives me absolutely nothing, still, won't the whole journey yield at least two or three days that I shall remember all my life, with rapture or with bitterness? And so on, and so on. That's how it is, sir. All this is unconvincing, but neither do your arguments convince me. You say, for instance, that Sakhalin is of no use and no interest to anybody. But is that so? Sakhalin can be of no use or interest only to a country that does not exile thousands of people there and does not spend millions on it. After Australia in the past and Cayenne,[3] Sakhalin is the only place where you can study colonization by criminals. All Europe is interested in it, and it is of no use to us? No longer ago than twenty-five or thirty years, our own compatriots in exploring Sakhalin performed amazing feats that make man worthy of deification, and yet that's of no use to us, we know nothing about those men, we sit within four walls and complain that God made a botch of man. Sakhalin is a place of unbearable sufferings, such as only human beings, free or bond, can endure. The men directly or indirectly connected with it solved terrible, grave problems and are still solving them. If I were sentimental—I am sorry I am not—I would say that to places like Sakhalin we should make pilgrimages, like the Turks who travel to Mecca, and navy men and criminologists in particular should regard Sakhalin as military men do Sevastopol. From the books I have been reading it is clear that we have let *millions* of people rot in prison, destroying them carelessly, thoughtlessly, barbarously; we drove people in chains through the cold across thousands of miles, infected them with syphilis, depraved them, multiplied criminals, and placed the blame for all this on red-nosed prison wardens. All civilized Europe knows now that it is not the wardens who are to blame, but all of us, yet this is no concern of ours, we are not interested. The vaunted '60s did *nothing* for the sick and the prisoners, thus violating the basic commandment of Christian civilization. In our time something is being done for the sick, but for prisoners nothing; prison problems don't interest our jurists at all. No, I assure you, we need Sakhalin, and it is important to us, and the only thing to be regretted is that I am the one to go

---

[3]The French deported convicts to Cayenne, and because of the high mortality, the place became known as "the dry guillotine."

there and not someone else who is better equipped for the task and is more capable of arousing public interest. As for me, I go after trifles.* * *

We have been having student riots on a large scale. They began at the Petrovsky Academy, where the authorities forbade the students to bring young women into their rooms, suspecting not only prostitution but also the political corruption of the girls. From the Academy the trouble spread to the university, where, now surrounded by heavily armed Hectors and Achilleses on horseback and with lances, the students make the following demands:

1. Complete autonomy of the universities.
2. Complete freedom of instruction.
3. Free admission to the universities without distinction of creed, nationality, sex, or social status.
4. Admission of Jews to the universities without any restrictions and granting them the same rights as other students.
5. Freedom of assemblage and recognition of student organizations.
6. Establishment of university and student tribunals.
7. Abolition of the police function of inspection.
8. Reduction of tuition.

I have copied this with some abbreviations from a proclamation. I think the fire is blazing strongest in a crowd of [. . .] of the sex which is eager to get admission to the University, while its preparation for this is five times as bad as that of the male, whose preparation is wretched and who, with rare exceptions, does miserably at the university.

* * * And now permit me out of respect for you to throw myself into an abyss and smash my head.

Your A. Chekhov

TO M. I. TCHAIKOVSKY

Moscow, March 16, 1890

Dear Modest Ilyich,
* * * I sit at home without venturing out and read about how much Sakhalin coal cost per ton in 1863 and the cost per ton of coal in Shanghai; I read about amplitudes and NE, NW, SE, and other winds which will be buffeting me as I observe my own seasickness near the shores of Sakhalin. I

read about soil and subsoil, about sandy clay and clayey sand. However, I haven't gone out of my mind yet, and yesterday I actually sent off a story to *New Times;* will send *The Wood-Sprite* to *The Northern Herald* shortly—will do so most unwillingly, since I don't like to see my plays in print.

In one and a half or two weeks my book[1]—the one I have dedicated to Pyotr Ilyich—will be coming out. I am ready to stand day and night as guard of honor near the entrance to the house where Pyotr Ilyich lives. In Yekaterinburg I received a telegram from Tyumen: "The first steamer from Tomsk leaves May 18." That meant that willy-nilly I had to race along in a carriage. I did so. I left Tyumen on May 3, having spent two or three days in Yekaterinburg, using them to repair my coughing and hemorrhoiding person.

Both post and private coachmen are available for travel in Siberia. I hired the latter: it was all the same to me. Your humble servant was placed in a wicker basket drawn by a pair of horses. You sit in this vehicle, look on God's world like a little siskin, without a thought in your head. The Siberian plain commences at Yekaterinburg and ends the devil knows where. I would say that it looks very much like our southern steppe, were it not for the small birch groves here and there and the cold wind pricking your cheeks. Spring hasn't arrived here as yet. There is no trace of greenery, the forests are bare, only some of the snow has melted, the lakes are under lackluster ice. On May 9, St. Nicholas' Day, there was a frost, and today, the 14th, there was a snowfall of over three inches. Only the ducks speak of spring. Oh, how many ducks! Never before in my life have I seen such a multitude of ducks. They fly over your head, flutter by the side of the carriage, swim in the ice holes of the lake and in puddles. In short, I could have shot a thousand of them in one day with a poor fowling-piece. Wild geese are heard honking. They too are numerous here. Files of cranes and swans often catch the eye. In the birch groves heathcocks and hazel-hens are seen flying. Hares, which are not shot and eaten here, stand up nonchalantly on their hind legs, with their ears pricked up, their eyes inquisitively following all comers. They run across the road so often that this is not considered a bad omen.

Traveling is a cold business. I have my sheepskin on. My body is comfortable, but my feet and legs are freezing. I wrap them in my leather overcoat, but it doesn't help. I am wearing two pairs of trousers. Well, you ride and ride. Mileposts flash by, puddles, birch groves. We pass tramping settlers, a file of convicts under guard. We have met vagabonds with pots

[1]*Gloomy People.*

on their backs; these gents roam the Siberian highway freely. On occasion they will do in an old woman in order to use her skirt for puttees, or they'll remove from a milepost a metal sign with a number on it, just on the chance that it may come in handy. Again, they will bash in the head of a beggar they meet or gouge out the eyes of their fellow deportee, but they won't touch a traveler. As far as robbery is concerned, travel hereabouts is entirely safe. From Tyumen to Tomsk neither the coachmen on the post vehicles nor the self-employed drivers can recall that anything has been stolen from a traveler. When you enter a station you leave your things in the courtyard; when you ask if they won't be stolen, the reply is a smile. It is even bad form to mention burglaries and murders on the highway. It seems to me that were I to lose my money at a station or in a vehicle, if the coachman found it, he would return it to me without fail, and wouldn't brag about the matter.

Generally speaking, people here are good, kindly, and with pleasing folkways. The rooms are tidy and the furniture simple, with some pretensions to luxury; the sleeping accommodations are soft, with featherbeds and big pillows; the floors are painted or covered with home-made linen rugs. All this is due to the general prosperity, to the fact that a family has an allowance of 43 acres of excellent black earth which produces rich crops of wheat (30 copecks is the price of 36 pounds of wheat flour). However, not everything is explained by material welfare, the people's way of life must not be overlooked. On entering a Siberian bedroom at night you are not assailed by the peculiar Russian stench. True, handing me a teaspoon, an old woman wiped it on her behind, but then they will not serve you tea without a tablecloth, people don't belch in your presence, don't search for insects in their hair; when they hand you water or milk, they don't put their fingers in the glass; the plates and dishes are clean, kvas is as transparent as beer. In sum, such cleanliness as there is here can be only dreamed of by the Khokhols, who are cleaner than Katzaps.[2] The bread they bake here is delicious; the first days I could not get my fill of it. Equally tasty are the pies, tarts, and turnovers; family bread resembles Ukrainian spongy rolls. Pancakes are thin. The rest of Siberian cookery is not for the European stomach.* * *

By evening the puddles and roads begin freezing and at night there is a full-fledged frost, calling for a fur coat. Brrr!

The mud having become hillocks, the carriage jolts, turning your innards inside out. By daybreak you are worn out by the cold, the bouncing, the jingling of the bells on the harness; you yearn for warmth and bed. While

---

[2]The familiar, somewhat derogatory name of the Great Russians.

the horses are being changed, you curl up in a corner and fall asleep immediately, but a minute later your coachman tugs at your sleeve and says, "Get up, friend, it's time!" On the second night I developed a sharp toothache in my heels. It was intolerable. I asked myself: aren't they frostbitten?

I can't go on writing. The district police officer has arrived. We get acquainted, start talking. Until tomorrow.

Tomsk, May 16

It was my jack boots that caused the pain in the heels. The backs are too narrow.* * * In Ishim I had to buy felt boots and traveled in them until they fell apart from dampness and mud.

Tea in the peasant hut in the small hours. On the road tea is a true blessing. Now I know its value and I drink it frantically. It warms you up, banishes sleep, you eat a lot of bread with it. You sip it, and you talk with the peasant women, who are sensible, fond of children, kind-hearted, diligent, and freer than they are in Europe. Their husbands do not scold and beat them because they are as tall and strong and intelligent as their masters. When their husbands are absent, the women do the driving. They like punning. The children are pampered and allowed to sleep long hours. They take tea and eat with the adults, and repay it in kind if the latter tease them.

There is diphtheria. Smallpox is widespread, but, oddly enough, it is not as infectious as it is elsewhere; two or three patients will die—and that's the end of the epidemic. There are no hospitals or doctors. The sick are treated by male nurses. Bloodletting and cupping are practiced on a grandiose, brutal scale. On the road I examined a Jew with cancer of the liver. He was emaciated and scarcely breathing, but this did not prevent the nurse from placing twelve cupping glasses on him. By the way, a word about the Jews. Here they till the soil, work as coachmen, run ferryboats, trade, and are called peasants, because they are peasants *de jure* and *de facto*. They are universally respected and, according to the police officer, are not rarely elected village elders. I saw a tall, lean Jew scowling with distaste and spitting when the policeman was telling risqué stories, an undefiled soul; his wife cooked a delicious fish soup. The wife of the Jew with cancer regaled me with pike roe and excellent white bread. Exploitation by Jews is unheard of. I might as well say something about the Poles. Some of them are exiles, deported from Poland after 1864. They are kind, hospitable, and most urbane people. Some of them are well-to-do, others are poor and work as clerks at the stations. At Ishim, for an excellent dinner and a room where I had a good sleep I paid one ruble to Pan Zaleski, a Polish nobleman who kept a tavern. A conscienceless moneygrubber to the marrow of his bones, the table he set, his manners, were those of a gentleman.* * *

Would you like me to tell you something about the Tartars, too? Here you are. There are not many of them here. Good people. In the Kazan province even priests speak well of them, and in Siberia they are "better than the Russians"—that's what I was told by the police officer in the presence of Russians, who confirmed this opinion by silence. My God, how rich Russia is in good people! Were it not for the cold that robs Siberia of the summer, and were it not for the officials who corrupt the peasants and the exiles, Siberia would be the richest and happiest land.* * *

During the first three days of my journey my collarbones, shoulders, vertebrae, and coccyx began to ache, what with the shaking and jolting. There was no sitting, walking, lying down. To make up for all that, my headaches and chest pains vanished, my appetite grew beyond belief, and the hemorrhoids modestly effaced themselves. The tension, the exertion of lifting heavy luggage, and perhaps also the farewell drinking parties in Moscow made me spit blood in the morning, and this caused me to be despondent and exposed me to dismal thoughts. All this ceased by the end of the trip; it's a long time since I have coughed as little as now, after a fortnight spent outdoors. Indeed, after the first three days on the road my body grew used to the jolts, and the time came when I stopped noticing how morning gave way to midday, followed in its turn by evening and night. The days flashed by rapidly, as in a lingering illness. You think that morning has not gone yet, but the driver advises me to stay overnight, to avoid losing the way in the dark. And indeed, I glance at the watch and find that it's past 7 P.M.

The driving is fast, though less so in spring than in winter. Uphill the horses go at a gallop, and before the coachman is seated on his box and the carriage leaves the courtyard, it takes two or three men to hold the horses. They resemble those used by Moscow firemen. On one occasion we almost ran over several old women, another time we all but dashed into a file of prisoners.

Now here is an adventure that I owe to Siberian driving. Only I beg Mamasha not to "oh" and "ah" and lament, because it all ended happily. In the small hours of May 6 a very nice old man was driving me in my tarantas drawn by a pair of horses. I was drowsy and, having nothing to do, watched snakelike flames sparkling in the fields and the birch groves: it was the burning of last year's grass, which is set on fire here. Suddenly I hear a drumming noise of wheels. A posting station troika is dashing at top speed, heading for us like a bird. My old man hastens to turn right and the troika flies past us, and in the uncertain light I make out someone driving a huge, heavy coach. It is followed by another coach also going at full speed. We hasten to turn right. . . . To my bewilderment and horror, it turns not right, but left. I barely have time to think. "My God, we'll collide!" when a terrible crash is heard, the horses tangle, a dark mass, the yokes fall, my carriage rears up, and I am on the ground with my luggage on top of me. But that is not all. A third troika is bearing down on us. In the natural course of events, this last troika should have crushed me and smashed my bags, but God be praised. I was not asleep, broke no bones in tumbling and jumped up so fast that I was able to yell "Stop!" at the third troika. It came to a halt, but not before it had landed into the other. . . . Of course, if I had been asleep in my carriage, or if the third coach had followed hard on the second, I would have returned home either an invalid or a headless horseman. Results of the collision: broken shafts, torn harness, yokes and baggage scattered on the ground, dazed, wornout horses, the thought of a narrow escape. It appears that the first driver had lashed his horses, but the drivers of the other two troikas were asleep and their horses just followed the first coach. Having recovered from the stupefaction, my old man and the other three drivers engaged in ferocious cursing. Oh, how they cursed! I thought it would come to blows. You cannot imagine how alone I felt in the midst of this savage, cursing horde, in the field, before dawn, within sight of fires near and far consuming the grass but failing to warm the cold night air even slightly. Oh, how oppressive it was! You hear the cursing, look at the broken shafts and at your smashed luggage, and it seems to you that you are in another world, and that you will be trampled to bits. . . . After an hour's cursing my old man began to tie the shafts and the harness together with a little rope—my belt came in handy. Somehow we dragged ourselves to the station, halting now and then.

Early in the morning there was a downpour with a high wind. It rained day and night. I put on my leather overcoat, which protected me from rain and wind. A wonderful overcoat. The mud became unconquerable. Coachmen were reluctant to drive at night. But what was worst and what I shall not forget my whole life was fording the river at night. The coachman and you begin to shout. Rain, wind, ice floes crawl downstream, splashing is heard. . . . Suddenly, joy: a bittern calls. These birds inhabit the shores of Siberian waterways. Seemingly, geography means more to them than climate. Well, an hour later, there appears a huge ferry, shaped like a barge, with enormous oars resembling lobster claws. Ferrymen are nasty folk, mostly deportees, sent here for vicious behavior, by order of the peasant communes to which they belong. Unbearably foul-mouthed, they shout and beg money for vodka. The crossing is slow, intolerably so! The ferry crawls. . . . Again a sense of aloneness, and the bittern seems to call on purpose, as if to say, "Don't be afraid, uncle, I am here. The Lintvarevs sent me here from the shores of the Psel."

On May 7 a private coachman whom I asked for horses said that the Irtysh had flooded the fields, that yesterday Kuzma, having driven out, was barely able to return, and that it was necessary to wait. I ask: how long? The answer is: the Lord knows.* * * Well, suspecting that the Irtysh flood was invented only so as not to drive me at night through the mud, I protested and ordered the horses to be hitched up. The peasant, who had heard about the flood from Kuzma and had not seen it himself, scratched his head and agreed; the old drivers encouraged him, saying that in their youth they had feared nothing. We are off. . . . Mud, rain, fierce wind, cold, and I am wearing felt boots. Do you know what such boots are when wet? They are made of jelly. We drive on and on, and before my eyes there stretches a vast lake dotted with tiny islands, and with small bushes sticking out here and there—the flooded meadows. Far off there is the steep opposite shore of the Irtysh, white with snow. . . . We begin to make our way across the lake. What prevented me from turning back was stubbornness and an incomprehensible daring ardor, the same ardor that made me jump from a yacht to bathe in the Black Sea, and indulge in not a few other follies. Perhaps a psychotic attack. We drive, selecting islets and strips of land. The direction of the road is indicated by the washed-out bridges. To drive along the strips of land it is necessary to lead the horses one by one. The coachman unhitches them and I jump into the water in my felt boots and hold on to the horses. Entertaining! With it all, rain and wind . . . save us, Queen of Heaven! Finally we reach an island with a roofless hut on it. Wet horses wandering over wet manure. A peasant with a long stick comes out of the hut and undertakes to guide us. He measures the depth of the water with the stick and tests the ground. May God give him health, he led us to a long tongue of land that he called a "ridge" and told us to turn right or left—I don't remember which—to reach another ridge. We followed his advice.

We're driving on. . . . The felt boots are as wet as a latrine. They squelch, my socks blow their noses. The coachman is silent, and clicks his tongue despondently. He would gladly drive back, but it's too late, darkness is falling. . . . Finally, oh joy! We reach the Irtysh. The bank is gullied, slippery, disgusting, not a trace of vegetation; muddy water with whitecaps lashes it and angrily jumps back as though averse to touch a bank that apparently can only be inhabited by toads and the souls of murderers. The river neither booms nor roars, but it seems as though on its bed it were knocking on coffins. A damnable impression! The other bank is steep, brown, barren.

A hut occupied by ferrymen. One of them comes out and announces that the weather is too bad for the ferry to leave. The river is wide, he says, and the wind high. And so I had to spend the night in the hut. I remember the night, the snoring of the ferrymen and of my driver, the howling of the wind, the drumbeat of the rain, the growling of the Irtysh.* * *

In the morning they would not ferry me because of the wind. We crossed the river in a rowboat. The rain lashes, the wind blows, the baggage is soaked; the felt boots, which at night were drying on the stove, again turn to jelly. Oh, my dear leather overcoat! If I didn't catch cold, I owe this to it alone. When I come home, rub it with suet or castor oil. Once ashore, I sat on my luggage a whole hour waiting for horses, which were to be brought up from the village. I remember how slippery it was climbing up the bank. In the village I warmed up and had tea. The deportees came to beg alms. Every day each family in the village leavens a pood of wheaten flour to bake bread for the deportees. It is a kind of tax.

The deportees take the bread and barter it for vodka. One of them, a raggedy, shaven old man, whose eyes had been gouged out by his fellow deportees in a tavern, having heard that a traveler was in the house and taking me for a merchant, began reciting and chanting prayers. He chanted prayers for health and for the repose of the dead, and an Easter canticle. What didn't he chant! Then he started lying to the effect that he came from a merchant family in Moscow. I noticed the contempt in which this boozer held the peasants on whom he sponged.

On the 11th I obtained post horses. Out of boredom I read the complaint books at the stations. I made a discovery that struck: the entries of the postal stations are provided with privies. They are invaluable in damp and rainy weather. Oh, you can't appreciate this!

On the 12th they would not let me have any horses. I was told that travel was impossible, since the Ob was in flood and had inundated the meadowland. I was advised to take a side road to Krasnyi Yar, thence to go by rowboat to Dubrovino, where post horses would be available. I started for Krasnyi Yar with horses hired from a private coachman. I reach it in the morning and am told that there is a rowboat, but that I shall have to wait a while, because grandfather had sent a workman off in it to row the district policeman's clerk to Dubrovino. Well, I'll wait. One hour passes, a second hour, a third. . . . Noon comes, evening. . . . *Allah kerim,* how much tea did I drink, how much bread did I eat, how many thoughts did I think! And how long I slept! Night comes, then dawn, no boat. Finally the workman returns in the boat at 9 o'clock. We're off. Thank heaven! How smoothly we move! There is no wind, the rowers are skilled, the islands we pass beautiful. The flood had caught cattle and people off guard. And I see peasant women going out in boats to the islands to milk the cows. These cows are lean, despondent; because of the cold there is no fodder at all to be had.

We covered eight miles. At the Dubrovino posthouse I had tea and with it was served—just imagine!—waffles. The woman who runs the place must be a deportee or the wife of one. At the next station the clerk, an old Pole, to whom I gave antipyrin to relieve his headache, complained of his poverty and told me that Count Saphieha, Chamberlain of the Court of Austria and a Pole, who helped Poles, had recently passed through Siberia. "He stopped near this station," the clerk told me, "but I never knew it! Holy Mother of God! He would have helped me. I wrote to him in Vienna, but got no reply—" and so on. Why am I not Sapieha? I would send this poor fellow back to his native land.

On May 14 I was again refused horses. The Tom is in flood. What a nuisance! Not a nuisance, but a calamity! Tomsk thirty-five miles away, and then this, so unexpectedly! In my place a woman would have burst into sobs. Some kind folks found a way out for me: "You go as far as the Tom, Your Honor—it's only four miles from here; there they'll row you across to Yar, and from there Ilya Markovich will drive you to Tomsk." I hire a private coach and go to the Tom, to the spot where the boat ought to be. I drive up: no boat. It has just gone off with the mail and isn't likely to come back soon, since there's a gale blowing. I begin my wait. The ground is covered with snow, the rain is mixed with granulated snow, and then there's the wind. . . . An hour passes, then another, no boat. Fate is mocking me! I go back to the station. Here three troikas and a postman are getting ready to set out in the direction of the Tom. I tell them there is no boat. They remain. Fate rewards me: the clerk, in answer to my hesitant query as to the chances of getting a bite to eat, tells me that the stationmaster's wife has cabbage soup. Oh rapture! Oh, most radiant day! And the woman's daughter actually brings me excellent cabbage soup, with wonderful meat, roast potatoes, and a cucumber. I have not dined so well since the meal I had at Pan Zaleski's inn. Having downed the victuals, I went the limit and made coffee for myself. A spree!

At dusk the mailman, an elderly fellow, who had obviously been through thick and thin and who dared not sit in my presence, started getting ready to drive to the Tom. So did I. We were off. As soon as we reāched the river, an incredibly long boat came into view. While the mail was being loaded onto the boat I witnessed a strange phenomenon: thunder, and at the same time snow and a cold wind. We finished loading and cast off. Sweet Misha, forgive me for being glad that I didn't take you with me! How clever I was not to have taken anyone with me! At first our boat moved over the meadow close to shrub willows. As often happens before or during a storm, a gust of wind suddenly swept over the water, raising mighty waves. The boatman seated at the rudder thought that we should weather the storm among the willow shrubs, but others disagreed, saying that if the storm grew more violent, we would spend the night in the shrubs and drown anyway. The matter was put to a vote and it was decided to move on. My ill luck that so mocks me! What was the point of all these jokes? The men were rowing silently, concentrating on their task. . . . I remember the figure of the mailman, who had had such a tough time. I remember a soldier who suddenly turned as purple as cherry juice. . . . The thought flashed through my mind that if the boat should capsize, I would first of all jettison my sheepskin and my leather overcoat—then the felt boots, then, etc. But now the shore looms closer and closer. . . . You relax more and more, the heart contracts with joy, you take a deep breath as though you have suddenly finished a heavy task, and you jump onto the wet, slippery bank. . . . Thank God!

At Ilya Markovich's we are told that the road is too bad for driving after dark and that we must stay the night. Well, I do. After tea I sit down to go on writing this letter, interrupted by the arrival of the police officer. He is a thick mixture of Nozdryov, Khlestakov,[3] and dog. He is a drunkard, a lecher, a liar, a singer, a raconteur, and with all that a goodhearted fellow. He brought with him a large chest stuffed with dossiers, a bed with a mattress, a gun, and a clerk. The clerk is an intellectual who studied in Petersburg, a fine, outspoken liberal, a man with nothing against him, who got to Siberia for some unknown reason, infected to the marrow of his bones with all diseases, owing his alcoholism to his superior, who called him Kolya. The man in power sends for a cordial. "Doctor!" he yells. "Drink another glass and I'll bow down at your feet!" Of course, I drink. The man in power guzzles mightily, lies recklessly, indulges shamelessly in ribaldry. We go to bed. In the morning they again send for liquor. They swill vodka till 10 o'clock, and finally we leave. Ilya Markovich, the convert, whom the peasants here worship gives me horses to take me as far as Tomsk.

[3]The bully in Gogol's *Dead Souls,* and the braggart in his *Inspector General,* respectively.

I, the police officer, and the clerk got into one carriage. As long as we were together on the road the police officer was telling whoppers, swilling liquor from a bottle, bragging that he did not take bribes, admiring nature, and shaking his fist at the tramps we passed. After covering ten miles, we halted at the village of Brovkino. . . . We stopped at a Jew's shop and stepped down for a "rest." He ran to get liquor, his wife cooked the soup I have already mentioned. The police officer called for his two village subalterns and the local road contractor, and in his drunken state began giving them a tongue-lashing, not embarrassed in the slightest by my presence. He swore like a Tartar.

I soon parted company with the police officer and his clerk and reached Tomsk the evening of May 15. You can judge what the road was like from the fact that in the last two days I covered only some fifty miles.

Tomsk is sunk in mud. About that city and the life there I'll write you shortly. Meanwhile farewell.* * * I embrace, kiss, and bless you all.

Your A. Chekhov

P.S. Forgive me that this letter is like vinaigrette sauce. Incoherent. What could I do? Sitting in a hotel room, one couldn't do better. Excuse with smugglers of gold—isn't this interesting? I run to board the *Yermak*. Good-bye. Thanks for the news of your family.

Your A. Chekhov

TO A. S. SUVORIN
Aboard the Baikal, *Tartar Strait,*
September 11, 1890

Greetings!

I am sailing through the Tartar Strait, from North Sakhalin to South Sakhalin. I am writing this letter without knowing when it will reach you. I am well, even though I have staring at me from every direction the green eyes of cholera, which has set a trap for me. In Vladivostok, Japan, Shanghai, Chefoo, Suez, and, it seems, even on the moon—cholera everywhere, everywhere quarantines and fear. Sakhalin is expecting cholera and vessels are quarantined. In short, it's a bad business. There are Europeans dying in Vladivostok; one of the deaths, incidentally, was that of a general's lady.

I lived on North Sakhalin for exactly two months. I was received with extraordinary courtesy by the local administration, even though Galkin[1] hadn't written a single word about me. Neither Galkin, nor Baroness Muskrat,[2] nor the other geniuses whom I was foolish enough to turn to for help, rendered me any help whatsoever; it became necessary to act at my own risk.

General Kononovich, the administrator of Sakhalin, is an educated and decent fellow. We hit the right note quickly enough and everything went well. I'll bring back certain papers showing you that the circumstances in which I was placed from the very beginning were most propitious. I saw *everything;* ergo, the question no longer consists of *what* I saw but *how* I saw it.

I don't know what I'll wind up with, but what I have done is not a little. It would suffice for three dissertations. I got up daily at five in the morning, went to bed late, and all my days were passed under the severe pressure of the thought that there was still a great deal that I had not done; but now that I have finished with penal servitude I have the feeling that apparently I saw everything but failed to notice the elephant.

Incidentally, I had the patience to take a census of the entire population of Sakhalin. I made the circuit of all the settlements, stopped in at all the huts and talked with all and sundry; in taking the census I employed a card system, and I have already recorded about ten thousand convicts and settlers. In other words, there is not a solitary convict or settler who hasn't had a talk with me. I was particularly successful with a census of the children and am pinning quite a few hopes on it.

I had dinner with Landsberg,[3] I sat in ex-Baroness Hembruck's[4] "kitchen." . . . I called on all the celebrities. I was present at a flogging, and for three or four nights afterward I dreamt of the executioner and the revolting "mare."[5] I had talks with those whose chains were forged to their wheelbarrows. Once, when I was having tea down in a mine, Borodavkin, a quondam merchant from St. Petersburg, deported here for

---

[1]Mikhail Nikolayevich Galkin-Vrasky, head of the Main Prison Board. On January 26, 1890, Chekhov petitioned him for assistance with his visit to Sakhalin for "scientific and literary purposes." The Sakhalin administration granted him the freedom of the island, but he was strictly forbidden to have any contact with political prisoners. Galkin, on his part, not only failed to give Chekhov the help for which he petitioned, but tried to interfere with the publication of his book on Sakhalin.

[2]In Russian, *Vykhukhol,* Chekhov's jesting reference to Baroness Ikskul von Hildeband.

[3]Karl Khristoforovich Landsberg, a convict, formerly an officer of the Guard.

[4]A convict.

[5]A board to which a man to be flogged was tied.

arson, took a teaspoon out of his pocket and proffered it to me. But, in sum, my nerves were shattered and I have vowed not to take any more trips to Sakhalin.

I would write you more, if it weren't for a lady who is sitting in the cabin and laughing loudly and chattering away with no let-up. I haven't the strength to write. She has been behaving this way since last evening. . . .* * *

Tomorrow from afar I shall see Japan, the island Matsmai. It is now midnight. The sea is blacked out, a wind is blowing. I don't understand how the steamer can navigate through the pitch darkness in the wild, little-known waters of the Tartar strait.

When I recall that I am separated from the world by more than sixty-five hundred miles I am overcome by apathy. It seems to me that it will take a hundred years for me to get home.* * *

Your A. Chekhov

It's tedious.

TO A. F. KONI[1]

Petersburg, January 26, 1891

Gracious sir, Anatoly Fyodorovich!

* * * My brief Sakhalin past appears to me so huge that when I want to talk about it, I do not know with what to begin, and every time it seems to me I don't say what should be said.

I shall try to describe in detail the condition of the Sakhalin children and adolescents. It is extraordinary. I saw hungry children, thirteen-year-old girls who were prostitutes, fifteen-year-old pregnant girls. Girls start in as prostitutes at the age of twelve, sometimes before menstruation. Church and school exist only on paper, it is the convict environment, the convict set-up that shape the children. Among other things I set down a conversation with a ten-year-old boy. I was taking a census in Upper Armudan, a village: the settlers are one and all beggars and have the reputation of desperate card players. I come into a hut; no one at home but a white-

---

[1]A. F. Koni (1844-1927), a jurist and public figure of the liberal persuasion, counted Turgenev, among other literary men, as a friend, and was himself a writer.

haired, hunched, barefoot little boy sitting on a bench. He is deep in thought about something. We start a conversation:

I: What's your father's name?

He: Don't know.

I: How is that? You live with your father and don't know his name? Shame.

HE: He isn't my real father.

I: What do you mean: not real?

HE: He just lives with Ma.

I: Is your mother married or a widow?

HE: A widow. She came because of him.

I: Because—What does it mean: because of him?

HE: Killed.

I: You remember your father?

HE: No. I'm unlawful. I was born in Kara.[1]

One of my fellow passengers on the steamer that took me to Sakhalin was a prisoner in leg irons who had killed his wife. With him was his daughter, a child of about six. I noticed that when the father was going down from the upper deck to where a latrine was located he was followed by several soldiers, and his daughter. While the prisoner was in the latrine, a soldier carrying a rifle stood at the door with the little girl. When the prisoner, returning, walked up the stairs, she climbed behind him, holding on to his fetters. At night the little girl slept in a heap with the prisoners and the soldiers.

I remember that when I was in Sakhalin I attended a funeral. The wife of a settler who had gone to Nikolayevsk was being buried. At the freshly dug grave stood four convict porters—ex officio, I and a local official who wandered through the cemetery in the capacity of Hamlet and Horatio, a Circassian who had roomed with the deceased, also a woman convict: out of pity she had brought the dead woman's two children—one an infant, the other a four-year-old boy by the name of Alyosha. He wore a woman's jacket and blue pants with bright patches on the knees. Cold, damp, water in the grave, the convicts laugh. The sea is within sight. Alyosha peers into the grave with curiosity; he wants to wipe his chilled nose but the long sleeves of his jacket interfere. When the grave is filled up, I ask him, "Alyoshka, where is Ma?" He waves his hand like a landowner who has lost his money gambling, laughs, and says, "Shovelled under."

The convicts laugh; the Circassian turns to us and asks what he should do with the children—he is not obliged to feed them.

[1]An infamous gold-mining district.

I did not find any contagious diseases in Sakhalin; there is very little inherited syphilis, but I saw blind children, filthy, covered with sores—all conditions caused by negligence.

Of course, I shall not settle the problem of the children. I do not know what should be done. It seems to me that charity and remnants of sums allotted to prisons and the like will not do. I believe it is wrong to rely on philanthropy, which in Russia is fortuitous, and on remnants which don't materialize. I prefer the State Treasury.* * *

Allow me to thank you for your cordiality and for your promise to visit me, and also to remain

Yours sincerely, respectfully, and devotedly,

A. Chekhov

OLIVER WENDELL HOLMES
*The Young Practitioner**

———— ❧ ————

The occasion which calls us together reminds us not a little of that other ceremony which unites a man and woman for life. The banns have already been pronounced which have wedded our young friends to the profession of their choice. It remains only to address to them some friendly words of cheering counsel, and to bestow upon them the parting benediction.

This is not the time for rhetorical display or ambitious eloquence. We must forget ourselves, and think only of them. To us it is an occasion; to them it is an epoch. The spectators at the wedding look curiously at the bride and bridegroom; at the bridal veil, the orange-flower garland, the giving and receiving of the ring; they listen for the tremulous "I will," and wonder what are the mysterious syllables the clergyman whispers in the ear of the married maiden. But to the newly-wedded pair what meaning in those words, "for better, for worse," "in sickness and in health," "till death us do part!" To the father, to the mother, who knows too well how often the deadly nightshade is interwoven with the wreath of orange-blossoms, how empty the pageant, how momentous the reality!

You will not wonder that I address myself chiefly to those who are just leaving academic life for the sterner struggle and the larger tasks of matured and instructed manhood. The hour belongs to them; if others find patience to listen, they will kindly remember that, after all, they are but as the spectators at the wedding, and that the priest is thinking less of them than of their friends who are kneeling at the altar.

I speak more directly to you, then, gentlemen of the graduating class. The days of your education, as pupils of trained instructors, are over. Your first harvest is all garnered. Henceforth you are to be sowers as well as reapers, and your field is the world. How does your knowledge stand to-day?

What have you gained as a permanent possession? What must you expect to forget? What remains for you yet to learn? These are questions which it may interest you to consider.

* A Valedictory Address delivered to the Graduating Class of the Bellevue Hospital College, March 2, 1871.

There is another question which must force itself on the thoughts of many among you: "How am I to obtain patients and to keep their confidence?" You have chosen a laborious calling, and made many sacrifices to fit yourselves for its successful pursuit. You wish to be employed that you may be useful, and that you may receive the reward of your industry. I would take advantage of these most receptive moments to give you some hints which may help you to realize your hopes and expectations. Such is the outline of the familiar talk I shall offer you.

Your acquaintance with some of the accessory branches is probably greater now than it will be in a year from now,—much greater than it will be ten years from now. The progress of knowledge, it may be feared, or hoped, will have outrun the text-books in which you studied these branches. Chemistry, for instance, is very apt to spoil on one's hands. "*Nous avons changé tout celà*" might serve as the standing motto of many of our manuals. Science is a great traveller, and wears her shoes out pretty fast, as might be expected.

You are now fresh from the lecture-room and the laboratory. You can pass an examination in anatomy, physiology, chemistry, materia medica, which the men in large practice all around you would find a more potent sudorific than any in the Pharmacopoeia. These masters of the art of healing were once as ready with their answers as you are now, but they have got rid of a great deal of the less immediately practical part of their acquisitions, and you must undergo the same depleting process. Hard work will train it off, as sharp exercise trains off the fat of a prize-fighter.

Yet, pause a moment before you infer that your teachers must have been in fault when they furnished you with mental stores not directly convertible to practical purposes, and likely in a few years to lose their place in your memory. All systematic knowledge involves much that is not practical, yet it is the only kind of knowledge which satisfies the mind, and systematic study proves, in the long-run, the easiest way of acquiring and retaining facts which are practical. There are many things which we can afford to forget, which yet it was well to learn. Your mental condition is not the same as if you had never known what you now try in vain to recall. There is a perpetual metempsychosis of thought, and the knowledge of to-day finds a soil in the forgotten facts of yesterday. You cannot see anything in the new season of the guano you placed last year about the roots of your climbing plants, but it is blushing and breathing fragrance in your trellised roses; it has scaled your porch in the bee-haunted honey-suckle; it has found its way where the ivy is green; it is gone where the woodbine expands its luxuriant foliage.

Your diploma seems very broad to-day with your list of accomplishments, but it begins to shrink from this hour like the Peau de Chagrin of Balzac's story. Do not worry about it, for all the while there will be making out for you an ampler and fairer parchment, signed by old Father Time himself as President of that great University in which experience is the one perpetual and all-sufficient professor.

Your present plethora of acquirements will soon cure itself. Knowledge that is not wanted dies out like the eyes of the fishes of the Mammoth Cave. When you come to handle life and death as your daily business, your memory will of itself bid good-by to such inmates as the well-known foramina of the sphenoid bone and the familiar oxides of methyl-ethyl-amyl-phenyl-ammonium. Be thankful that you have once known them, and remember that even the learned ignorance of a nomenclature is something to have mastered, and may furnish pegs to hang facts upon which would otherwise have strewed the floor of memory in loose disorder.

But your education has, after all, been very largely practical. You have studied medicine and surgery, not chiefly in books, but at the bedside and in the operating amphitheatre. It is the special advantage of large cities that they afford the opportunity of seeing a great deal of disease in a short space of time, and of seeing many cases of the same kind of disease brought together. Let us not be unjust to the claims of the schools remote from the larger centres of population.

*   *   *

I am afraid we do not always do justice to our country brethren, whose merits are less conspicuously exhibited than those of the great city physicians and surgeons, such especially as have charge of large hospitals. There are modest practitioners living in remote rural districts who are gifted by nature with such sagacity and wisdom, trained so well in what is most essential to the practice of their art, taught so thoroughly by varied experience, forced to such manly self-reliance by their comparative isolation, that, from converse with them alone, from riding with them on their long rounds as they pass from village to village, from talking over cases with them, putting up their prescriptions, watching their expedients, listening to their cautions, marking the event of their predictions, hearing them tell of their mistakes, and now and then glory a little in the detection of another's blunder, a young man would find himself better fitted for his real work than many who have followed long courses of lectures and passed a showy examination. But the young man is exceptionally fortunate who enjoys the intimacy of such a teacher. And it must be confessed that the great hospitals, infirmaries, and dispensaries of large cities, where men of well-sifted reputations are in constant attendance, are the true centres of medical education. No students, I believe, are more thoroughly aware of this than those who have graduated at this institution. Here, as in all our larger city schools, the greatest pains are taken to teach things as well as names. You have entered into the inheritance of a vast amount of transmitted skill and wisdom, which you have taken, warm, as it were, with the life of your well-schooled instructors. You have not learned all that art has to teach you, but you are safer practitioners to-day than were many of those whose names we hardly mention without a genuflection. I had rather be cared for in a fever by the best-taught among you than by the renowned Fernelius or the illustrious Boerhaave, could they come back to us from that better world where there are no physicians needed, and, if the old adage can be trusted, not many within call. I had rather have one of you exercise his surgical skill upon me than find myself in the hands of a resuscitated Fabricius Hildanus, or even of a wise Ambroise Paré, revisiting earth in the light of the nineteenth century.

You will not accuse me of underrating your accomplishments. You know what to do for a child in a fit, for an alderman in an apoplexy, for a girl that has fainted, for a woman in hysterics, for a leg that is broken, for an arm that is out of joint, for fevers of every color, for the sailor's rheumatism, and the tailor's cachexy. In fact you do really know so much at this very hour, that nothing but the searching test of time can fully teach you the limitations of your knowledge.

Of some of these you will permit me to remind you. You will never have outgrown the possibility of new acquisitions, for Nature is endless in her variety. But even the knowledge which you may be said to possess will be a different thing after long habit has made it a part of your existence. The *tactus eruditus* extends to the mind as well as to the finger-ends. Experience means the knowledge gained by habitual trial, and an expert is one who has been in the habit of trying. This is the kind of knowledge that made Ulysses wise in the ways of men. Many cities had he seen, and known the minds of those who dwelt in them. This knowledge it was that Chaucer's Shipman brought home with him from the sea:

"In many a tempest had his berd be shake."

This is the knowledge we place most confidence in, in the practical affairs of life.

Our training has two stages. The first stage deals with our intelligence, which takes the idea of what is to be done with the most charming ease and readiness. Let it be a game of billiards, for instance, which the marker is going to teach us. We have nothing to do but to make this ball glance from that ball and hit that other ball, and to knock that ball with this ball into a certain caecal *sacculus* or *diverticulum* which our professional friend calls a pocket. Nothing can be clearer; it is as easy as "playing upon this pipe," for which Hamlet gives Guildenstern such lucid directions. But this intelligent *Me,* who steps forward as the senior partner in our dual personality, turns out to be a terrible bungler. He misses those glancing hits which the hard-featured young professional person calls "carroms," and insists on pocketing his own ball instead of the other one.

It is the *un*intelligent *Me,* stupid as an idiot, that has to try a thing a thousand times before he can do it, and then never knows how he does it, that at last does it well. We have to educate ourselves through the pretentious claims of intellect, into the humble accuracy of instinct, and we end at last by acquiring the dexterity, the perfection, the certainty, which those masters of arts, the bee and the spider, inherit from Nature.

Book-knowledge, lecture-knowledge, examination-knowledge, are all in the brain. But work-knowledge is not only in the brain, it is in the senses, in the muscles, in the ganglia of the sympathetic nerves,—all over the man, as one may say, as instinct seems diffused through every part of those lower animals that have no such distinct organ as a brain. See a skilful surgeon handle a broken limb; see a wise old physician smile away a case that looks to a novice as if the sexton would soon be sent for; mark what a large experience has done for those who were fitted to profit by it, and you will feel convinced that, much as you know, something is still left for you to learn.

*   *   *

New ideas build their nests in young men's brains. "Revolutions are not made by men in spectacles," as I once heard it remarked, and the first whispers of a new truth are not caught by those who begin to feel the need of an ear-trumpet. Granting all these advantages to the young man, he ought, nevertheless, to go on improving, on the whole, as a medical practitioner, with every year, until he has ripened into a well-mellowed maturity. But, to improve, he must be good for something at the start. If you ship a poor cask of wine to India and back, if you keep it a half a century, it only grows thinner and sharper.

You are soon to enter into relations with the public, to expend your skill and knowledge for its benefit, and find your support in the rewards of your labor. What kind of a constituency is this which is to look to you as its authorized champions in the struggle of life against its numerous enemies?

In the first place, the persons who seek the aid of the physician are very honest and sincere in their wish to get rid of their complaints, and, generally speaking, to live as long as they can. However attractively the future is painted to them, they are attached to the planet with which they are already acquainted. They are addicted to the daily use of this empirical and unchemical mixture which we call air, and would hold on to it as a tippler does to his alcoholic drinks. There is nothing men will not do, there is nothing they have not done, to recover their health and save their lives. They have submitted to be half-drowned in water, and half-choked with gases, to be buried up to their chins in earth, to be seared with hot irons like galley-slaves, to be crimped with knives, like cod-fish, to have needles thrust into their flesh, and bonfires kindled on their skin, to swallow all sorts of abominations, and to pay for all this, as if to be singed and scalded were a costly privilege, as if blisters were a blessing, and leeches were a luxury. What more can be asked to prove their honesty and sincerity?

This same community is very intelligent with respect to a great many subjects—commerce, mechanics, manufactures, politics. But with regard to medicine it is hopelessly ignorant and never finds it out. I do not know that it is any worse in this country than in Great Britain, where Mr. Huxley speaks very freely of "the utter ignorance of the simplest laws of their own animal life, which prevails among even the most highly-educated persons." If the community could only be made aware of its own utter ignorance, and incompetence to form opinions on medical subjects, difficult enough to those who give their lives to the study of them, the practitioner would have an easier task. But it will form opinions of its own, it cannot help it, and we cannot blame it, even though we know how slight and deceptive are their foundations.

This is the way it happens: Every grown-up person has either been ill himself or had a friend suffer from illness, from which he has recovered. Every sick person has done something or other by somebody's advice, or of his own accord, a little before getting better. There is an irresistible tendency to associate the thing done, and the improvement which followed it, as cause and effect. This is the great source of fallacy in medical practice. But the physician has some chance of correcting his hasty inference. He thinks his prescription cured a single case of a particular complaint; he tries it in twenty similar cases without effect, and sets down the first as probably nothing more than a coincidence. The unprofessional experimenter or observer has no large experience to correct his hasty generalization. He wants to believe that the means he employed effected his cure. He feels grateful to the person who advised it, he loves to praise the pill or potion which helped him, and he has a kind of monumental pride in himself as a living testimony to its efficacy. So it is that you will find the community in which you live, be it in town or country, full of brands plucked from the burning, as they believe, by some agency which, with your better training, you feel reasonably confident had nothing to do with it. Their disease went out of itself, and the stream from the medical fire-annihilator had never even touched it.

You cannot and need not expect to disturb the public in the possession of its medical superstitions. A man's ignorance is as much his private property, and as precious in his own eyes, as his family Bible. You have only to open your own Bible at the ninth chapter of St. John's Gospel, and you will find that the logic of a restored patient was very simple then, as it is now, and very hard to deal with. My clerical friends will forgive me for poaching on their sacred territory, in return for an occasional raid upon the medical domain of which they have now and then been accused.

A blind man was said to have been restored to sight by a young person whom the learned doctors of the Jewish law considered a sinner, and, as such, very unlikely to have been endowed with a divine gift of healing. They visited the patient repeatedly, and evidently teased him with their questions about the treatment, and their insinuations about the young man, until he lost his temper. At last he turned sharply upon them: "Whether he be a sinner or no, I know not: one thing I know, that, whereas I was blind, now I see."

This is the answer that always has been and always will be given by most persons when they find themselves getting well after doing anything, no matter what,—recommended by anybody, no matter whom. Lord Bacon, Robert Boyle, Bishop Berkeley, all put their faith in panaceas which we should laugh to scorn. They had seen people get well after using them. Are we any wiser than those great men? Two years ago, in a lecture before the Massachusetts Historical Society, I mentioned this recipe of Sir Kenelm Digby for fever and ague: Pare the patient's nails; put the parings in a little bag, and hang the bag round the neck of a live eel, and place him in a tub of water. The eel will die, and the patient will recover.

Referring to this prescription in the course of the same lecture, I said: "You smiled when I related Sir Kenelm Digby's prescription, with the live eel in it; but if each of you were to empty his or her pockets, would there not roll out, from more than one of them, a horse-chestnut, carried about as a cure for rheumatism?'' Nobody saw fit to empty his or her pockets, and my question brought no response. But two months ago I was in a company of educated persons, college graduates every one of them, when a gentleman, well known in our community, a man of superior ability and strong common-sense, on the occasion of some talk arising about rheumatism, took a couple of very shiny horse-chestnuts from his breeches-pocket, and laid them on the table, telling us how, having suffered from the complaint in question, he had, by the advice of a friend, procured these two horse-chestnuts on a certain time a year or more ago, and carried them about him ever since; from which very day he had been entirely free from rheumatism.

This argument, from what looks like cause and effect, whether it be so or not, is what you will have to meet wherever you go, and you need not think you can answer it. In the natural course of things some thousands of persons must be getting well or better of slight attacks of colds, of rheumatic pains, every week, in this city alone. Hundreds of them do something or other in the way of remedy, by medical or other advice, or of their own motion, and the last thing they do gets the credit of the recovery. Think what a crop of remedies this must furnish, if it were all harvested!

Experience has taught, or will teach you, that most of the wonderful stories patients and others tell of sudden and signal cures are like Owen Glendower's story of the portents that announced his birth. The earth shook at your nativity, did it? Very likely, and

> "So it would have done,
> At the same season, if your mother's cat
> Had kittened, though yourself had ne'er been born.''

You must listen more meekly than Hotspur did to the babbling Welshman, for ignorance is a solemn and sacred fact, and, like infancy, which it resembles, should be respected. Once in a while you will have a patient of sense, born with the gift of observation, from whom you may learn something. When you find yourself in the presence of one who is fertile of medical opinions, and affluent in stories of marvellous cures,—of a member of Congress whose name figures in certificates to the value of patent medicines, of a voluble dame who discourses on the miracles she has wrought or seen wrought with the little jokers of the sugar-of-milk globule-box, take out your watch and count the pulse; also note the time of day, and charge the price of a visit for every extra fifteen, or, if you are not very busy, every twenty minutes. In this way you will turn what seems a serious dispensation into a double blessing, for this class of patients loves dearly to talk, and it does them a deal of good, and you feel as if you had earned your money by the dose you have taken, quite as honestly as by any dose you may have ordered.

You must take the community just as it is, and make the best of it. You wish to obtain its confidence; there is a short rule for doing this which you will find useful,—*deserve it*. But, to deserve it in full measure, you must unite many excellences, natural and acquired.

As the basis of all the rest, you must have all those traits of character which fit you to enter into the most intimate and confidential relations with the families of which you are the privileged friend and counsellor. Medical Christianity, if I may use such a term, is of very early date. By the oath of Hippocrates, the practitioner of ancient times bound himself to enter his patient's house with the sole purpose of doing him good, and so to conduct himself as to avoid the very appearance of evil. Let the physician of to-day begin by coming up to this standard, and add to it all the more recently discovered virtues and graces.

A certain amount of natural ability is requisite to make you a good physician, but by no means that disproportionate development of some special faculty which goes by the name of genius. A just balance of the mental powers is a great deal more likely to be useful than any single talent, even were it the power of observation, in excess. For a mere observer is liable to be too fond of facts for their own sake, so that, if he told the real truth, he would confess that he takes more pleasure in a post-mortem examination which shows him what was the matter with a patient, than in a case which insists on getting well and leaving him in the dark as to its nature. Far more likely to interfere with the sound practical balance of the mind is that speculative, theoretical tendency which has made so many men noted in their day, whose fame has passed away with their dissolving theories. Read Dr. Bartlett's comparison of the famous Benjamin Rush with his modest fellow-townsman Dr. William Currie, and see the dangers into which a passion for grandiose generalizations betrayed a man of many admirable qualities.

I warn you against all ambitious aspirations outside of your profession. Medicine is the most difficult of sciences and the most laborious of arts. It will task all your powers of body and mind if you are faithful to it. Do not dabble in the muddy sewer of politics, nor linger by the enchanted streams of literaure, nor dig in far-off fields for the hidden waters of alien sciences. The great practitioners are generally those who concentrate all their powers on their business. If there are here and there brilliant exceptions, it is only in virtue of extraordinary gifts, and industry to which very few are equal.

To get business a man must really want it; and do you suppose that when you are in the middle of a heated caucus, or half-way through a delicate analysis, or in the spasm of an unfinished ode, your eyes rolling in the fine frenzy of poetical composition, you want to be called to a teething infant, or an ancient person groaning under the griefs of a lumbago? I think I have known more than one young man whose doctor's sign proclaimed his readiness to serve mankind in that capacity, but who hated the sound of a patient's knock, and as he sat with his book or his microscope, felt exactly as the old party expressed himself in my friend Mr. Brownell's poem—

"All I axes is, let me alone."

The community soon finds out whether you are in earnest, and really mean business, or whether you are one of those diplomaed dilettanti who like the amusement of *quasi* medical studies, but have no idea of wasting their precious time in putting their knowledge in practice for the benefit of their suffering fellow-creatures.

The public is a very incompetent judge of your skill and knowledge, but it gives its confidence most readily to those who stand well with their professional brethren, whom they call upon when they themselves or their families are sick, whom they choose to honorable offices, whose writings and teachings they hold in esteem. A man may be much valued by the profession and yet have defects which prevent his becoming a favorite practitioner, but no popularity can be depended upon as permanent which is not sanctioned by the judgment of professional experts, and with these you will always stand on your substantial merits.

*   *   *

No matter how hard he stares at your countenance, he should never be able to read his fate in it. It should be cheerful as long as there is hope, and serene in its gravity when nothing is left but resignation. The face of a physician, like that of a diplomatist, should be impenetrable. Nature is a benevolent old hypocrite; she cheats the sick and the dying with illusions better than any anodynes. If there are cogent reasons why a patient should be undeceived, do it deliberately and advisedly, but do not betray your apprehensions through your tell-tale features.

We had a physician in our city whose smile was commonly reckoned as being worth five thousand dollars a year to him, in the days, too, of moderate incomes. You cannot put on such a smile as that any more than you can get sunshine without sun; there was a tranquil and kindly nature under it that irradiated the pleasant face it made one happier to meet on his daily rounds. But you can cultivate the disposition, and it will work its way through to the surface,—nay, more,—you can try to wear a quiet and encouraging look, and it will react on your disposition and make you like what you seem to be, or at least bring you nearer to its own likeness.

Your patient has no more right to all the truth you know than he has to all the medicine in your saddlebags, if you carry that kind of cartridge-box for the ammunition that slays disease. He should get only just so much as is good for him. I have seen a physician examining a patient's chest stop all at once, as he brought out a particular sound with a tap on the collar-bone, in the attitude of a pointer who has just come on the scent or sight of a woodcock. You remember the Spartan boy, who, with unmoved countenance, hid the fox that was tearing his vitals beneath his mantle. What he could do in his own suffering you must learn to do for others on whose vital organs disease has fastened its devouring teeth. It is a terrible thing to take away hope, even earthly hope, from a fellow-creature. Be very careful what names you let fall before your patient. He knows what it means when you tell him he has tubercles or Bright's disease, and, if he hears the word carcinoma, he will certainly look it out in a medical dictionary, if he does not interpret its dread significance on the instant. Tell him he has asthmatic symptoms, or a tendency to the gouty diathesis, and he will at once think of all the asthmatic and gouty old patriarchs he has ever heard of, and be comforted. You need not be so cautious in speaking of the health of rich and remote relatives, if he is in the line of succession.

Some shrewd old doctors have a few phrases always on hand for patients that will insist on knowing the pathology of their complaints without the slightest capacity of understanding the scientific explanation. I have known the term "spinal irritation" serve well on such occasions, but I think nothing on the whole has covered so much ground, and meant so little, and given such profound satisfaction to all parties, as the magnificent phrase "congestion of the portal system."

Once more, let me recommend you, as far as possible, to keep your doubts to yourself, and give the patient the benefit of your decision. Firmness, gentle firmness, is absolutely necessary in this and certain other relations. Mr. Rarey with Cruiser, Richard with Lady Anne, Pinel with his crazy people, show what steady nerves can do with the most intractable of animals, the most irresistible of despots, and the most unmanageable of invalids.

If you cannot acquire and keep the confidence of your patient, it is time for you to give place to some other practitioner who can. If you are wise and diligent, you can establish relations with the best of them which they will find it very hard to break. But, if they wish to employ another person, who, as they think, knows more than you do, do not take it as a personal wrong. A patient believes another man can save his life, can restore him to health, which, as he thinks, you have not the skill to do. No matter whether the patient is right or wrong, it is a great impertinence to think you have any property in him. Your estimate of your own ability is not the question, it is what the patient thinks of it. All your wisdom is to him like the lady's virtue in Raleigh's song:—

> "If she seem not chaste to me,
> What care I how chaste she be?"

What I call a good patient is one who, having found a good physician, sticks to him till he dies. But there are many very good people who are not what I call good patients. I was once requested to call on a lady suffering from nervous and other symptoms. It came out in the preliminary conversational skirmish, half medical, half social, that I was the *twenty-sixth* member of the faculty into whose arms, professionally speaking, she had successively thrown herself. Not being a believer in such a rapid rotation of scientific crops, I gently deposited the burden, commending it to the care of number twenty-seven, and, him, whoever he might be, to the care of Heaven.

If there happened to be among my audience any person who wished to know on what principles the patient should choose his physician, I should give him these few precepts to think over:—

Choose a man who is personally agreeable, for a daily visit from an intelligent, amiable, pleasant, sympathetic person will cost you no more than one from a sloven or a boor, and his presence will do more for you than any prescription the other will order.

Let him be a man of recognized good sense in other matters, and the chance is that he will be sensible as a practitioner.

Let him be a man who stands well with his professional brethren, whom they approve as honest, able, courteous.

Let him be one whose patients are willing to die in his hands, not one whom they go to for trifles, and leave as soon as they are in danger, and who can say, therefore, that he never loses a patient.

Do not leave the ranks of what is called the regular profession, unless you wish to go farther and fare worse, for you may be assured that its members recognize no principle which hinders their accepting any remedial agent proved to be useful, no matter from what quarter it comes. The difficulty is that the stragglers, organized under fantastic names in pretentious associations, or lurking in solitary dens behind doors left ajar, make no real contributions to the art of healing. When they bring forward a remedial agent like chloral, like the bromide of potassium, like ether, used as an anaesthetic, they will find no difficulty in procuring its recognition.

Some of you will probably be more or less troubled by the pretensions of that parody of mediaeval theology which finds its dogma of hereditary depravity in the doctrine of *psora*, its miracle of transubstantiation in the mystery of its triturations and dilutions, its church in the people who have mistaken their century, and its priests in those who have mistaken their calling. You can do little with persons who are disposed to accept these curious medical superstitions. The saturation-point of individual minds with reference to evidence, and especially medical evidence, differs, and must always continue to differ, very widely. There are those whose minds are satisfied with the decillionth dilution of a scientific proof. No wonder they believe in the efficacy of a similar attenuation of bryony or pulsatilla. You have no fulcrum you can rest upon to lift an error out of such minds as these, often highly endowed with knowledge and talent, sometimes with genius, but commonly richer in the imaginative than the observing and reasoning faculties.

Let me return once more to the young graduate. Your relations to your professional brethren may be a source of lifelong happiness and growth in knowledge and character, or they may make you wretched and end by leaving you isolated from those who should be your friends and counsellors. The life of a physician becomes ignoble when he suffers himself to feed on petty jealousies and sours his temper in perpetual quarrels. You will be liable to meet an uncomfortable man here and there in the profession,—one who is so fond of being in hot water that it is a wonder all the albumen in his body is not coagulated. There are common barrators among doctors as there are among lawyers,—stirrers up of strife under one pretext and another, but in reality because they like it. They are their own worst enemies, and do themselves a mischief each time they assail their neighbors. In my student-days I remember a good deal of this Donnybrook-Fair style of quarrelling, more especially in Paris, where some of the noted surgeons were always at logger-heads, and in one of our lively Western cities. Soon after I had set up an office, I had a trifling experience which may serve to point a moral in this direction. I had placed a lamp behind the glass in the entry to indicate to the passer-by where relief from all curable infirmities was to be sought and found. Its brilliancy attracted the attention of a devious youth, who dashed his fist through the glass and upset my modest luminary. All he got by his vivacious assault was that he left portions of integument from his knuckles upon the glass, had a lame hand, was very easily identified, and had to pay the glazier's bill. The moral is that, if the brilliancy of another's reputation excites your belligerent instincts, it is not worth your while to strike at it, without calculating which of you is likely to suffer most, if you do.

*   *   *

And now, gentlemen of the graduating class, nothing remains but for me to bid you, in the name of those for whom I am commissioned and privileged to speak, farewell as students, and welcome as practitioners. I pronounce the two benedictions in the same breath, as the late king's demise and the new king's accession are proclaimed by the same voice at the same moment. You would hardly excuse me if I stooped to any meaner dialect than the classical and familiar language of your prescriptions, the same in which your title to the name of physician is, if, like our own institution, you follow the ancient usage, engraved upon your diplomas.

Valete, JUVENES, *artis medicoe studiosi; valete, discipuli, valete, filii!*

Salvete, VIRI, *medicoe magistri; salvete, amici; salvete, fratres!*

WILLIAM CARLOS WILLIAMS
Autobiography

It's the humdrum, day-in, day-out, everyday work that is the real satisfaction of the practice of medicine; the patients a man has seen on his daily visits over a forty-year period of weekdays and Sundays that make up his life. I have never had a money practice; it would have been impossible for me. But the actual calling on people, at all times and under all conditions, the coming to grips with the intimate conditions of their lives, when they were being born, when they were dying, watching them die, watching them get well when they were ill, has always absorbed me.

I lost myself in the very properties of their minds: for the moment at least I actually became *them,* whoever they should be, so that when I detached myself from them at the end of a half hour of intense concentration over some illness which was affecting them, it was as though I were reawakening from a sleep. For the moment I myself did not exist; nothing of myself affected me. As a consequence I came back to myself, as from any other sleep, rested.

Time after time I have gone out into my office in the evening feeling as if I couldn't keep my eyes open a moment longer. I would start out on my morning calls after only a few hours' sleep, sit in front of some house waiting to get the courage to climb the steps and push the front-door bell. But once I saw the patient, all that would disappear. In a flash the details of case would begin to formulate themselves into a recognizable outline, the diagnosis would unravel itself or would refuse to make itself plain, and the hunt was on. Along with that, the patient himself would shape up into something that called for attention, his peculiarities, her reticences or candors. And though I might be attracted or repelled, the professional attitude which every physician must call on would steady me, dictate the terms on which I was to proceed. Many a time a man must watch the patient's mind as it watches him, distrusting him, ready to fly off at a tangent at the first opportunity; sees himself distrusted, sees the patient turn to someone else, rejected.

More than once we have all seen ourselves rejected, seen some hard-pressed mother or husband go to some other adviser when we know that the advice we have given him has been correct. That, too, is part of the game. But in general it is the rest, the peace of mind that comes from adopting the patient's condition as one's own to be struggled with toward a solution during those few minutes or that hour or those trying days when we are searching for causes, trying to relate this to that to build a reasonable basis for action which really gives us our peace. As I say, often after I have gone into my office harassed by personal perplexities of whatever sort, fatigued physically and mentally, after two hours of intense application to the work, I came out at the finish completely rested (and I mean rested), ready to smile and to laugh as if the day were just starting.

That is why as a writer I have never felt that medicine interfered with me but rather that it was my very food and drink, the very thing which made it possible for me to write. Was I not interested in man? There the thing was, right in front of me. I could touch it, smell it. It was myself, naked, just as it was, without a lie telling itself to me in its own terms. Oh, I knew it wasn't for the most part giving me anything very profound, but it was giving me terms, basic terms with which I could spell out matters as profound as I cared to think of.

I knew it was an elementary world that I was facing, but I have always been amazed at the authenticity with which the simpleminded often face that world when compared with the tawdriness of the public viewpoint exhibited in reports from the world at large. The public view which affects the behavior of so many is a very shabby thing when compared with what I see every day in my practice of medicine. I can almost say it is the interference of the public view of their lives with what I see which makes the difficulty, in most instances, between sham and a satisfactory basis of thought.

I don't care much about that, however, I don't care a rap what people are or believe. They come to me. I care for them and either they become my friends or they don't. That is their business. My business, aside from the mere physical diagnosis, is to make a different sort of diagnosis concerning them as individuals, quite apart from anything for which they seek my advice. That fascinates me. From the very beginning, that fascinated me even more than I myself knew. For no matter where I might find myself, every sort of individual that it is possible to imagine in some phase of his development, from the highest to the lowest, at some time exhibited himself to me. I am sure I have seen them all. And all have contributed to my pie. Let the successful carry off their blue ribbons; I have known the unsuccessful, far better persons than their more lucky brothers. One can laugh at them both, whatever the costumes they adopt. And when one is able to reveal them to themselves, high or low, they are always grateful as they are surprised that one can so have revealed the inner secrets of another's private motives. To do this is what makes a writer worth heeding: that somehow or other, whatever the source may be, he has gone to the base of the matter to lay it bare before us in terms which, try as we may, we cannot in the end escape. There is no choice then but to accept him and make him a hero.

All day long the doctor carries on this work, observing, weighing, comparing values of which neither he nor his patients may know the significance. He may be insensitive. But if in addition to actually being an accurate craftsman and a man of insight, he has the added quality of—some distress of mind, a restless concern with the . . . If he is not satisfied with mere cures, if he lacks ambition, if he is content to. . .If there is no content in him and likely to be none; if, in other words, without wishing to force it, since that would interfere with his lifelong observation, he allows himself to be called a name! What can one think of him?

He is half-ashamed to have people suspect him of carrying on a clandestine, a sort of underhand piece of spying on the public at large. They naïvely ask him, "How do you do it? How can you carry on an active business like that and at the same time find time to write? You must be superhuman. You must have at the very least the energy of two men." But they do not grasp that one occupation complements the other, that they are two parts of a whole, that it is not two jobs at all, that one rests the man when the other fatigues him. The only person to feel sorry for is his wife. She practically becomes a recluse. His only fear is that the source of his interest, his daily going about among human beings of all sorts, all ages, all conditions, will be terminated. That he will be found out.

As far as the writing itself is concerned, it takes next to no time at all. Much too much is written every day of our lives. We are overwhelmed by it. But when at times we see through the welter of evasive or interested patter, when by chance we penetrate to some moving detail of a life, there is always time to bang out a few pages. The thing isn't to find the time for it—we waste hours every day doing absolutely nothing at all—the difficulty is to catch the evasive life of the thing, to phrase the words in such a way that stereotype will yield a moment of insight. That is where the difficulty lies. We are lucky when that underground current can be tapped and the secret spring of all our lives will send up its pure water. It seldom happens. A thousand trivialities push themselves to the front, our lying habits of everyday speech and thought are foremost, telling us that *that* is what "they" want to hear. Tell them something else. You know you want to be a successful writer. This sort of chit-chat the daily practice of medicine tends drastically to cure.

Forget writing; it's a trivial matter. But day in, day out, when the inarticulate patient struggles to lay himself bare for you, or with nothing more than a boil on his back is so caught off balance that he reveals some secret twist of a whole community's pathetic way of thought, a man is suddenly seized again with a desire to speak of the underground stream which for a moment has come up just under surface. It is just a glimpse, an intimation of all that which the daily print misses or deliberately hides, but the excitement is intense and the rush to write is on again. It is then we see, by this constant feeling for a meaning, from the unselected nature of the material, just as it comes in over the phone or at the office door, that there is no better way to get an intimation of what is going on in the world.

We catch a glimpse of something, from time to time, which shows us that a presence has just brushed past us, some rare thing—just when the smiling little Italian woman has left us. For a moment we are dazzled. What was that? We can't name it; we know it never gets into any recognizable avenue of expression; men will be long dead before they can have so much as ever approached it. Whole lives are spent in the tremendous affairs of daily events without even approaching the great sights that I see every day. My patients do not know what is about them among their very husbands and children, their wives and acquaintances. But there is no need for us to be such strangers to each other, saving alone laziness, indifference, and age-old besotted ignorance.

So for me the practice of medicine has become the pursuit of a rare element which may appear at any time, at any place, at a glance. It can be most embarrassing. Mutual recognition is likely to flare up at a moment's notice. The relationship between physican and patient, if it were literally followed, would give us a world of extraordinary fertility of the imagination, which we can hardly afford. There's no use trying to multiply cases; it is there, it is magnificent, it fills my thoughts, it reaches to the farthest limits of our lives.

What is the use of reading the common news of the day, the tragic deaths and abuses of daily living, when for over half a lifetime we have known that they must have occurred just as they have occurred, given the conditions that cause them? There is no light in it. It is trivial fill-gap. We know the plane will crash, the train be derailed. And we know why. No one cares; no one can care. We get the news and discount it; we are quite right in doing so. It is trivial. But the hunted news I get from some obscure patients' eyes is not trivial. It is profound: whole academies of learning, whole ecclesiastical hierarchies are founded upon it and have developed what they call their dialectic upon nothing else, their lying dialectics. A dialectic is any arbitrary system, which, since all systems are mere inventions, is necessarily in each case a false premise, upon which a closed system is built, shutting those who confine themselves to it from the rest of the world. All men one way or another use a dialectic of some sort into which they are shut, whether it be an Argentina or a Japan. So each group is maimed. Each is enclosed in a dialectic cloud, incommunicado, and for that reason we rush into wars and prides of the most superficial natures.

Do we not see that we are inarticulate? That is what defeats us. It is our inability to communicate to another how we are locked within ourselves, unable to say the simplest thing of importance to one another, any of us, even the most valuable, that makes our lives like those of a litter of kittens in a woodpile. That gives the physician, and I don't mean the high-priced psychoanalyst, his opportunity; psychoanalysis amounts to no more than another dialectic into which to be locked.

The physician enjoys a wonderful opportunity actually to witness the words being born. Their actual colors and shapes are laid before him carrying their tiny burdens, which he is privileged to take into his care with their unspoiled newness. He may see the difficulty with which they have been born and what they are destined to do. No one else is present but the speaker and ourselves; we have been the words' very parents. Nothing is more moving.

But after we have run the gamut of the simple meanings that come to one over the years, a change gradually occurs. We have grown used to the range of communication which is likely to reach us. The girl who comes to me breathless, staggering into my office, in her underwear a still breathing infant, asking me to lock her mother out of the room; the man whose mind is gone—all of them finally say the same thing. And then a new meaning begins to intervene. For under that language to which we have been listening all our lives a new, a more profound language underlying all the dialectics offers itself. It is what they call poetry. That is the final phase.

It is that, we realize, which beyond all they have been saying is what they have been trying to say. They laugh (for are they not laughable?); they can think of nothing more useless (what else are they but the same?); something made of words (have they not been trying to use words all their lives?). We begin to see that the underlying meaning of all they want to tell us and have always failed to communicate is the poem, the poem which their lives are being lived to realize. No one will believe it. And it is the actual words, as we hear them spoken under all circumstances, which contain it. It is actually there, in the life before us, every minute that we are listening, a rarest element—not in our imaginations but there, there in fact. It is that essence which is hidden in the very words which are going in at our ears and from which we must recover underlying meaning as realistically as we recover metal out of ore.

The poem that each is trying actually to communicate to us lies in the words. It is at least the words that make it articulate. It has always been so. Occasionally that named person is born who catches a rumor of it, a Homer, a Villon, and his race and the world perpetuate his memory. Is it not plain why? The physician, listening from day to day, catches a hint of it in his preoccupation. By listening to the minutest variations of the speech, we begin to detect that today, as always, the essence is also to be found, hidden under the verbiage, seeking to be realized.

But one of the characteristics of this rare presence is that it is jealous of exposure and that it is shy and revengeful. It is not a name that is bandied about in the marketplace, no more than it is something that can be captured and exploited by the academy. Its face is a particular face; it is likely to appear under the most unlikely disguises. You cannot recognize it from past appearances—in fact it is always a new face. It knows all that we are in the habit of describing. It will not use the same appearance for any new materialization. And it is our very life. It is we ourselves, at our rarest moments, but inarticulate for the most part except when in the poem one man, every five or six hundred years, escapes to formulate a few gifted sentences.

The poem springs from the half-spoken words of such patients as the physician sees from day to day. He observes it in the peculiar, actual conformations in which its life is hid. Humbly he presents himself before it, and by long practice he strives as best he can to interpret the manner of its speech. In that the secret lies. This, in the end, comes perhaps to be the occupation of the physician after a lifetime of careful listening.

WILLIAM CARLOS WILLIAMS
The Use of Force

They were new patients to me, all I had was the name, Olson. Please come down as soon as you can, my daughter is very sick.

When I arrived I was met by the mother, a big startled looking woman, very clean and apologetic who merely said, Is this the doctor? and let me in. In the back, she added. You must excuse us, doctor, we have her in the kitchen where it is warm. It is very damp here sometimes.

The child was fully dressed and sitting on her father's lap near the kitchen table. He tried to get up, but I motioned for him not to bother, took off my overcoat and started to look things over. I could see that they were all very nervous, eyeing me up and down distrustfully. As often, in such cases, they weren't telling me more than they had to, it was up to me to tell them; that's why they were spending three dollars on me.

The child was fairly eating me up with her cold, steady eyes, and no expression to her face whatever. She did not move and seemed, inwardly, quiet; an unusually attractive little thing, and as strong as a heifer in appearance. But her face was flushed, she was breathing rapidly, and I realized that she had a high fever. She had magnificent blonde hair, in profusion. One of those picture children often reproduced in advertising leaflets and the photogravure sections of the Sunday papers.

She's had a fever for three days, began the father and we don't know what it comes from. My wife has given her things, you know, like people do, but it don't do no good. And there's been a lot of sickness around. So we tho't you'd better look her over and tell us what is the matter.

As doctors often do I took a trial shot at it as a point of departure. Has she had a sore throat?

Both parents answered me together, No . . . No, she says her throat don't hurt her.

Does your throat hurt you? added the mother to the child. But the little girl's expression didn't change nor did she move her eyes from my face.

Have you looked?

I tried to, said the mother, but I couldn't see.

As it happens we had been having a number of cases of diphtheria in the school to which this child went during that month and we were all, quite apparently, thinking of that, though no one had as yet spoken of the thing.

Well, I said, suppose we take a look at the throat first. I smiled in my best professional manner and asking for the child's first name I said, come on, Mathilda, open your mouth and let's take a look at your throat.

Nothing doing.

Aw, come on, I coaxed, just open your mouth wide and let me take a look. Look, I said opening both hands wide, I haven't anything in my hands. Just open up and let me see.

Such a nice man, put in the mother. Look how kind he is to you. Come on, do what he tells you to. He won't hurt you.

At that I ground my teeth in disgust. If only they wouldn't use the word ''hurt'' I might be able to get somewhere. But I did not allow myself to be hurried or disturbed but speaking quietly and slowly I approached the child again.

As I moved my chair a little nearer suddenly with one catlike movement both her hands clawed instinctively for my eyes and she almost reached them too. In fact she knocked my glasses flying and they fell, though unbroken, several feet away from me on the kitchen floor.

Both the mother and father almost turned themselves inside out in embarrassment and apology. You bad girl, said the mother, taking her and shaking her by one arm. Look what you've done. The nice man . . .

For heaven's sake, I broke in. Don't call me a nice man to her. I'm here to look at her throat on the chance that she might have diphtheria and possibly die of it. But that's nothing to her. Look here, I said to the child, we're going to look at your throat. You're old enough to understand what I'm saying. Will you open it now by yourself or shall we have to open it for you?

Not a move. Even her expression hadn't changed. Her breaths however were coming faster and faster. Then the battle began. I had to do it. I had to have a throat culture for her own protection. But first I told the parents that it was entirely up to them. I explained the danger but said that I would not insist on a throat examination so long as they would take the responsibility.

If you don't do what the doctor says you'll have to go to the hospital, the mother admonished her severely.

Oh yeah? I had to smile to myself. After all, I had already fallen in love with the savage brat, the parents were contemptible to me. In the ensuing struggle they grew more and more abject, crushed, exhausted while she surely rose to magnificent heights of insane fury of effort bred of her terror of me.

The father tried his best, and he was a big man but the fact that she was his daughter, his shame at her behavior and his dread of hurting her made him release her just at the critical moment several times when I had almost achieved success, till I wanted to kill him. But his dread also that she might have diphtheria made him tell me to go on, go on though he himself was almost fainting, while the mother moved back and forth behind us raising and lowering her hands in an agony of apprehension.

Put her in front of you on your lap, I ordered, and hold both her wrists.

But as soon as he did the child let out a scream. Don't, you're hurting me. Let go of my hands. Let them go I tell you. Then she shrieked terrifyingly, hysterically. Stop it! Stop it! You're killing me!

Do you think she can stand it, doctor! said the mother.

You get out, said the husband to his wife. Do you want her to die of diphtheria?

Come on now, hold her, I said.

Then I grasped the child's head with my left hand and tried to get the wooden tongue depressor between her teeth. She fought, with clenched teeth, desperately! But now I also had grown furious—at a child. I tried to hold myself down but I couldn't. I know how to expose a throat for inspection. And I did my best. When finally I got the wooden spatula behind the last teeth and just the point of it into the mouth cavity, she opened up for an instant but before I could see anything she came down again and gripping the wooden blade between her molars she reduced it to splinters before I could get it out again.

Aren't you ashamed, the mother yelled at her. Aren't you ashamed to act like that in front of the doctor?

Get me a smooth-handled spoon of some sort, I told the mother. We're going through with this. The child's mouth was already bleeding. Her tongue was cut and she was screaming in wild hysterical shrieks. Perhaps I should have desisted and come back in an hour or more. No doubt it would have been better. But I have seen at least two children lying dead in bed of neglect in such cases, and feeling that I must get a diagnosis now or never I went at it again. But the worst of it was that I too had got beyond reason. I could have torn the child apart in my own fury and enjoyed it. It was a pleasure to attack her. My face was burning with it.

The damned little brat must be protected against her own idiocy, one says to one's self at such times. Others must be protected against her. It is social necessity. And all these things are true. But a blind fury, a feeling of adult shame, bred of a longing for muscular release are the operatives. One goes on to the end.

In a final unreasoning assault I overpowered the child's neck and jaws. I forced the heavy silver spoon back of her teeth and down her throat till she gagged. And there it was—both tonsils covered with membrane. She had fought valiantly to keep me from knowing her secret. She had been hiding that sore throat for three days at least and lying to her parents in order to escape just such an outcome as this.

Now truly she *was* furious. She had been on the defensive before but now she attacked. Tried to get off her father's lap and fly at me while tears of defeat blinded her eyes.

HANS ZINSSER
As I Remember Him

———◆———

Some of the suicides were extremely ingenious; others were unbelievably maladroit. There seemed to be a sort of fashion in the technique of suicide. For a time, they were almost all illuminating gas. Then, in succession, it was carbolic acid or lysol, bichloride of mercury, hanging, shooting, and throat-cutting with amazingly inefficient utensils—jackknives, or even slivers of glass. The most sensible ones, I thought, were the illuminating-gas people. Many of them, however, made too little allowance for the fact that the odor of the gas would attract rescue. Only one man I found had taken precautions against this. He had done so by sticking an ordinary tin kitchen funnel into the gas hose and tying it over his face with a string above the ears. These people became unconscious rapidly, and if they were rescued before they died, some of them continued to live for five or six days in coma.

The carbolic-acid cases could often be rescued if the ambulance got there soon enough. All that was necessary was to get a stomach tube into them and wash them out with dilute alcohol or, if that was not available, with whiskey. Sometimes, however, it was difficult to get the stomach tube into them, since they had spasms of the diaphragm where the oesophagus enters the stomach. Then, occasionally, the stomach tube slipped into the larynx. In a case of this kind in which I had eventually reached the stomach in time to wash it out and save the patient, I had first slipped my tube into the larynx, and had pumped whiskey into the lung. This unfortunate, though he got over the carbolic acid, developed a pneumonia from which I am glad to say he recovered. While demonstrating the case to a class in my presence, Dr. James humiliated me deeply by saying that it was the only true alcoholic pneumonia he had ever encountered.

Another carbolic candidate, ignorant of course of the fact that alcohol is the antidote, walked into a saloon near the hospital one night, asked the barkeeper for a double whiskey, then pulled out a little bottle from his pocket and, saying to the bartender, "Well, Bill, this is the last drink I will ever take," swallowed the contents of the bottle and followed it with a large dose of bad whiskey. He than sank to the floor—purely because that seemed to be the proper thing to do. When I got there a few minutes later,

320

and washed out his stomach, he was considerably annoyed because I made so little fuss about him.

*   *   *

Related to this problem is that of the physician's duty of keeping patients alive for short periods of uncontrollable suffering, when all hope of even temporary improvement is gone. This question of "euthanasia" is one that is arousing a good deal of discussion among intelligent people. To put hopeless sufferers deliberately out of their agonies with lethal drugs may often be desirable, but to admit even a consideration of this implies the exercise of judgment that will inevitably be fallible in a small percentage of cases. It might be worked out under reliable boards in a limited number of conditions. But it would open the doors for dreadful possibilities. One can easily imagine these, if one considers the manner in which psychiatric experts—even in groups—can be induced to testify on both sides of cases where insanity is an issue, or the case with which lawyers can find doctors to testify in accident insurance cases and in matters of veterans' compensation. The average integrity of the medical profession is perhaps a little higher than that of the population as a whole, but not high enough for euthanasia.

It is quite another question, however, whether a doctor should continue to keep a hopeless case alive for a few weeks or months, when judicious inactivity would bring rest to the patient and peaceful resignation to his family and friends. This is a problem which has troubled me on a number of occasions. And always I have come to the conclusion that the safest principle—except in a few special instances, such as the last stages of cancer or of leukemia or of Hodgkin's disease—is to continue to work with all means at one's disposal as long as the pulse keeps going and the breathing continues. I remember the experiences of two of my young colleagues who purposely gave up—one, the case of his own father— with the compassionate thought of not prolonging a tragic situation. In both instances, I am sure their judgments were right. In both cases, however, they never entirely got over reproaching themselves. On the other hand, I have graven in my memory a typhus patient in a Serbian hospital, whom we had given up for dead. It was my job to do autopsies on such cases as soon after death as possible, in order to take material for culture before secondary post-mortem infections of the tissues could take place and before the responsible—then uncertain—virus could begin to die out. For in some infections—such, for instance, as syphilis—the infecting organisms die quite promptly when the body dies and the cells cease to respire. This patient was hardly breathing, and his pulse could be detected only with a stethoscope. He was in that state of final exhaustion which I have seen to a similar degree only in this disease and in typhoid fever. I postponed a short walk into the hills because I thought that this boy would be carried into my autopsy barrack at any minute. But my friend George Shattuck, who was the physician on the ward, kept working at him. His persistence fascinated me. He gave saline infusions; he stimulated him with camphor and strychnin; he covered him with hot blankets. Shattuck omitted nothing that might feed the little flame that still flickered. He was hopeless, as I was, but he kept on. We expected death by noon. At two o'clock the patient was unchanged, but still going. By four, we could begin to feel the pulse. By six, there was distinct hope. Six weeks later, the young warrior was lying in the sun near my autopsy barracks, drinking a glass of thin milk, and beginning to feel bloodthirsty again—hoping soon to kill an Austrian.

A girl with typhoid fever at the Roosevelt Hospital came back from the inner gates in just the same way. I was young enough then to ask her later whether she had had any sense of death, or any visions. She said she had no memories whatever. A year later, I went to her wedding, when she married a policeman. Were we wise in saving her, after all? At any rate, he was not a traffic officer.

*   *   *

I once brought a huge, buck Negro out of a poolroom, where he had been shot from across the table with a .45 army revolver. He was lying on the floor when I found him, but was in perfectly good condition. He had apparently fallen down either from the shock or because, when one is shot, it is a conventional thing to do. The bullet, by one of those fantastic accidents that happen to bullets, had entered the front of his throat, next to the larynx, and had skidded around under the fascia of the neck. I took it out easily from just under the skin of the back of his head.

The defenses of the neck in this respect are extraordinary, if things don't hit it squarely or with sufficient force. I once had a fencing épée enter my own neck in the same way, skid around on the fascia, bounce off the sternomastoid muscle, and come out again, without doing any damage to the large vessels.

Sometimes shooting was done with the old-fashioned pocket pistols of small calibre in such a way that the consequences were more amusing than tragic. A little man in one of the Irish tenement houses one evening shot his excessively fat and belligerent wife with a small .22 pistol. He managed to get in five shots before she fetched him a clap with something—I've forgotten whether it was a skillet or some other household weapon. By the time I got there, the little Irishman was completely laid out with a scalp wound. His wife said she had been shot twice, in both breasts. There were little holes in her enormous bosom, from which fat-globules oozed. I easily located the bullets, quite close under the skin, but when I had managed to remove these and clean out the wounds in the hospital emergency ward, she said she also had a pain in the place where she sat. Apparently, she had stooped over to pick up the weapon with which she laid out her peevish husband, and during that time he had taken another shot. She thought he had kicked her, but here, too, she was well defended and had almost forgotten the episode. She could hardly believe it when I managed to get another bullet out of the padding. It took a lot more trouble to bring her husband back to life.

*　　*　　*

Obstetrics is not the pleasantest of medical occupations, although it pays well and is one of the things that the young physician with any kind of practice can count on as a financial backlog. Yet it takes a great deal of time and means a lot of night work. While the statement may not be statistically correct, it does seem to the medical man as though the large majority of all babies were born at night. An observant medical student in my class once asked one of our instructors about this. "Dr. V., why is it that most children are born at night?" Dr. V., who was something of a wag, replied: "Well, my boy, that's simple. It takes just nine months."

*　　*　　*

My own first obstetrical case, however, did not come through Dr. T. It was sent me by a humbler colleague who was still himself taking all the obstetrics that came to him with money. Those who had little or nothing and wouldn't go to a hospital, he referred "for experience," as he called it, to beginners like myself. This one lived in a two-family frame house in East 173rd Street. My office was in 80th Street on the West Side. There were no automobiles—and if there had been, I could not have afforded one. To make my visits, I had to take the streetcar from 80th Street to 59th Street, another one across to the Third Avenue Elevated Railroad and proceed on this to 166th Street, whence I walked north and west fifteen minutes up a steep hill. I mention these details because the case, a "first delivery," was very nervous, although not more so than I was myself. In consequence, there were a great many false alarms during the two weeks preceding the actual event. Every time there was the slightest twinge, the grandfather was sent out to the neighboring drugstore to call me on the telephone. His usual formula was, "I don't think it's anything, but maybe you'd better come up." I made three round trips within twenty-four hours a week before the child was born. The unusual thing about the case was that both father and mother were deaf and dumb. They spoke to each other with their hands, making weird sea-lion noises, and it was only from the expressions on their faces that I could gather that I seemed far too young, that they didn't think much of me anyway, but that they couldn't afford anything better. When there was finally no doubt that things were beginning to happen, they were very much frightened; and the gesticulations and the noises of animal panic added to my tension. During the last forty-eight hours, I cancelled all other engagements and lived there, snatching an occasional nap on a horsehair sofa that seemed stuffed with steel wire and had leaked. In the early stages, when pains were not too frequent, I soothed my disturbed nerves by walking around the block, accompanied by the grandfather. He—good man—was much sorrier for me than he was for his daughter, and consoled me by saying: "Now, doctor, don't worry. Everything's going to come out all right. There've been lots of babies in our family, and nothing ever happened." Towards the end, I felt that the final stage was lasting much too long. I prepared a forceps by boiling it on the kitchen stove, and then went out to telephone to K. to come up and help me. He was out. It took five or six telephone calls in various directions to locate him. When I finally got back to the house, I was met in the hall by the beaming grandfather, who said: "Hurray, doctor! It's a fine big boy! He was born about five minutes after you left."

*   *   *

On one occasion a man whom he knew only slightly accosted him on the street and said: "Dr. Jacobi, I know you are busy, but I, too, am a very busy man. I've a little sore throat this morning, and wonder whether you would take a quick look at it to see if there is anything I ought to do about it. Maybe you will look at me right here on the street." Dr. Jacobi smiled at him and said: "All right. Come over and lean against this lamppost. Now stoop, open your mouth, close your eyes, and stick out your tongue." Then he walked away, and when he reached home said: "I guess the damn fool is standing there yet."

WOMEN AND HEALING

—◦⊗◦—

At a time when more than one-third of all medical
students are females, it may seem strange that the
woman doctor should ever have been regarded as an
oddity. Evidence of progress in medicine has not
been confined to advances in science that have
prolonged human life; perhaps the most significant
aspect of such progress has been in the vastly increased number of women who have become physicians and in the accompanying acceptance of, and
respect for, their enlarged roles as healers.

SIR ARTHUR CONAN DOYLE
The Doctors of Hoyland

Dr. James Ripley was always looked upon as an exceedingly lucky dog by all of the profession who knew him. His father had preceded him in a practice in the village of Hoyland, in the north of Hampshire, and all was ready for him on the very first day that the law allowed him to put his name at the foot of a prescription. In a few years the old gentleman retired, and settled on the South Coast, leaving his son in undisputed possession of the whole country side. Save for Dr. Horton, near Basingstoke, the young surgeon had a clear run of six miles in every direction, and took his fifteen hundred pounds a year, though, as is usual in country practices, the stable swallowed up most of what the consulting-room earned.

Dr. James Ripley was two-and-thirty years of age, reserved, learned, unmarried, with set, rather stern features, and a thinning of the dark hair upon the top of his head, which was worth quite a hundred a year to him. He was particularly happy in his management of ladies. He had caught the tone of bland sternness and decisive suavity which dominates without offending. Ladies, however, were not equally happy in their management of him. Professionally, he was always at their service. Socially, he was a drop of quicksilver. In vain the country mammas spread out their simple lures in front of him. Dances and picnics were not to his taste, and he preferred during his scanty leisure to shut himself up in his study, and to bury himself in Virchow's Archives and the professional journals.

Study was a passion with him, and he would have none of the rust which often gathers round a country practitioner. It was his ambition to keep his knowledge as fresh and bright as at the moment when he had stepped out of the examination hall. He prided himself on being able at a moment's notice to rattle off the seven ramifications of some obscure artery, or to give the exact percentage of any physiological compound. After a long day's work he would sit up half the night performing iridectomies and extractions upon the sheep's eyes sent in by the village butcher, to the horror of his housekeeper, who had to remove the *débris* next morning. His love for his work was the one fanaticism which found a place in his dry, precise nature.

It was the more to his credit that he should keep up to date in his knowledge, since he had no competition to force him to exertion. In the seven years during which he had practised in Hoyland three rivals had pitted themselves against him, two in the village itself and one in the neighbouring hamlet of Lower Hoyland. Of these one had sickened and wasted, being, as it was said, himself the only patient whom he had treated during his eighteen months of ruralising. A second had bought a fourth share of a Basingstoke practice, and had departed honourably, while a third had vanished one September night, leaving a gutted house and an unpaid drug bill behind him. Since then the district had become a monopoly, and no one had dared to measure himself against the established fame of the Hoyland doctor.

It was, then, with a feeling of some surprise and considerable curiosity that on driving through Lower Hoyland one morning he perceived that the new house at the end of the village was occupied, and that a virgin brass plate glistened upon the swinging gate which faced the high road. He pulled up his fifty guinea chestnut mare and took a good look at it. "Verrinder Smith, M.D.," was printed across it in very neat, small lettering. The last man had had letters half a foot long, with a lamp like a fire-station. Dr. James Ripley noted the difference, and deduced from it that the new-comer might possibly prove a more formidable opponent. He was convinced of it that evening when he came to consult the current medical directory. By it he learned that Dr. Verrinder Smith was the holder of superb degrees, that he had studied with distinction at Edinburgh, Paris, Berlin, and Vienna, and finally that he had been awarded a gold medal and the Lee Hopkins scholarship for original research, in recognition of an exhaustive inquiry into the functions of the anterior spinal nerve roots. Dr. Ripley passed his fingers through his thin hair in bewilderment as he read his rival's record. What on earth would so brilliant a man mean by putting up his plate in a little Hampshire hamlet.

But Dr. Ripley furnished himself with an explanation to the riddle. No doubt Dr. Verrinder Smith had simply come down there in order to pursue some scientific research in peace and quiet. The plate was up as an address rather than as an invitation to patients. Of course, that must be the true explanation. In that case the presence of this brilliant neighbour would be a splendid thing for his own studies. He had often longed for some kindred mind, some steel on which he might strike his flint. Chance had brought it to him, and he rejoiced exceedingly.

And this joy it was which led him to take a step which was quite at variance with his usual habits. It is the custom for a new-comer among medical men to call first upon the older, and the etiquette upon the subject is strict. Dr. Ripley was pedantically exact on such points, and yet he deliberately drove over next day and called upon Dr. Verrinder Smith.

Such a waiving of ceremony was, he felt, a gracious act upon his part, and a fit prelude to the intimate relations which he hoped to establish with his neighbour.

The house was neat and well appointed, and Dr. Ripley was shown by a smart maid into a dapper little consulting room. As he passed in he noticed two or three parasols and a lady's sun bonnet hanging in the hall. It was a pity that his colleague should be a married man. It would put them upon a different footing, and interfere with those long evenings of high scientific talk which he had pictured to himself. On the other hand, there was much in the consulting room to please him. Elaborate instruments, seen more often in hospitals than in the houses of private practitioners, were scattered about. A sphygmograph stood upon the table and a gasometer-like engine, which was new to Dr. Ripley, in the corner. A book-case full of ponderous volumes in French and German, paper-covered for the most part, and varying in tint from the shell to the yoke of a duck's egg, caught his wandering eyes, and he was deeply absorbed in their titles when the door opened suddenly behind him. Turning round, he found himself facing a little woman, whose plain, palish face was remarkable only for a pair of shrewd, humorous eyes of a blue which had two shades too much green in it. She held a *pince-nez* in her left hand, and the doctor's card in her right.

"How do you do, Dr. Ripley?" said she.

"How do you do, madam?" returned the visitor. "Your husband is perhaps out?"

"I am not married," said she simply.

"Oh, I beg your pardon! I meant the doctor—Dr. Verrinder Smith."

"I am Dr. Verrinder Smith."

Dr. Ripley was so surprised that he dropped his hat and forgot to pick it up again.

"What!" he gasped, "the Lee Hopkins prizeman! You!"

He had never seen a woman doctor before, and his whole conservative soul rose up in revolt at the idea. He could not recall any Biblical injunction that the man should remain ever the doctor and the woman the nurse, and yet he felt as if a blasphemy had been committed. His face betrayed his feelings only too clearly.

"I am sorry to disappoint you," said the lady drily.

"You certainly have surprised me," he answered, picking up his hat.

"You are not among our champions, then?"

"I cannot say that the movement has my approval."

"And why?"

"I should much prefer not to discuss it."

"But I am sure you will answer a lady's question."

"Ladies are in danger of losing their privileges when they usurp the place of the other sex. They cannot claim both."

"Why should a woman not earn her bread by her brains?"

Dr. Ripley felt irritated by the quiet manner in which the lady cross-questioned him.

"I should much prefer not to be led into a discussion, Miss Smith."

"Dr. Smith," she interrupted.

"Well, Dr. Smith! But if you insist upon an answer, I must say that I do not think medicine a suitable profession for women and that I have a personal objection to masculine ladies."

It was an exceedingly rude speech, and he was ashamed of it the instant after he had made it. The lady, however, simply raised her eyebrows and smiled.

"It seems to me that you are begging the question," said she. "Of course, if it makes women masculine that *would* be a considerable deterioration."

It was a neat little counter, and Dr. Ripley, like a pinked fencer, bowed his acknowledgment.

"I must go," said he.

"I am sorry that we cannot come to some more friendly conclusion since we are to be neighbours," she remarked.

He bowed again, and took a step towards the door.

"It was a singular coincidence," she continued, "that at the instant that you called I was reading your paper on 'Locomotor Ataxia,' in the *Lancet*."

"Indeed," said he drily.

"I thought it was a very able monograph."

"You are very good."

"But the views which you attribute to Professor Pitres, of Bordeaux, have been repudiated by him."

"I have his pamphlet of 1890," said Dr. Ripley angrily.

"Here is his pamphlet of 1891." She picked it from among a litter of periodicals. "If you have time to glance your eye down this passage—"

Dr. Ripley took it from her and shot rapidly through the paragraph which she indicated. There was no denying that it completely knocked the bottom out of his own article. He threw it down, and with another frigid bow he made for the door. As he took the reins from the groom he glanced round and saw that the lady was standing at her window, and it seemed to him that she was laughing heartily.

All day the memory of this interview haunted him. He felt that he had come very badly out of it. She had showed herself to be his superior on his own pet subject. She had been courteous while he had been rude, self-possessed when he had been angry. And then, above all, there was her presence, her monstrous intrusion to rankle in his mind. A woman doctor had been an abstract thing before, repugnant but distant. Now she was there in actual practice, with a brass plate up just like his own, competing for the same patients. Not that he feared competition, but he objected to this lowering of his ideal of womanhood. She could not be more than thirty; and had a bright, mobile face, too. He thought of her humorous eyes, and of her strong, well-turned chin. It revolted him the more to recall the details of her education. A man, of course, could come through such an ordeal with all his purity, but it was nothing short of shameless in a woman.

But it was not long before he learned that even her competition was a thing to be feared. The novelty of her presence had brought a few curious invalids into her consulting rooms, and, once there, they had been so impressed by the firmness of her manner and by the singular, new-fashioned instruments with which she tapped, and peered, and sounded, that it formed the core of their conversation for weeks afterwards. And soon there were tangible proofs of her powers upon the country side. Farmer Eyton, whose callous ulcer had been quietly spreading over his shin for years back under a gentle *régime* of zinc ointment, was painted round with blistering fluid, and found, after three blasphemous nights, that his sore was stimulated into healing. Mrs. Crowder, who had always regarded the birthmark upon her second daughter Eliza as a sign of the indignation of the Creator at a third helping of raspberry tart which she had partaken of during a critical period, learned that, with the help of two galvanic needles, the mischief was not irreparable. In a month Dr. Verrinder Smith was known, and in two she was famous.

Occasionally, Dr. Ripley met her as he drove upon his rounds. She had started a high dogcart, taking the reins herself, with a little tiger behind. When they met he invariably raised his hat with punctilious politeness, but the grim severity of his face showed how formal was the courtesy. In fact, his dislike was rapidly deepening into absolute detestation. "The unsexed woman," was the description of her which he permitted himself to give to those of his patients who still remained staunch. But, indeed, they were a rapidly-decreasing body, and every day his pride was galled by the news of some fresh defection. The lady had somehow impressed the country folk with almost superstitious belief in her power, and from far and near they flocked to her consulting room.

But what galled him most of all was, when she did something which he had pronounced to be impracticable. For all his knowledge he lacked nerve as an operator, and usually sent his worst cases up to London. The lady, however, had no weakness of the sort, and took everything that came in her way. It was agony to him to hear that she was about to straighten little Alec Turner's club foot, and right at the fringe of the rumour came a note from his mother, the rector's wife, asking him if he would be so good as to act as chloroformist. It would be inhumanity to refuse, as there was no other who could take the place, but it was gall and wormwood to his sensitive nature. Yet, in spite of his vexation, he could not but admire the dexterity with which the thing was done. She handled the little wax-like foot so gently, and held the tiny tenotomy knife as an artist holds his pencil. One straight insertion, one snick of a tendon, and it was all over without a stain upon the white towel which lay beneath. He had never seen anything more masterly, and he had the honesty to say so, though her skill increased his dislike of her. The operation spread her fame still further at his expense, and self-preservation was added to his other grounds for detesting her. And this very detestation it was which brought matters to a curious climax.

One winter's night, just as he was rising from his lonely dinner, a groom came riding down from Squire Faircastle's, the richest man in the district, to say that his daughter had scalded her hand, and that medical help was needed on the instant. The coachman had ridden for the lady doctor, for it mattered nothing to the Squire who came as long as it were speedily. Dr. Ripley rushed from his surgery with the determination that she should not effect an entrance into this stronghold of his if hard driving on his part could prevent it. He did not even wait to light his lamps, but sprang into his gig and flew off as fast as hoof could rattle. He lived rather nearer to the Squire's than she did, and was convinced that he could get there well before her.

And so he would but for that whimsical element of chance, which will for ever muddle up the affairs of this world and dumbfound the prophets. Whether it came from the want of his lights, or from his mind being full of the thoughts of his rival, he allowed too little by half a foot in taking the sharp turn upon the Basingstoke road. The empty trap and the frightened horse clattered away into the darkness, while the Squire's groom crawled out of the ditch into which he had been shot. He struck a match, looked down at his groaning companion, and then, after the fashion of rough, strong men when they see what they have not seen before, he was very sick.

The doctor raised himself a little on his elbow in the glint of the match. He caught a glimpse of something white and sharp bristling through his trouser leg half way down the shin.

"Compound!" he groaned. "A three months' job," and fainted.

When he came to himself the groom was gone, for he had scudded off to the Squire's house for help, but a small page was holding a gig-lamp in front of his injured leg, and a woman, with an open case of polished instruments gleaming in the yellow light, was deftly slitting up his trouser with a crooked pair of scissors.

"It's all right, doctor," said she soothingly. "I am so sorry about it. You can have Dr. Horton to-morrow, but I am sure you will allow me to help you to-night. I could hardly believe my eyes when I saw you by the roadside."

"The groom has gone for help," groaned the sufferer.

"When it comes we can move you into the gig. A little more light, John! So! Ah, dear, dear, we shall have laceration unless we reduce this before we move you. Allow me to give you a whiff of chloroform, and I have no doubt that I can secure it sufficiently to—"

Dr. Ripley never heard the end of that sentence. He tried to raise a hand and to murmur something in protest, but a sweet smell was in his nostrils, and a sense of rich peace and lethargy stole over his jangled nerves. Down he sank, through clear, cool water, ever down and down into the green shadows beneath, gently, without effort, while the pleasant chiming of a great belfry rose and fell in his ears. Then he rose again, up and up, and ever up, with a terrible tightness about his temples, until at last he shot out of those green shadows and was in the light once more. Two bright, shining, golden spots gleamed before his dazed eyes. He blinked and blinked before he could give a name to them. They were only the two brass balls at the end posts of his bed, and he was lying in his own little room, with a head like a cannon ball, and a leg like an iron bar. Turning his eyes, he saw the calm face of Dr. Verrinder Smith looking down at him.

"Ah, at last!" said she. "I kept you under all the way home, for I knew how painful the jolting would be. It is in good position now with a strong side splint. I have ordered a morphia draught for you. Shall I tell your groom to ride for Dr. Horton in the morning?"

"I should prefer that you should continue the case," said Dr. Ripley feebly, and then, with a half hysterical laugh,—"You have all the rest of the parish as patients, you know, so you may as well make the thing complete by having me also."

It was not a very gracious speech, but it was a look of pity and not of anger which shone in her eyes as she turned away from his bedside.

Dr. Ripley had a brother, William, who was assistant surgeon at a London hospital, and who was down in Hampshire within a few hours of his hearing of the accident. He raised his brows when he heard the details.

"What! You are pestered with one of those!" he cried.

"I don't know what I should have done without her."

"I've no doubt she's an excellent nurse."

"She knows her work as well as you or I."

"Speak for yourself, James," said the London man with a sniff. "But apart from that, you know that the principle of the thing is all wrong."

"You think there is nothing to be said on the other side?"

"Good heavens! do you?"

"Well, I don't know. It struck me during the night that we may have been a little narrow in our views."

"Nonsense, James. It's all very fine for women to win prizes in the lecture room, but you know as well as I do that they are no use in an emergency. Now I warrant that this woman was all nerves when she was setting your leg. That reminds me that I had better just take a look at it and see that it is all right."

"I would rather that you did not undo it," said the patient. "I have her assurance that it is all right."

Brother William was deeply shocked.

"Of course, if a woman's assurance is of more value than the opinion of the assistant surgeon of a London hospital, there is nothing more to be said," he remarked.

"I should prefer that you did not touch it," said the patient firmly, and Dr. William went back to London that evening in a huff.

The lady, who had heard of his coming, was much surprised on learning his departure.

"We had a difference upon a point of professional etiquette," said Dr. James, and it was all the explanation he would vouchsafe.

For two long months Dr. Ripley was brought in contact with his rival every day, and he learned many things which he had not known before. She was a charming companion, as well as a most assiduous doctor. Her short presence during the long, weary day was like a flower in a sand waste. What interested him was precisely what interested her, and she could meet him at every point upon equal terms. And yet under all her learning and her firmness ran a sweet, womanly nature, peeping out in her talk, shining in her greenish eyes, showing itself in a thousand subtle ways which the dullest of men could read. And he, though a bit of a prig and a pedant, was by no means dull, and had honesty enough to confess when he was in the wrong.

"I don't know how to apologise to you," he said in his shame-faced fashion one day, when he had progressed so far as to be able to sit in an arm-chair with his leg upon another one; "I feel that I have been quite in the wrong."

"Why, then?"

"Over this woman question. I used to think that a woman must inevitably lose something of her charm if she took up such studies."

"Oh, you don't think they are necessarily unsexed, then?" she cried, with a mischievous smile.

"Please don't recall my idiotic expression."

"I feel so pleased that I should have helped in changing your views. I think that it is the most sincere compliment that I have ever had paid me."

"At any rate, it is the truth," said he, and was happy all night at the remembrance of the flush of pleasure which made her pale face look quite comely for the instant.

For, indeed, he was already far past the stage when he would acknowledge her as the equal of any other woman. Already he could not disguise from himself that she had become the one woman. Her dainty skill, her gentle touch, her sweet presence, the community of their tastes, had all united to hopelessly upset his previous opinions. It was a dark day for him now when his convalescence allowed her to miss a visit, and darker still that other one which he saw approaching when all occasion for her visits would be at an end. It came round at last, however, and he felt that his whole life's fortune would hang upon the issue of that final interview. He was a direct man by nature, so he laid his hand upon hers as it felt for his pulse, and he asked her if she would be his wife.

"What, and unite the practices?" said she.

He started in pain and anger.

"Surely you do not attribute any such base motive to me!" he cried. "I love you as unselfishly as ever a woman was loved."

"No, I was wrong, it was a foolish speech," said she, moving her chair a little back, and tapping her stethoscope upon her knee. "Forget that I ever said it. I am so sorry to cause you any disappointment, and I appreciate most highly the honour which you do me, but what you ask is quite impossible."

With another woman he might have urged the point, but his instincts told him that it was quite useless with this one. Her tone of voice was conclusive. He said nothing, but leaned back in his chair a stricken man.

"I am so sorry," she said again. "If I had known what was passing in your mind I should have told you earlier that I intended to devote my life entirely to science. There are many women with a capacity for marriage, but few with a taste for biology. I will remain true to my own line, then. I came down here while waiting for an opening in the Paris Physiological Laboratory. I have just heard that there is a vacancy for me there, and so you will be troubled no more by my intrusion upon your practice. I have done you an injustice just as you did me one. I thought you narrow and pedantic, with no good quality. I have learned during your illness to appreciate you better, and the recollection of our friendship will always be a very pleasant one to me.''

And so it came about that in a very few weeks there was only one doctor in Hoyland. But folks noticed that the one had aged many years in a few months, that a weary sadness lurked always in the depths of his blue eyes, and that he was less concerned than ever with the eligible young ladies whom chance, or their careful country mammas, placed in his way.

WILLIAM ERNEST HENLEY
In Hospital

———❦———

WILLIAM ERNEST HENLEY (1849-1903) was a poet, playwright, and
editor of the *National Observer*. He is notable for publishing and
promoting the early works of Hardy, Kipling, Yeats, and Robert Louis
Stevenson. Henley was crippled from youth by tuberculosis, having
one foot amputated, and was hospitalized intermittently throughout his
life.

The greater masters of the commonplace,
REMBRANDT and good SIR WALTER—only these
Could paint her all to you: experienced ease
And antique liveliness and ponderous grace;
The sweet old roses of her sunken face;
The depth and malice of her sly, gray eyes;
The broad Scots tongue that flatters, scolds, defies;
The thick Scots wit that fells you like a mace,
These thirty years has she been nursing here,
Some of them under SYME, her hero still.
Much is she worth, and even more is made of her.
Patients and students hold her very dear.
The doctors love her, tease her, use her skill.
They say 'The Chief' himself is half-afraid of her.

*　　*　　*

BLUE-EYED and bright of face but waning fast
Into the sere of virginal decay,
I view her as she enters, day by day,
As a sweet sunset almost overpast.
Kindly and calm, patrician to the last,
Superbly falls her gown of sober gray,
And on her chignon's elegant array
The plainest cap is somehow touched with caste.

She talks BEETHOVEN; frowns disapprobation
At BALZAC's name, sighs it at 'poor GEORGE SAND's';
Knows that she has exceeding pretty hands;
Speaks Latin with a right accentuation;
And gives at need (as one who understands)
Draught, counsel, diagnosis, exhortation.

WILLIAM DEAN HOWELLS
Dr. Breen's Practice

—◆◇◆—

WILLIAM DEAN HOWELLS (1837-1920) wrote prolific novels, plays, stories, and essays in an easy, popular style. As editor of the *Atlantic Monthly* he was influential in promoting new writers, particularly Mark Twain and Henry James.

The driver stopped his horses, and leaned out of the side of the wagon with a little package in his hand. He read the superscription, and then glanced consciously at the girl. "You're Miss Breen, ain't you?"

"Yes," she said, with lady-like sweetness and a sort of business-like alertness.

"Well," suggested the driver, "this is for Miss Grace Breen, *M.D.*"

"For me, thank you," said the young lady. "I'm Dr. Breen." She put out her hand for the little package from the homœopathic pharmacy in Boston; and the driver yielded it with a blush that reddened him to his hair. "Well," he said slowly, staring at the handsome girl, who did not visibly share his embarrassment, "they *told* me you was the *one*; but I could n't seem to get it through me. I thought it must be the *old* lady."

"My mother is *Mrs.* Breen," the young lady briefly explained, and walked rapidly away, leaving the driver stuck in the heavy sand of Sea-Glimpse Avenue.

"Why, *get* up!" he shouted to his horses. "Goin' to stay here all *day*?" He craned his neck round the side of the wagon for a sight of her. "Well, dumn 'f I don't wish *I* was sick! Steps along," he mused, watching the swirl and ripple of her skirt, "like—*I* dunno what."

With her face turned from him Dr. Breen blushed, too; she was not yet so used to her quality of physician that she could coldly bear the confusion to which her being a doctor put men. She laughed a little to herself at the helplessness of the driver, confronted probably for the first time with a graduate of the New York homœopathic school; but she believed that she had reasons for taking herself seriously in every way, and she had not entered upon this career without definite purpose. When she was not yet out of her teens, she had an unhappy love affair, which was always darkly referred to as a disappointment by people who knew of it at the time.

Though the particulars of the case do not directly concern this story, it may be stated that the recreant lover afterwards married her dearest girl-friend, whom he had first met in her company. It was cruel enough, and the hurt went deep; but it neither crushed nor hardened her. It benumbed her for a time; she sank out of sight; but when she returned to the knowledge of the world she showed no mark of the blow except what was thought a strange eccentricity in a girl such as she had been. The world which had known her—it was that of an inland New England city—heard of her definitely after several years as a student of medicine in New York. Those who had more of her intimacy understood that she had chosen this work with the intention of giving her life to it, in the spirit in which other women enter convents, or go out to heathen lands; but probably this conception had its exaggerations. What was certain was that she was rich enough to have no need of her profession as a means of support, and that its study had cost her more than the usual suffering that it brings to persons of sensitive nerves. Some details were almost insuperably repugnant; but in schooling herself to them she believed that she was preparing to encounter anything in the application of her science.

Her first intention had been to go back to her own town after her graduation, and begin the practice of her profession among those who had always known her, and whose scrutiny and criticism would be hardest to bear, and therefore, as she fancied, the most useful to her in the formation of character. But afterwards she relinquished her purpose in favor of a design which she thought would be more useful to others: she planned going to one of the great factory towns, and beginning practice there, in company with an older physician, among the children of the operatives. Pending the completion of this arrangement, which was waiting upon the decision of the other lady, she had come to Jocelyn's with her mother, and with Mrs. Maynard, who had arrived from the West, aimlessly sick and unfriended, just as they were about leaving home. There was no resource but to invite her with them, and Dr. Breen was finding her first patient in this unexpected guest. She did not wholly regret the accident; this, too, was useful work, though not that she would have chosen; but her mother, after a fortnight, openly repined, and could not mention Mrs. Maynard without some rebellious murmur. She was an old lady, who had once kept a very vigilant conscience for herself; but after making her life unhappy with it for some three-score years, she now applied it entirely to the exasperation and condemnation of others. She especially devoted it to fretting a New England girl's naturally morbid sense of duty in her daughter, and keeping it is the irritation of perpetual self-question. She had never actively opposed her studying medicine; that ambition had harmonized very well with certain radical tendencies of her own, and it was at least not marriage, which she had found tolerable only in its modified form of widowhood; but at every step after the decisive step was taken she was beset with misgivings lest Grace was not fully alive to the grave responsibilities of her office, which she accumulated upon the girl in proportion as she flung off all responsibilities of her own. She was doubtless deceived by that show of calm which sometimes deceived Grace herself, who, in tutoring her soul to bear what it had to bear, mistook her tense effort for spiritual repose, and scarcely realized through her tingling nerves the strain she was undergoing. In spite of the bitter experience of her life, she was still very ardent in her hopes of usefulness, very scornful of distress or discomfort to herself, and a little inclined to exact the heroism she was ready to show. She had a child's severe morality, and she had hardly learned to understand that there is much evil in the world that does not characterize the perpetrators: she held herself as strictly to account for every word and deed as she held others, and she had an almost passionate desire to meet the consequence of her errors; till that was felt, an intolerable doom hung over her. She tried not to be impulsive; that was criminal in one of her calling; and she struggled for patience with an endeavor that was largely successful.

As to the effect of her career outside of herself, and of those whom her skill was to benefit, she tried to think neither arrogantly nor meanly. She would not entertain the vanity that she was serving what is called the cause of woman, and she would not assume any duties or responsibilities toward it. She thought men were as good as women; at least one man had been no worse than one woman; and it was in no representative or exemplary character that she had chosen her course. At the same time that she held these same opinions, she believed that she had put away the hopes with the pleasures that might once have taken her as a young girl. In regard to what had changed the current of her life, she mentally asserted her mere nullity, her absolute non-existence. The thought of it no longer rankled, and that interest could never be hers again. If it had not been so much like affectation, and so counter to her strong aesthetic instinct, she might have made her dress somehow significant of her complete abeyance in such matters; but as it was she only studied simplicity, and as we have seen from the impression of the barge-driver she did not finally escape distinction in dress and manner. In fact, she could not have escaped that effect if she would; and it was one of the indomitable contradictions of her nature that she would not.

MADNESS

———— ∞ ————

No disease has been more of a challenge to physicians over the centuries than mental illness. There is no precise point, like water turning into steam, where irrational behavior clearly becomes a sickness. Yet the zone of irrationality knows no limits and its population can be mammoth. Madness affects not just individuals but entire societies, as contemporary history readily attests. Novels or plays—such as Maxwell Anderson's *The Bad Seed* or Charlotte Brontë's *Jane Eyre* are only a few examples of the affinity of the writer for the torments of soul that afflict almost all human beings at one time or another—and writers more than most.

FYODOR DOSTOEVSKI
Notes from Underground

---❧---

FYODOR MIKHAILOVICH DOSTOEVSKI (1821-1881), one of the nineteenth century's premier Russian novelists, was the son of a physician and grew up on the grounds of a hospital. He suffered frequent epileptic seizures, and it is not difficult to conclude that his own ill-health and later exile gave him a bleak outlook on life. The angst of modern man is expressed in *Notes from Underground*.

UNDERGROUND[1]

I

I am a sick man . . . I am a spiteful man. I am an unpleasant man. I think my liver is diseased. However, I don't know beans about my disease, and I am not sure what is bothering me. I don't treat it and never have, though I respect medicine and doctors. Besides, I am extremely superstitious, let's say sufficiently so to respect medicine. (I am educated enough not to be superstitious, but I am.) No, I refuse to treat it out of spite. You probably will not understand that. Well, but *I* understand it. Of course, I can't explain to you just whom I am annoying in this case by my spite. I am perfectly well aware that I cannot "get even" with the doctors by not consulting them. I know better than anyone that I thereby injure only myself and no one else. But still, if I don't treat it, it is out of spite. My liver is bad, well then—let it get even worse!

I have been living like that for a long time now—twenty years. I am forty now. I used to be in the civil service, but no longer am. I was a spiteful official. I was rude and took pleasure in being so. After all, I did not accept

[1]The author of these notes and the "Notes" themselves are, of course, imaginary. Nevertheless, such persons as the writer of these notes, not only may, but positively must, exist in our society, considering those circumstances under which our society was in general formed. I wanted to expose to the public more clearly than it is done usually, one of the characters of the recent past. He is one of the representatives of the current generation. In this excerpt, entitled "Underground," this person introduces himself, his views, and, as it were, tries to explain the reasons why he appeared and was bound to appear in our midst. In the following excerpt, the actual notes of this person about several events in his life, will appear. (*Fyodor Dostoevski*)

bribes, so I was bound to find a compensation in that, at least. (A bad joke but I will not cross it out. I wrote it thinking it would sound very witty; but now that I see myself that I only wanted to show off in a despicable way, I will purposely not cross it out!) When petitioners would come to my desk for information I would gnash my teeth at them, and feel intense enjoyment when I succeeded in distressing some one. I was almost always successful. For the most part they were all timid people—of course, they were petitioners. But among the fops there was one officer in particular I could not endure. He simply would not be humble, and clanked his sword in a disgusting way. I carried on a war with him for eighteen months over that sword. At last I got the better of him. He left off clanking it. However, that happened when I was still young. But do you know, gentlemen, what the real point of my spite was? Why, the whole trick, the real vileness of it lay in the fact that continually, even in moments of the worst spleen, I was inwardly conscious with shame that I was not only not spiteful but not even an embittered man, that I was simply frightening sparrows at random and amusing myself by it. I might foam at the mouth, but bring me some kind of toy, give me a cup of tea with sugar, and I would be appeased. My heart might even be touched, though probably I would gnash my teeth at myself afterward and lie awake that night with shame for months after. That is the way I am.

*   *   *

Gentlemen, you must excuse me for philosophizing; it's the result of forty years underground! Allow me to indulge my fancy for a minute. You see, gentlemen, reason, gentlemen, is an excellent thing, there is no disputing that, but reason is only reason and can only satisfy man's rational faculty, while will is a manifestation of all life, that is, of all human life including reason as well as all impulses. And although our life, in this manifestation of it, is often worthless, yet it is life nevertheless and not simply extracting square roots. After all, here I, for instance, quite naturally want to live, in order to satisfy all my faculties for life, and not simply my rational faculty, that is, not simply one-twentieth of all my faculties for life. What does reason know? Reason only knows what it has succeeded in learning (some things it will perhaps never learn; while this is nevertheless no comfort, why not say so frankly?) and human nature acts as a whole, with everything that is in it, consciously or unconsciously, and, even if it goes wrong, it lives. I suspect, gentlemen, that you are looking at me with compassion; you repeat to me that an enlightened and developed man, such, in short, as the future man will be, cannot knowingly desire anything disadvantageous to himself, that this can be proved mathematically. I thoroughly agree, it really can—by mathematics. But I repeat for the hundredth time, there is one case, one only, when man may purposely, consciously, desire what is injurious to himself, what is stupid, very stupid—simply in order *to have the right* to desire for himself even what is very stupid and not to be bound by an obligation to desire only what is rational. After all, this very stupid thing, after all, this caprice of ours, may really be more advantageous for us, gentlemen, than anything else on earth, especially in some cases. And in particular it may be more advantageous than any advantages even when it does us obvious harm, and contradicts the soundest conclusions of our reason about our advantage—because in any case it preserves for us what is most precious and most important—that is, our personality, our individuality. Some, you see, maintain that this really is the most precious thing for man; desire can, of course, if it desires, be in agreement with reason; particularly if it does not abuse this practice but does so in moderation, it is both useful and sometimes even praiseworthy. But very often, and even most often, desire completely and stubbornly opposes reason, and . . . and . . . and do you know that that, too, is useful and sometimes even praiseworthy? Gentlemen, let us suppose that man is not stupid. (Indeed, after all, one cannot say that about him anyway, if only for the one consideration that, if man is stupid, then, after all, who is wise?) But if he is not stupid, he is just the same monstrously ungrateful! Phenomenally ungrateful. I even believe that the best definition of man is—a creature that walks on two legs and is ungrateful. But that is not all, that is not his worst defect; his worst defect is his perpetual immorality, perpetual—from the days of the Flood to the Schleswig-Holstein period of human destiny. Immorality, and consequently lack of good sense; for it has long been accepted that lack of good sense is due to no other cause than immorality. Try it, and cast a look upon the history of mankind. Well, what will you see? Is it a grand spectacle? All right, grand, if you like. The Colossus of Rhodes, for instance, that is worth something. Mr. Anaevsky may well testify that some say it is the work of human hands, while others maintain that it was created by Nature herself. Is it variegated? Very well, it may be variegated too. If one only took the dress uniforms, military and civilian, of all peoples in all ages—that alone is worth something, and if you take the undress uniforms you will never get to the end of it; no historian could keep up with it. Is it monotonous? Very well. It may be monotonous, too; they fight and fight; they are fighting now, they fought first and they fought last—you will admit that it is almost too monotonous. In short, one may say anything about the history of the world—anything that might enter the most disordered imagination. The only thing one cannot say is that it is rational. The very word sticks in one's throat. And, indeed, this is even the kind of thing that continually happens. After all, there are continually turning up in life moral and rational people, sages, and lovers of humanity, who make it their goal for life to live as morally and rationally as possible, to be, so to speak, a light to their neighbors, simply in order to show them that it is really possible to live morally and rationally in this world. And so what? We all know that those very people sooner or later toward the end of their lives have been false to themselves, playing some trick, often a most indecent one. Now I ask you: What can one expect from man since he is a creature endowed with such strange qualities? Shower upon him every earthly blessing, drown him in bliss so that nothing but bubbles would dance on the surface of his bliss, as on a sea; give him such economic prosperity that he would have nothing else to do but sleep, eat cakes and busy himself with ensuring the continuation of world history and even then man, out of sheer ingratitude, sheer libel, would play you some loathsome trick. He would even risk his cakes and would deliberately desire the most fatal rubbish, the most uneconomical absurdity, simply to introduce into all this positive rationality his fatal fantastic element. It is just his fantastic dreams, his vulgar folly, that he will desire to retain, simply in order to prove to himself (as though that were so necessary) that men still are men and not piano keys, which even if played by the laws of nature themselves threaten to be controlled so completely that soon one will be able to desire nothing but by the calendar. And, after all, that is not all: even if man really were nothing but a piano key, even if this were proved to him by natural science and mathematics, even then he would not become reasonable, but would purposely do something perverse out of sheer ingratitude, simply to have his own way. And if he does not find any means he will devise destruction and chaos, will devise sufferings of all sorts, and will thereby have his own way. He will launch a curse upon the world, and, as only man can curse (it is his privilege, the primary distinction between him and other animals) then, after all, perhaps only by his curse will he attain his object, that is, really convince himself that he is a man and not a piano key! If you say that all this, too, can be calculated and tabulated, chaos and darkness and curses, so that the mere possibility of calculating it all beforehand would stop it all, and reason would reassert itself—then man would purposely go mad in order to be rid of reason and have his own way! I believe in that, I vouch for it, because, after all, the whole work of man seems really to consist in nothing but proving to himself continually that he is a man and not an organ stop. It may be at the cost of his skin! But he has proved it; he may become a caveman, but he will have proved it. And after that can one help sinning, rejoicing that it has not yet come, and that desire still depends on the devil knows what!

You will shout at me (that is, if you will still favor me with your shout) that, after all, no one is depriving me of my will, that all they are concerned with is that my will should somehow of itself, of its own free will, coincide with my own normal interests, with the laws of nature and arithmetic.

Bah, gentlemen, what sort of free will is left when we come to tables and arithmetic, when it will all be a case of two times two makes four? Two times two makes four even without my will. As if free will meant that!

* * *

Gentlemen, I am joking, of course, and I know myself that I'm joking badly, but after all you know, one can't take everything as a joke. I am, perhaps, joking with a heavy heart. Gentlemen, I am tormented by questions; answer them for me. Now you, for instance, want to cure men of their old habits and reform their will in accordance with science and common sense. But how do you know, not only that it is possible, but also that it is *desirable*, to reform man in that way? And what leads you to the conclusion that it is so *necessary* to reform man's desires? In short, how do you know that such a reformation will really be advantageous to man? And to go to the heart of the matter, why are you so *sure* of your conviction that not to act against his real normal advantages guaranteed by the conclusions of reason and arithmetic is always advantageous for man and must be a law for all mankind? After all, up to now it is only your supposition. Let us assume it to be a law of logic, but perhaps not a law of humanity at all. You gentlemen perhaps think that I am mad? Allow me to defend myself. I agree that man is pre-eminently a creative animal, predestined to strive consciously toward a goal, and to engage in engineering; that is, eternally and incessantly, to build new roads, *wherever they may lead*. But the reason why he sometimes wants to swerve aside may be precisely that he is *forced* to make that road, and perhaps, too, because however stupid the straightforward practical man may be in general, the thought nevertheless will sometimes occur to him that the road, it would seem, almost always does lead *somewhere*, and that the destination it leads to is less important than the process of making it, and that the chief thing is to save the well-behaved child from despising engineering, and so giving way to the fatal idleness, which, as we all know, is the mother of all vices. Man likes to create and build roads, that is beyond dispute. But why does he also have such a passionate love for destruction and chaos? Now tell me that! But on that point I want to say a few special words myself. May it not be that he loves chaos and destruction (after all, he sometimes unquestionably likes it very much, that is surely so) because he is instinctively afraid of attaining his goal and completing the edifice he is constructing? How do you know, perhaps he only likes that edifice from a distance, and not at all at close range, perhaps he only likes to build it and does not want to live in it, but will leave it, when completed, *aux animaux domestiques*—such as the ants, the sheep, and so on, and so on. Now the ants have quite a different taste. They have an amazing edifice of that type, that endures forever—the anthill.

With the anthill, the respectable race of ants began and with the anthill they will probably end, which does the greatest credit to their perseverance and staidness. But man is a frivolous and incongruous creature, and perhaps, like a chessplayer, loves only the process of the game, not the end of it. And who knows (one cannot swear to it), perhaps the only goal on earth to which mankind is striving lies in this incessant process of attaining, or in other words, in life itself, and not particularly in the goal which of course must always be two times two makes four, that is a formula, and after all, two times two makes four is no longer life, gentlemen, but is the beginning of death. Anyway, man has always been somehow afraid of this two times two makes four, and I am afraid of it even now. Granted that man does nothing but seek that two times two makes four, that he sails the oceans, sacrifices his life in the quest, but to succeed, really to find it—he is somehow afraid, I assure you. He feels that as soon as he has found it there will be nothing for him to look for. When workmen have finished their work they at least receive their pay, they go to the tavern, then they wind up at the police station—and there is an occupation for a week. But where can man go? Anyway, one can observe a certain awkwardness about him every time he attains such goals. He likes the process of attaining, but does not quite like to have attained, and that, of course, is terribly funny. In short, man is a comical creature; there seems to be a kind of pun in it all. But two times two makes four is, after all, something insufferable. Two times two makes four seems to me simply a piece of insolence. Two times two makes four is a fop standing with arms akimbo barring your path and spitting. I admit that two times two makes four is an excellent thing, but if we are going to praise everything, two times two makes five is sometimes also a very charming little thing.

And why are you so firmly, so triumphantly convinced that only the normal and the positive—in short, only prosperity—is to the advantage of man? Is not reason mistaken about advantage? After all, perhaps man likes something besides prosperity? Perhaps he likes suffering just as much? Perhaps suffering is just as great an advantage to him as prosperity? Man is sometimes fearfully, passionately in love with suffering and that is a fact. There is no need to appeal to universal history to prove that; only ask yourself, if only you are a man and have lived at all. As far as my own personal opinion is concerned, to care only for prosperity seems to me somehow even ill-bred. Whether it's good or bad, it is sometimes very pleasant to smash things, too. After all, I do not really insist on suffering or on prosperity either. I insist on my caprice, and its being guaranteed to me when necessary. Suffering would be out of place in vaudevilles, for instance; I know that. In the crystal palace it is even unthinkable; suffering means doubt, means negation, and what would be the good of a crystal palace if there could be any doubt about it? And yet I am sure man will never renounce real suffering, that is, destruction and chaos. Why, after all, suffering is the sole origin of consciousness. Though I stated at the beginning that consciousness, in my opinion, is the greatest misfortune for man, yet I know man loves it and would not give it up for any satisfaction. Consciousness, for instance, is infinitely superior to two times two makes four. Once you have two times two makes four, there is nothing left to do or to understand. There will be nothing left but to bottle up your five senses and plunge into contemplation. While if you stick to consciousness, even though you attain the same result, you can at least flog yourself at times, and that will, at any rate, liven you up. It may be reactionary, but corporal punishment is still better than nothing.

F. SCOTT FITZGERALD
Tender is the Night

Nicole was in the salon wearing a strange expression.

"Read that," she said.

He opened the letter. It was from a woman recently discharged, though with skepticism on the part of the faculty. It accused him in no uncertain terms of having seduced her daughter, who had been at her mother's side during the crucial stage of the illness. It presumed that Mrs. Diver would be glad to have this information and learn what her husband was "really like."

Dick read the letter again. Couched in clear and concise English he yet recognized it as the letter of a maniac. Upon a single occasion he had let the girl, a flirtatious little brunette, ride into Zurich with him, upon her request, and in the evening had brought her back to the clinic. In an idle, almost indulgent way, he kissed her. Later, she tried to carry the affair further, but he was not interested and subsequently, probably consequently, the girl had come to dislike him, and taken her mother away.

"This letter is deranged," he said. "I had no relations of any kind with that girl. I didn't even like her."

"Yes, I've tried thinking that," said Nicole.

"Surely you don't believe it?"

"I've been sitting here."

He sank his voice to a reproachful note and sat beside her.

"This is absurd. This is a letter from a mental patient."

"I was a mental patient."

He stood up and spoke more authoritatively.

"Suppose we don't have any nonsense, Nicole. Go and round up the children and we'll start."

In the car, with Dick driving, they followed the little promontories of the lake, catching the burn of light and water in the windshield, tunnelling through cascades of evergreen. It was Dick's car, a Renault so dwarfish that they all stuck out of it except the children, between whom Mademoiselle towered mast-like in the rear seat. They knew every kilometer of the road—where they would smell the pine needles and the black stove smoke. A high sun with a face traced on it beat fierce on the straw hats of the children.

Nicole was silent; Dick was uneasy at her straight hard gaze. Often he felt lonely with her, and frequently she tired him with the short floods of personal revelations that she reserved exclusively for him, "I'm like this—I'm more like that," but this afternoon he would have been glad had she rattled on in staccato for a while and given him glimpses of her thoughts. The situation was always most threatening when she backed up into herself and closed the doors behind her.

At Zug Mademoiselle got out and left them. The Divers approached the Agiri Fair through a menagerie of mammoth steamrollers that made way for them. Dick parked the car, and as Nicole looked at him without moving, he said: "Come on, darl." Her lips drew apart into a sudden awful smile, and his belly quailed, but as if he hadn't seen it he repeated: "Come on. So the children can get out."

"Oh, I'll come all right," she answered, tearing the words from some story spinning itself out inside her, too fast for him to grasp. "Don't worry about that. I'll come—"

"Then come."

She turned from him as he walked beside her but the smile still flickered across her face, derisive and remote. Only when Lanier spoke to her several times did she manage to fix her attention upon an object, a Punch-and-Judy show, and to orient herself by anchoring to it.

Dick tried to think what to do. The dualism in his views of her—that of the husband, that of the psychiatrist—was increasingly paralyzing his faculties. In these six years she had several times carried him over the line with her, disarming him by exciting emotional pity or by a flow of wit, fantastic and disassociated, so that only after the episode did he realize with the consciousness of his own relaxation from tension, that she had succeeded in getting a point against his better judgment.

A discussion with Topsy about the guignol—as to whether the Punch was the same Punch they had seen last year in Cannes—having been settled, the family walked along again between the booths under the open sky. The women's bonnets, perching over velvet vests, the bright, spreading skirts of many cantons, seemed demure against the blue and orange paint of the wagons and displays. There was the sound of a whining, tinkling hootchy-kootchy show.

Nicole began to run very suddenly, so suddenly that for a moment Dick did not miss her. Far ahead he saw her yellow dress twisting through the crowd, an ochre stitch along the edge of reality and unreality, and started after her. Secretly she ran and secretly he followed. As the hot afternoon went shrill and terrible with her flight he had forgotten the children; then he wheeled and ran back to them, drawing them this way and that by their arms, his eyes jumping from booth to booth.

"Madame," he cried to a young woman behind a white lottery wheel,

"Est-ce que je peux laisser ces petits avec vous deux minutes? C'est très urgent—je vous donnerai dix francs."

"Mais oui."

He headed the children into the booth. "Alors—restez avec cette gentille dame."

"Oui, Dick."

He darted off again but he had lost her; he circled the merry-go-round keeping up with it till he realized he was running beside it, staring always at the same horse. He elbowed through the crowd in the buvette; then remembering a predilection of Nicole's he snatched up an edge of a fortuneteller's tent and peered within. A droning voice greeted him, "La septième fille d'une septième fille née sur les rives du Nil—entrez, Monsieur—"

Dropping the flap he ran along toward where the plaisance terminated at the lake and a small ferris wheel revolved slowly against the sky. There he found her.

She was alone in what was momentarily the top boat of the wheel, and as it descended he saw that she was laughing hilariously; he slunk back in the crowd, a crowd which, at the wheel's next revolution, spotted the intensity of Nicole's hysteria.

"Regardez-moi ça!"

"Regarde donc cette Anglaise!"

Down she dropped again—this time the wheel and its music were slowing and a dozen people were around her car, all of them impelled by the quality of her laughter to smile in sympathetic idiocy. But when Nicole saw Dick her laughter died—she made a gesture of slipping by and away from him but he caught her arm and held it as they walked away.

"Why did you lose control of yourself like that?"

"You know very well why."

"No, I don't."

"That's just preposterous—let me loose—that's an insult to my intelligence. Don't you think I saw that girl look at you—that little dark girl. Oh, this is farcical—a child, not more than fifteen. Don't you think I saw?"

"Stop here a minute and quiet down."

They sat at a table, her eyes in a profundity of suspicion, her hand moving across her line of sight as if it were obstructed. "I want a drink—I want a brandy."

"You can't have brandy—you can have a bock if you want it."

"Why can't I have a brandy?"

"We won't go into that. Listen to me—this business about a girl is a delusion, do you understand that word?"

"It's always a delusion when I see what you don't want me to see."

He had a sense of guilt as in one of those nightmares where we are accused of a crime which we recognize as something undeniably experienced, but which upon waking we realize we have not committed. His eyes wavered from hers.

"I left the children with a gypsy woman in a booth. We ought to get them."

"Who do you think you are?" she demanded. "Svengali?"

Fifteen minutes ago they had been a family. Now as she was crushed into a corner by his unwilling shoulder, he saw them all, child and man, as a perilous accident.

"We're going home."

"Home!" she roared in a voice so abandoned that its louder tones wavered and cracked. "And sit and think that we're all rotting and the children's ashes are rotting in every box I open? That filth!"

Almost with relief he saw that her words sterilized her, and Nicole, sensitized down to the corium of the skin, saw the withdrawal in his face. Her own face softened and she begged, "Help me, help me, Dick!"

A wave of agony went over him. It was awful that such a fine tower should not be erected, only suspended, suspended from him. Up to a point that was right: men were for that, beam and idea, girder and logarithm; but somehow Dick and Nicole had become one and equal, not apposite and complementary; she was Dick too, the drought in the marrow of his bones. He could not watch her disintegrations without participating in them. His intuition rilled out of him as tenderness and compassion—he could only take the characteristically modern course, to interpose—he would get a nurse from Zurich, to take her over to-night.

"You *can* help me."

Her sweet bullying pulled him forward off his feet. "You've helped me before—you can help me now."

"I can only help you the same old way."

"Some one can help me."

"Maybe so. You can help yourself most. Let's find the children."

There were numerous lottery booths with white wheels—Dick was startled when he inquired at the first and encountered blank disavowals. Evil-eyed, Nicole stood apart, denying the children, resenting them as part of a downright world she sought to make amorphous. Presently Dick found them, surrounded by women who were examining them with delight like fine goods, and by peasant children staring.

"Merci, Monsieur, ah Monsieur est trop généreux. C'était un plaisir, M'sieur, Madame. Au revoir, mes petits."

They started back with a hot sorrow streaming down upon them; the car was weighted with their mutual apprehension and anguish, and the children's mouths were grave with disappointment. Grief presented itself in its terrible, dark unfamiliar color. Somewhere around Zug, Nicole, with a convulsive effort, reiterated a remark she had made before about a misty yellow house set back from the road that looked like a painting not yet dry, but it was just an attempt to catch at a rope that was playing out too swiftly.

Dick tried to rest—the struggle would come presently at home and he might have to sit a long time, restating the universe for her. A "schizophrêne" is well named as a split personality—Nicole was alternately a person to whom nothing need be explained and one to whom nothing *could* be explained. It was necessary to treat her with active and affirmative insistence, keeping the road to reality always open, making the road to escape harder going. But the brilliance, the versatility of madness is akin to the resourcefulness of water seeping through, over and around a dike. It requires the united front of many people to work against it. He felt it necessary that this time Nicole cure herself; he wanted to wait until she remembered the other times, and revolted from them. In a tired way, he planned that they would again resume the rêgime relaxed a year before.

He had turned up a hill that made a short cut to the clinic, and now as he stepped on the accelerator for a short straightaway run parallel to the hillside the car swerved violently left, swerved right, tipped on two wheels and, as Dick, with Nicole's voice screaming in his ear, crushed down the mad hand clutching the steering wheel, righted itself, swerved once more and shot off the road; it tore through low underbrush, tipped again and settled slowly at an angle of ninety degrees against a tree.

The children were screaming and Nicole was screaming and cursing and trying to tear at Dick's face. Thinking first of the list of the car and unable to estimate it Dick bent away Nicole's arm, climbed over the top side and lifted out the children; then he saw the car was in a stable position. Before doing anything else he stood there shaking and panting.

"You—!" he cried.

She was laughing hilariously, unashamed, unafraid, unconcerned. No one coming on the scene would have imagined that she had caused it; she laughed as after some mild escape of childhood.

"You were scared weren't you?" she accused him. "You wanted to live!"

She spoke with such force that in his shocked state Dick wondered if he had been frightened for himself—but the strained faces of the children, looking from parent to parent, made him want to grind her grinning mask into jelly.

Directly above them, half a kilometer by the winding road but only a hundred yards climbing, was an inn; one of its wings showed through the wooded hill.

"Take Topsy's hand," he said to Lanier, "like that, tight, and climb up that hill—see the little path? When you get to the inn tell them 'La voiture Divare est cassée.' Some one must come right down."

Lanier, not sure what had happened, but suspecting the dark and unprecedented, asked:

"What will you do, Dick?"

"We'll stay here in the car."

Neither of them looked at their mother as they started off. "Be careful crossing the road up there! Look both ways!" Dick shouted after them.

He and Nicole looked at each other directly, their eyes like blazing windows across a court of the same house. Then she took out a compact, looked in its mirror, and smoothed back the temple hair. Dick watched the children climbing for a moment until they disappeared among the pines half way up; then he walked around the car to see the damage and plan how to get it back on the road. In the dirt he could trace the rocking course they had pursued for over a hundred feet; he was filled with a violent disgust that was not like anger.

In a few minutes the proprietor of the inn came running down.

"My God!" he exclaimed. "How did it happen, were you going fast? What luck! Except for that tree you'd have rolled down hill!"

Taking advantage of Emile's reality, the wide black apron, the sweat upon the rolls of his face, Dick signalled to Nicole in a matter-of-fact way to let him help her from the car; whereupon she jumped over the lower side, lost her balance on the slope, fell to her knees and got up again. As she watched the men trying to move the car her expression became defiant. Welcoming even that mood Dick said:

"Go and wait with the children, Nicole."

Only after she had gone did he remember that she had wanted cognac, and that there was cognac available up there—he told Emile never mind about the car; they would wait for the chauffeur and the big car to pull it up onto the road. Together they hurried up to the inn.

WILLIAM SHAKESPEARE
King Lear

ACT V, SCENE VI

Edg. The safer sense will ne'er accommodate His master thus.

Lear. No, they cannot touch me for coining; I am the king himself.

Edg. Oh thou side-piercing sight!

Lear. Nature's above art in that respect. There's your press-money. That fellow handles his bow like a crow-keeper; draw me a clothier's yard. Look, look! a mouse. Peace, peace! this piece of toasted cheese will do't. There's my gauntlet; I'll prove it on a giant. Bring up the brown bills. O! well flown, bird; i' the clout, i' the clout; hewgh! Give the word.

Edg. Sweet marjoram.

Lear. Pass.

Glou. I know that voice.

Lear. Ha! Goneril, with a white beard! They flattered me like a dog, and told me I had white hairs in my beard ere the black ones were there. To say "ay" and "no" to ever thing I said! "Ay" and "no" too was no good divinity. When the rain came to wet me once and the wind to make me chatter, when the thunder would not peace at my bidding, there I found 'em, there I smelt 'em out. Go to, they are not men o' their words; they told me I was every thing; 'tis a lie. I am not ague-proof.

Glou. The trick of that voice I do well remember; Is't not the king?

Lear. Ay, every inch a king;

When I do stare, see how the subject quakes.

I pardon that man's life. What was thy cause?

Adultery?

Thou shalt not die; die for adultery! No;

The wren goes to't, and the small gilded fly

Does lecher in my sight,

Let copulation thrive; for Gloucester's bastard son

Was kinder to his father than my daughters

Got 'tween the lawful sheets.

To't luxury pell-mell! for I lack soldiers.

Behold yond simpering dame,

Whose face between her forks presageth snow;

That minces virtue, and does shake the head

To hear of pleasure's name;

358

The fitchew nor the soiled horse goes to't
With a more riotous appetite.
Down from the waist they are Centaurs,
Though women all above;
But to the girdle do the gods inherit.
Beneath is all the fiend's;
There's hell, there's darkness, there's the sulphurous pit,
Burning, scalding, stench, consumption; fie, fie,
fie! pah, pah! Give me an ounce of civet,
good apothecary, to sweeten my imagination:
there's money for thee.

Glou. O! let me kiss that hand.

Lear. Let me wipe it first; it smells of mortality.

Glou. Oh ruin'd piece of nature! This great world
Shall so wear out to naught. Dost thou know me?

Lear. I remember thine eyes well enough. Dost thou squint at me? No, do thy worst, blind Cupid; I'll not love. Read thou this challenge; mark but the penning of it.

Glou. Were all thy letters suns, I could not see one.

Edg. [*Aside*] I would not take this from report; it is,
And my heart breaks at it.

Lear. Read.

Glou. What! with the case of eyes?

Lear. Oh, ho! are you there with me? No eyes in your head, nor no money in your purse? Your eyes are in a heavy case, your purse in a light: yet you see how this world goes.

Glou. I see it feelingly.

Lear. What! art mad? A man may see how this world goes with no eyes. Look with thine ears: see how yond justice rails upon yond simple thief. Hark, in thine ear: change places, and, handy-dandy, which is the justice, which is the thief? Thou hast seen a farmer's dog bark at a beggar?

Glou. Ay, sir.

Lear. And the creature run from the cur? There thou might'st behold the great image of authority; a dog's obeyed in office,
Thou rascal beadle, hold thy bloody hand!
Why dost thou lash that whore? Strip thine own back;
Thou hotly lusts to use her in that kind
For which thou whipp'st her. The usurer hangs the cozener.
Through tatter'd clothes small vices do appear;

Robes and furr'd gowns hide all. Plate sin with gold,
And the strong lance of justice hurtless breaks;
Arm it in rags, a pigmy's straw does pierce it.
None does offend, none, I say, none; I'll able 'em:
Take that of me, my friend, who have the power
To seal the accuser's lips. Get thee glass eyes;
And, like a scurvy politician, seem
To see the things thou dost not. Now, now, now, now;
Pull off my boots; harder, harder; so.
Edg. [*Aside*] O! matter and impertinency mix'd;
Reason in madness.
Lear. If thou wilt weep my fortunes, take my eyes;
I know thee well enough; thy name is Gloucester;
Thou must be patient; we came crying hither:
Thou know'st the first time that we smell the air
We waul and cry. I will preach to thee: mark.
Glou. Alack, alack the day!
Lear. When we are born, we cry that we are come
To this great stage of fools. This' a good block!
It were a delicate strategem to shoe
A troop of horse with felt; I'll put 't in proof,
And when I have stol'n upon these sons-in-law,
Then, kill, kill, kill, kill, kill, kill!

Enter a Gentleman, with Attendants.

Gent. Oh! here he is; lay hand upon him. Sir, Your most dear daughter—
Lear. No rescue? What! a prisoner? I am even
The natural fool of fortune. Use me well;
You shall have ransom. Let me have surgeons;
I am cut to the brains.
Gent. You shall have any thing.
Lear. No seconds? all myself?
Why this would make a man a man of salt,
To use his eyes for garden water-pots,
Ay, and for laying autumn's dust.
Gent.   Good sir,—
Lear. I will die bravely, like a bridegroom. What!
I will be jovial; come, come; I am a king,
My masters, know you that?

Gent. You are a royal one, and we obey you.

Lear. Then there's life in't. Nay, an you get it, you shall get it by running.
Sa, sa, sa, sa.

[*Exit running. Attendants follow.*

Gent. A sight most pitiful in the meanest wretch,
Past speaking of in a king! Thou hast one daughter,
Who redeems nature from the general curse
Which twain have brought her to.

Edg. Hail, gentle sir!

Gent.   Sir, speed you; what's your will?

Edg. Do you hear aught, sir, of a battle toward?

Gent. Most sure and vulgar; every one hears that,
Which can distinguish sound.

Edg.   But, by your favour,
How near's the other army?

Gent. Near, and on speedy foot; the main descry
Stands on the hourly thought.

Edg.   I thank you, sir: that's all.

Gent. Though that the queen on special cause is here,
Her army is moved on.

Edg.   I thank you, sir. [*Exit Gentleman.*

Glou. You ever-gentle gods, take my breath from me:
Let not my worser spirit tempt me again
To die before you please!

Edg.   Well pray you, father.

Glou. Now, good sir, what are you?

Edg. A most poor man, made tame to fortune's blows;
Who, by the art of known and feeling sorrows,
Am pregnant to good pity. Give me your hand,
I'll lead you to some biding.

Glou.   Hearty thanks:
The bounty and the benison of heaven
To boot, and boot!

Enter OSWALD.

Osw.   A proclaim'd prize! Most happy!
That eyeless head of thine was first framed flesh
To raise my fortunes. Thou old unhappy traitor,

Briefly thyself remember: the sword is out
That must destroy thee.
Glou.   Now let thy friendly hand
Put strength enough to 't.   [*Edgar interposes.*
Osw.   Wherefore, bold peasant
Darest thou support a publish'd traitor? Hence;
Lest that the infection of his fortune take
Like hold on thee. Let go his arm.
Edg. Chill not let go, zur, without vurther 'casion.
Osw. Let go, slave, or thou diest.
Edg. Good gentleman, go your gait, and let poor volk pass. An chud ha'bin
zwaggered out of my life, 'twould not ha'bin zo long as 'tis by a vortnight.
Nay, come not near th' old man; keep out, che vor ye, or ise try whither
your costard or my ballow be the harder. Chill be plain with you.
Osw. Out, dunghill!
Edg. Chill pick your teeth, zir. Come; no matter vor your foins.
                    [*They fight, and Edgar knocks him down.*
Osw. Slave, thou hast slain me. Villain, take my purse.
If ever thou wilt thrive, bury my body;
And give the letters which thou find'st about me
To Edmund Earl of Gloucester; seek him out
Upon the English party; O! untimely death
Death!
                                              [*Dies.*

Edg. I know thee well: a serviceable villain;
As duteous to the vices of thy mistress
As badness would desire.
Glou.   What! is he dead?
Edg. Sit you down, father; rest you.
Let's see these pockets; the letters that he speaks of
May be my friends. He's dead; I am only sorry
He had no other deathsman. Let us see:
Leave, gentle wax; and, manners, blame us not:
To know our enemies' minds, we'd rip their hearts;
Their papers is more lawful.

*Let us reciprocal vows be remembered. You have many opportunities
to cut him off; if your will want not, time and place will be fruitfully
offered. There is nothing done if he return the conqueror; then am I the*

*prisoner, and his bed my gaol; from the loathed warmth whereof deliver
me, and supply the place for your labour.*

Your—wife, so I would say—

Affectionate Servant,

GONERIL.

O undistinguish'd space of woman's will!
A plot upon her virtuous husband's life,
And the exchange my brother! Here, in the sands,
Thee I'll rake up, the post unsanctified
Of murderous lechers; and in the mature time
With this ungracious paper strike the sight
Of the death-practised duke. For him 'tis well
That of thy death and business I can tell.

Glou. The king is mad; how stiff is my vile sense
That I stand up, and have ingenious feeling
Of my huge sorrows! Better I were distract:
So should my thoughts be sever'd from my griefs,
And woes by wrong imaginations lose
The knowledge of themselves.   [*A drum afar off.*

Edg.   Give me your hand:
Far off, methinks, I hear the beaten drum.
Come, father, I'll bestow you with a friend.   [*Exeunt.*

SCENE VII.—*A Tent in the French Camp.*

Enter CORDELIA, KENT, *Doctor, and Gentleman.*

Cor. Oh thou good Kent! how shall I live and work
To match thy goodness? My life will be too short,
And every measure fail me.

Kent. To be acknowledg'd, madam, is o'er-paid.
All my reports go with the modest truth,
Nor more nor clipp'd, but so.

Cor.   Be better suited:
These weeds are memories of those worser hours:
I prithee, put them off.

Kent.   Pardon me, dear madam;
Yet to be known shortens my made intent;
My boon I make it that you know me not
Till time and I think meet.

Cor. Then be't so, my good lord. [*To the Doctor.*] How does the king?

Doct. Madam, sleeps still.

Cor. O you kind gods,
Cure this great breach in his abused nature!
The untuned and jarring senses, O! wind up
Of this child-changed father.

Doct.   So please your majesty
That we may wake the king? he hath slept long.

Cor. Be govern'd by your knowledge, and proceed
I' the sway of your own will. Is he array'd?

Enter LEAR *in a chair carried by Servants.*

Doct. Ay, madam; in the heaviness of sleep
We put fresh garments on him.

Kent. Be by, good madam, when we do awake him;
I doubt not of his temperance.

Cor.   Very well. [*Music.*

Doct. Please you, draw near. Louder the music there!

Cor. O my dear father! Restoration hang
Thy medicine on my lips, and let this kiss
Repair those violent harms that my two sisters
Have in thy reverence made!

Kent.   Kind and dear princess!

Cor. Had you not been their father, these white flakes
Had challenged pity of them. Was this a face
To be opposed against the warring winds?
To stand against the deep dread-bolted thunder?
In the most terrible and nimble stroke
Of quick, cross lightning? to watch—poor perdu!
With this thin helm? Mine enemy's dog,
Though he had bit me, should have stood that night
Against my fire. And wast thou fain, poor father,
To hovel thee with swine and rogues forlorn,
In short and musty straw? Alack, alack!
'Tis wonder that thy life and wits at once
Had not concluded all. He wakes; speak to him.

Doct. Madam, do you 'tis fittest.

Cor. How does my royal lord? How fares your majesty?

Lear. You do me wrong to take me out o' the grave;
Thou art a soul in bliss; but I am bound

Upon a wheel of fire that mine own tears
Do scald like molten lead.
Cor.   Sir, do you know me?
Lear. You are a spirit, I know; when did you die?
Cor. Still, still, far wide.
Doct. He's scarce awake; let him alone awhile.
Lear. Where have I been? Where am I? Fair day,
light?
  I am mightily abused. I should e'en die with pity
  To see another thus. I know not what to say.
  I will not swear these are my hands; let's see;
  I feel this pin prick. Would I were assured
  Of my condition!
Cor.   O! look upon me, sir,
  And hold your hands in benediction o'er me.
  No, sir, you must not kneel.
Lear.   Pray, do not mock me;
  I am a very foolish fond old man,
  Fourscore and upward, not an hour more nor less;
  And, to deal plainly,
  I fear I am not in my perfect mind.
  Methinks I should know you and know this man;
  Yet I am doubtful: for I am mainly ignorant
  What place this is, and all the skill I have
  Remembers not these garments; nor I know not
  Where I did lodge last night. Do not laugh at me;
  For, as I am a man, I think this lady
  To be my child Cordelia.
Cor.   And so I am, I am.
Lear. Be your tears wet? Yes, faith. I pray, weep not:
  If you have poison for me, I will drink it.
  I know you do not love me; for your sisters
  Have, as I do remember, done me wrong;
  You have some cause, they have not.
Cor.   No cause, no cause.
Lear. Am I in France?
Kent.   In your own kingdom, sir.
Lear. Do not abuse me.
Doct. Be comforted, good madam; the great rage,
  You see, is kill'd him; and yet it is danger

To make him even o'er the time he has lost.
Desire him to go in; trouble him no more
Till further settling.

Cor. Will't please your highness walk?

Lear.   You must bear with me.
Pray you now, forget and forgive: I am old and foolish.

[Exeunt Lear, Cordelia, Doctor, and Attendants.

Gent. Holds it true, sir, that the Duke of Cornwall was so slain?

Kent. Most certain, sir.

Gent. Who is conductor of his people?

Kent. As 'tis said, the bastard son of Gloucester.

Gent. They say Edgar, his banished son, is with the Earl of Kent in Germany.

Kent. Report is changeable. 'Tis time to look about; the powers of the kingdom approach apace.

Gent. The arbitrement is like to be bloody. Fare you well, sir.   [*Exit.*

Kent. My point and period will be throughly wrought,
Or well or ill, as this day's battle's fought.   [*Exit.*

VIRGINIA WOOLF
Mrs. Dalloway

VIRGINIA WOOLF (1882-1940) was an outstanding literary critic, essayist, and novelist in the stream-of-consciousness style. She was plagued with manic bouts of madness, reproduced hauntingly in the portrait of the shell-shocked veteran in *Mrs. Dalloway*.

Nothing could rouse him. Rezia put him to bed. She sent for a doctor—Mrs. Filmer's Dr. Holmes. Dr. Holmes examined him. There was nothing whatever the matter, said Dr. Holmes. Oh, what a relief! What a kind man, what a good man! thought Rezia. When he felt like that he went to the Music Hall, said Dr. Holmes. He took a day off with his wife and played golf. Why not try two tabloids of bromide dissolved in a glass of water at bedtime? These old Bloomsbury houses, said Dr. Holmes, tapping the wall, are often full of very fine panelling, which the landlords have the folly to paper over. Only the other day, visiting a patient, Sir Somebody Something in Bedford Square—

So there was no excuse; nothing whatever the matter, except the sin for which human nature had condemned him to death; that he did not feel. He had not cared when Evans was killed; that was worst; but all the other crimes raised their heads and shook their fingers and jeered and sneered over the rail of the bed in the early hours of the morning at the prostrate body which lay realising its degradation; how he had married his wife without loving her; had lied to her; seduced her; outraged Miss Isabel Pole, and was so pocked and marked with vice that women shuddered when they saw him in the street. The verdict of human nature on such a wretch was death.

Dr. Holmes came again. Large, fresh coloured, handsome, flicking his boots, looking in the glass, he brushed it all aside—headaches, sleeplessness, fears, dreams—nerve symptoms and nothing more, he said. If Dr. Holmes found himself even half a pound below eleven stone six, he asked his wife for another plate of porridge at breakfast. (Rezia would learn to cook porridge.) But, he continued, health is largely a matter in our own control. Throw yourself into outside interests; take up some hobby. He opened Shakespeare—*Antony and Cleopatra;* pushed Shakespeare aside.

Some hobby, said Dr. Holmes, for did he not owe his own excellent health (and he worked as hard as any man in London) to the fact that he could always switch off from his patients on to old furniture? And what a very pretty comb, if he might say so, Mrs. Warren Smith was wearing!

When the damned fool came again, Septimus refused to see him. Did he indeed? said Dr. Holmes, smiling agreeably. Really he had to give that charming little lady, Mrs. Smith, a friendly push before he could get past her into her husband's bedroom.

"So you're in a funk," he said agreeably, sitting down by his patient's side. He had actually talked of killing himself to his wife, quite a girl, a foreigner, wasn't she? Didn't that give her a very odd idea of English husbands? Didn't one owe perhaps a duty to one's wife? Wouldn't it be better to do something instead of lying in bed? For he had forty years' experience behind him; and Septimus could take Dr. Holmes's word for it—there was nothing whatever the matter with him. And next time Dr. Holmes came he hoped to find Smith out of bed and not making that charming little lady his wife anxious about him.

Human nature, in short, was on him—the repulsive brute, with the blood-red nostrils. Holmes was on him. Dr. Holmes came quite regularly every day. Once you stumble, Septimus wrote on the back of a postcard, human nature is on you. Holmes is on you. Their only chance was to escape, without letting Holmes know; to Italy—anywhere, anywhere, away from Dr. Holmes.

But Rezia could not understand him. Dr. Holmes was such a kind man. He was so interested in Septimus. He only wanted to help them, he said. He had four little children and he had asked her to tea, she told Septimus.

So he was deserted. The whole world was clamouring: Kill yourself, kill yourself, for our sakes. But why should he kill himself for their sakes? Food was pleasant; the sun hot; and this killing oneself, how does one set about it, with a table knife, uglily, with floods of blood,—by sucking a gaspipe? He was too weak; he could scarcely raise his hand. Besides, now that he was quite alone, condemned, deserted, as those who are about to die are alone, there was a luxury in it, an isolation full of sublimity; a freedom which the attached can never know. Holmes had won of course; the brute with the red nostrils had won. But even Holmes himself could not touch his last relic straying on the edge of the world, this outcast, who gazed back at the inhabited regions, who lay, like a drowned sailor, on the shore of the world.

It was at that moment (Rezia gone shopping) that the great revelation took place. A voice spoke from behind the screen. Evans was speaking. The dead were with him.

"Evans, Evans!" he cried.

Mr. Smith was talking aloud to himself, Agnes the servant girl cried to Mrs. Filmer in the kitchen. "Evans, Evans," he had said as she brought in the tray. She jumped, she did. She scuttled downstairs.

And Rezia came in, with her flowers, and walked across the room, and put the roses in a vase, upon which the sun struck directly, and it went laughing, leaping round the room.

She had had to buy the roses, Rezia said, from a poor man in the street. But they were almost dead already, she said, arranging the roses.

So there was a man outside; Evans presumably; and the roses, which Rezia said were half dead, had been picked by him in the fields of Greece. "Communication is health; communication is happiness, communication—" he muttered.

"What are you saying, Septimus?" Rezia asked, wild with terror, for he was talking to himself.

She sent Agnes running for Dr. Holmes. Her husband, she said, was mad. He scarcely knew her.

"You brute! You brute!" cried Septimus, seeing human nature, that is Dr. Holmes, enter the room.

"Now what's all this about?" said Dr. Holmes in the most amiable way in the world. "Talking nonsense to frighten your wife?" But he would give him something to make him sleep. And if they were rich people, said Dr. Holmes, looking ironically around the room, by all means let him go to Harley Street; if they had no confidence in him, said Dr. Holmes, looking not quite so kind.

It was precisely twelve o'clock; twelve by Big Ben; whose stroke was wafted over the northern part of London; blent with that of other clocks, mixed in a thin ethereal way with the clouds and wisps of smoke, and died up there among the seagulls—twelve o'clock struck as Clarissa Dalloway laid her green dress on her bed, and the Warren Smiths walked down Harley Street. Twelve was the hour of their appointment. Probably, Rezia thought, that was Sir William Bradshaw's house with the grey motor car in front of it. The leaden circles dissolved in the air.

Indeed it was—Sir William Bradshaw's motor car; low, powerful, grey with plain initials interlocked on the panel, as if the pomps of heraldry were incongruous, this man being the ghostly helper, the priest of science; and, as the motor car was grey, so to match its sober suavity, grey furs, silver grey rugs were heaped in it, to keep her ladyship warm while she waited. For often Sir William would travel sixty miles or more down into the country to visit the rich, the afflicted, who could afford the very large fee which Sir William very properly charged for his advice. Her ladyship waited with the rugs about her knees an hour or more, leaning back, thinking sometimes of the patient, sometimes, excusably, of the wall of gold, mounting minute by minute while she waited; the wall of gold that was mounting between them and all shifts and anxieties (she had borne them bravely; they had had their struggles) until she felt wedged on a calm ocean, where only spice winds blow; respected, admired, envied, with scarcely anything left to wish for, though she regretted her stoutness; large dinner-parties every Thursday night to the profession; an occasional bazaar to be opened; Royalty greeted; too little time, alas, with her husband, whose work grew and grew; a boy doing well at Eton; she would have liked a daughter too; interests she had, however, in plenty; child welfare; the after-care of the epileptic, and photography, so that if there was a church building, or a church decaying, she bribed the sexton, got the key and took photographs, which were scarcely to be distinguished from the work of professionals, while she waited.

Sir William himself was no longer young. He had worked very hard; he had won his position by sheer ability (being the son of a shopkeeper); loved his profession; made a fine figurehead at ceremonies and spoke well—all of which had by the time he was knighted given him a heavy look, a weary look (the stream of patients being so incessant, the responsibilities and privileges of his profession so onerous), which weariness, together with his grey hairs, increased the extraordinary distinction of his presence and gave him the reputation (of the utmost importance in dealing with nerve cases) not merely of lightning skill, and almost infallible accuracy in diagnosis but of sympathy; tact; understanding of the human soul. He could see the first moment they came into the room (the Warren Smiths they were called); he was certain directly he saw the man; it was a case of extreme gravity. It was a case of complete breakdown—complete physical and nervous breakdown, with every symptom in an advanced stage, he ascertained in two or three minutes (writing answers to questions, murmured discreetly, on a pink card).

How long had Dr. Holmes been attending him?

Six weeks.

Prescribed a little bromide? Said there was nothing the matter? Ah yes (those general practitioners! thought Sir William. It took half his time to undo their blunders. Some were irreparable).

"You served with great distinction in the War?"

The patient repeated the word "war" interrogatively.

He was attaching meanings to words of a symbolical kind. A serious symptom, to be noted on the card.

"The War?" the patient asked. The European War—that little shindy of schoolboys with gunpowder? Had he served with distinction? He really forgot. In the War itself he had failed.

"Yes, he served with the greatest distinction," Rezia assured the doctor; "he was promoted."

"And they have the very highest opinion of you at your office?" Sir William murmured, glancing at Mr. Brewer's very generously worded letter. "So that you have nothing to worry you, no financial anxiety, nothing?"

He had committed an appalling crime and been condemned to death by human nature.

"I have—I have," he began, "committed a crime—"

"He had done nothing wrong whatever," Rezia assured the doctor. If Mr. Smith would wait, said Sir William, he would speak to Mrs. Smith in the next room. Her husband was very seriously ill, Sir William said. Did he threaten to kill himself?

Oh, he did, she cried. But he did not mean it, she said. Of course not. It was merely a question of rest, said Sir William; of rest, rest, rest; a long rest in bed. There was a delightful home down in the country where her husband would be perfectly looked after. Away from her? she asked. Unfortunately, yes; the people we care for most are not good for us when we are ill. But he was not mad, was he? Sir William said he never spoke of "madness"; he called it not having a sense of proportion. But her husband did not like doctors. He would refuse to go there. Shortly and kindly Sir William explained to her the state of the case. He had threatened to kill himself. There was no alternative. It was a question of law. He would lie in bed in a beautiful house in the country. The nurses were admirable. Sir William would visit him once a week. If Mrs. Warren Smith was quite sure she had no more questions to ask—he never hurried his patients—they would return to her husband. She had nothing more to ask—not of Sir William.

So they returned to the most exalted of mankind; the criminal who faced his judges; the victim exposed on the heights; the fugitive; the drowned sailor; the poet of the immortal ode; the Lord who had gone from life to death; to Septimus Warren Smith, who sat in the arm-chair under the skylight staring at a photograph of Lady Bradshaw in Court dress, muttering messages about beauty.

"We have had our little talk," said Sir William.

"He says you are very, very ill," Rezia cried.

"We have been arranging that you should go into a home," said Sir William.

"One of Holmes's homes?" sneered Septimus.

The fellow made a distasteful impression. For there was in Sir William, whose father had been a tradesman, a natural respect for breeding and clothing, which shabbiness nettled; again, more profoundly, there was in Sir William, who had never had time for reading, a grudge, deeply buried, against cultivated people who came into his room and intimated that doctors, whose profession is a constant strain upon all the highest faculties, are not educated men.

"One of *my* homes, Mr. Warren Smith," he said, "where we will teach you to rest."

And there was just one thing more.

He was quite certain that when Mr. Warren Smith was well he was the last man in the world to frighten his wife. But he had talked of killing himself.

"We all have our moments of depression," said Sir William.

Once you fall, Septimus repeated to himself, human nature is on you. Holmes and Bradshaw are on you. They scour the desert. They fly screaming into the wilderness. The rack and the thumbscrew are applied. Human nature is remorseless.

"Impulses came upon him sometimes?" Sir William asked, with his pencil on a pink card.

That was his own affair, said Septimus.

"Nobody lives for himself alone," said Sir William, glancing at the photograph of his wife in Court dress.

"And you have a brilliant career before you," said Sir William. There was Mr. Brewer's letter on the table. "An exceptionally brilliant career."

But if he confessed? If he communicated? Would they let him off then, his tortures?

"I—I—" he stammered.

But what was his crime? He could not remember it.

"Yes?" Sir William encouraged him. (But it was growing late.)

Love, trees, there is no crime—what was his message?

He could not remember it.

"I—I" Septimus stammered.

"Try to think as little about yourself as possible," said Sir William kindly. Really, he was not fit to be about.

Was there anything else they wished to ask him? Sir William would make all arrangements (he murmured to Rezia) and he would let her know between five and six that evening he murmured.

"Trust everything to me," he said, and dismissed them.

Never, never had Rezia felt such agony in her life! She had asked for help and been deserted! He had failed them! Sir William Bradshaw was not a nice man.

The upkeep of that motor car alone must cost him quite a lot, said Septimus, when they got out into the street.

She clung to his arm. They had been deserted.

But what more did she want?

To his patients he gave three-quarters of an hour; and if in this exacting science which has to do with what, after all, we know nothing about—the nervous system, the human brain—a doctor loses his sense of proportion, as a doctor he fails. Health we must have; and health is proportion; so that when a man comes into your room and says he is Christ (a common delusion), and has a message, as they mostly have, and threatens, as they often do, to kill himself, you invoke proportion; order rest in bed; rest in solitude; silence and rest; rest without friends, without books, without messages; six months' rest; until a man who went in weighing seven stone six comes out weighing twelve.

Proportion, divine proportion, Sir William's goddess, was acquired by Sir William walking hospitals, catching salmon, begetting one son in Harley Street by Lady Bradshaw, who caught salmon herself and took photographs scarcely to be distinguished from the work of professionals. Worshipping proportion, Sir William not only prospered himself but made England prosper, secluded her lunatics, forbade childbirth, penalised despair, made it impossible for the unfit to propagate their views until they, too, shared his sense of proportion—his, if they were men, Lady Bradshaw's if they were women (she embroidered, knitted, spent four nights out of seven at home with her son), so that not only did his colleagues respect him, his subordinates fear him, but the friends and relations of his patients felt for him the keenest gratitude for insisting that these prophetic Christs and Christesses, who prophesied the end of the world, or the advent of God, should drink milk in bed, as Sir William ordered; Sir William with his thirty years' experience of these kinds of cases, and his infallible instinct, this is madness, this sense; in fact, his sense of proportion.

But Proportion has a sister, less smiling, more formidable, a Goddess even now engaged—in the heat and sands of India, the mud and swamp of Africa, the purlieus of London, wherever in short the climate or the devil tempts men to fall from the true belief which is her own—is even now engaged in dashing down shrines, smashing idols, and setting up in their place her own stern countenance. Conversion is her name and she feasts on the wills of the weakly, loving to impress, to impose, adoring her own features stamped on the face of the populace. At Hyde Park Corner on a tub she stands preaching; shrouds herself in white and walks penitentially disguised as brotherly love through factories and parliaments; offers help, but desires power; smites out of her way roughly the dissentient, or dissatisfied; bestows her blessing on those who, looking upward, catch submissively from her eyes the light of their own. This lady too (Rezia Warren Smith divined it) had her dwelling in Sir William's heart, though concealed, as she mostly is, under some plausible disguise; some venerable name; love, duty, self sacrifice. How he would work—how toil to raise funds, propagate reforms, initiate institutions! But conversion, fastidious Goddess, loves blood better than brick, and feasts most subtly on the human will. For example, Lady Bradshaw. Fifteen years ago she had gone under. It was nothing you could put your finger on; there had been no scene, no snap; only the slow sinking, water-logged, of her will into his. Sweet was her smile, swift her submission; dinner in Harley Street, numbering eight or nine courses, feeding ten or fifteen guests of the professional classes, was smooth and urbane. Only as the evening wore on a very slight dullness, or uneasiness perhaps, a nervous twitch, fumble, stumble and confusion indicated, what it was really painful to believe—that the poor lady lied. Once, long ago, she had caught salmon freely: now, quick to minister to the craving which lit her husband's eye so oilily for dominion, for power, she cramped, squeezed, pared, pruned, drew back, peeped through; so that without knowing precisely what made the evening disagreeable, and caused this pressure on the top of the head (which might well be imputed to the professional conversation, or the fatigue of a great doctor whose life, Lady Bradshaw said, "is not his own but his patients' ") disagreeable it was: so that guests, when the clock struck ten, breathed in the air of Harley Street even with rapture; which relief, however, was denied to his patients.

There in the grey room, with the pictures on the wall, and the valuable furniture, under the ground glass skylight, they learnt the extent of their transgressions; huddled up in arm-chairs, they watched him go through, for their benefit, a curious exercise with the arms, which he shot out, brought sharply back to his hip, to prove (if the patient was obstinate) that Sir William was master of his own actions, which the patient was not. There some weakly broke down; sobbed, submitted; others, inspired by Heaven knows what intemperate madness, called Sir William to his face a damnable humbug; questioned, even more impiously, life itself. Why live? they demanded. Sir William replied that life was good. Certainly Lady Bradshaw in ostrich feathers hung over the mantelpiece, and as for his income it

was quite twelve thousand a year. But to us, they protested, life has given
no such bounty. He acquiesced. They lacked a sense of proportion. And
perhaps, after all, there is no God? He shrugged his shoulders. In short, this
living or not living is an affair of our own? But there they were mistaken. Sir
William had a friend in Surrey where they taught, what Sir William frankly
admitted was a difficult art—a sense of proportion. There were, moreover,
family affection; honour; courage; and a brilliant career. All of these had in
Sir William a resolute champion. If they failed him, he had to support police
and the good of society, which, he remarked very quietly, would take care,
down in Surrey, that these unsocial impulses, bred more than anything by
the lack of good blood, were held in control. And then stole out from her
hiding-place and mounted her throne that Goddess whose lust is to override
opposition, to stamp indelibly in the sanctuaries of others the image of
herself. Naked, defenceless, the exhausted, the friendless received the
impress of Sir William's will. He swooped; he devoured. He shut people
up. It was his combination of decision and humanity that endeared Sir
William so greatly to the relations of his victims.

DYING

———◆———

There are few greater challenges to a writer's ability to use words than the fact of death—universal, omnipresent, incomprehensible. The doctor is called upon to combat it more than any other, but his greatest victory can only be a deferral. Yet even deferrals are great prizes to a species for which life is only an interim arrangement. The writer therefore observes the physician closely in his role adjacent to that of philosopher and theologian, a role which is as difficult for the physician to accept explicitly as it is for him to shun or deny.

> No life that breathes with human breath
> Has ever truly longed for death.
>
> *Tennyson.*

> Let death be daily before your eyes, and you will never entertain any abject thought, nor too eagerly covet anything.
>
> *Epictetus.*

> We sometimes congratulate ourselves at the moment of waking from a troubled dream; it may be so the moment after death.
>
> *Hawthorne.*

> Death is the liberator of him whom freedom cannot release; the physician of him whom medicine cannot cure; the comforter of him whom time cannot console.
>
> *Colton.*

> Death,
> The undiscover'd country, from whose bourne
> No traveller returns.
>
> *Shakespeare.*

W. H. AUDEN
Give Me a Doctor

Give me a doctor, partridge-plump,
Short in the leg and broad in the rump,
An endomorph with gentle hands,
Who'll never make absurd demands
That I abandon all my vices,
Nor pull a long face in a crisis,
But with a twinkle in his eye
Will tell me that I have to die.

ERNEST HEMINGWAY
Indian Camp

————◁∞▷————

ERNEST HEMINGWAY (1899-1961), the son of a doctor, is even more highly regarded around the world than in the United States. Most literary critics agree that Hemingway and William Faulkner are the pre-eminent literary figures of their time. His work is wide-ranging, both in form and subject matter. The source of his broad appeal to readers is his narrative prose. Few writers handle dialogue as skillfully as he has done. Despite all the acclaim, he was terribly unsure of himself as a writer. His insecurity was never more manifest than in his attitude towards money. With assured royalties from his books running into the millions, he agonized constantly over his financial future. He was in the hands of psychiatrists almost constantly in the last few years of his life. "Indian Camp," and all of the other Nick Adams stories, are largely autobiographical.

At the lake shore there was another rowboat drawn up. The two Indians stood waiting.

Nick and his father got in the stern of the boat and the Indians shoved it off and one of them got in to row. Uncle George sat in the stern of the camp rowboat. The young Indian shoved the camp boat off and got in to row Uncle George.

The two boats started off in the dark. Nick heard the oarlocks of the other boat quite a way ahead of them in the mist. The Indians rowed with quick choppy strokes. Nick lay back with his father's arm around him. It was cold on the water. The Indian who was rowing them was working very hard, but the other boat moved further ahead in the mist all the time.

"Where are we going, Dad?" Nick asked.

"Over to the Indian camp. There is an Indian lady very sick."

"Oh," said Nick.

Across the bay they found the other boat beached. Uncle George was smoking a cigar in the dark. The young Indian pulled the boat way up on the beach. Uncle George gave both the Indians cigars.

They walked up from the beach through a meadow that was soaking wet with dew, following the young Indian who carried a lantern. Then they

went into the woods and followed a trail that led to the logging road that ran
back into the hills. It was much lighter on the logging road as the timber was
cut away on both sides. The young Indian stopped and blew out his lantern
and they all walked on along the road.

They came around a bend and a dog came out barking. Ahead were the
lights of the shanties where the Indian barkpeelers lived. More dogs rushed
out at them. The two Indians sent them back to the shanties. In the shanty
nearest the road there was a light in the window. An old woman stood in the
doorway holding a lamp.

Inside on a wooden bunk lay a young Indian woman. She had been trying
to have her baby for two days. All the old women in the camp had been
helping her. The men had moved off up the road to sit in the dark and smoke
out of range of the noise she made. She screamed just as Nick and the two
Indians followed his father and Uncle George into the shanty. She lay in the
lower bunk, very big under a quilt. Her head was turned to one side. In the
upper bunk was her husband. He had cut his foot very badly with an ax
three days before. He was smoking a pipe. The room smelled very bad.

Nick's father ordered some water to be put on the stove, and while it was
heating he spoke to Nick.

"This lady is going to have a baby, Nick," he said.

"I know," said Nick.

"You don't know," said his father. "Listen to me. What she is going
through is called being in labor. The baby wants to be born and she wants it
to be born. All her muscles are trying to get the baby born. That is what is
happening when she screams."

"I see," Nick said.

Just then the woman cried out.

"Oh, Daddy, can't you give her something to make her stop screaming?"
asked Nick.

"No. I haven't any anaesthetic," his father said. "But her screams are
not important. I don't hear them because they are not important."

The husband in the upper bunk rolled over against the wall.

The woman in the kitchen motioned to the doctor that the water was hot.
Nick's father went into the kitchen and poured about half of the water out of
the big kettle into a basin. Into the water left in the kettle he put several
things he unwrapped from a handkerchief.

"Those must boil," he said, and began to scrub his hands in the basin of
hot water with a cake of soap he had brought from the camp. Nick watched
his father's hands scrubbing each other with the soap. While his father
washed his hands very carefully and thoroughly, he talked.

"You see, Nick, babies are supposed to be born head first but sometimes they're not. When they're not they make a lot of trouble for everybody. Maybe I'll have to operate on this lady. We'll know in a little while."

When he was satisfied with his hands he went in and went to work.

"Pull back that quilt, will you, George?" he said. "I'd rather not touch it."

Later when he started to operate Uncle George and three Indian men held the woman still. She bit Uncle George on the arm and Uncle George said, "Damn squaw bitch!" and the young Indian who had rowed Uncle George over laughed at him. Nick held the basin for his father. It all took a long time.

His father picked the baby up and slapped it to make it breathe and handed it to the old woman.

"See, it's a boy, Nick," he said. "How do you like being an interne?"

Nick said, "All right." He was looking away so as not to see what his father was doing.

"There. That gets it," said his father and put something into the basin. Nick didn't look at it.

"Now," his father said, "there's some stitches to put in. You can watch this or not, Nick, just as you like. I'm going to sew up the incision I made."

Nick did not watch. His curiosity had been gone for a long time.

His father finished and stood up. Uncle George and the three Indian men stood up. Nick put the basin out in the kitchen.

Uncle George looked at his arm. The young Indian smiled reminiscently.

"I'll put some peroxide on that, George," the doctor said.

He bent over the Indian woman. She was quiet now and her eyes were closed. She looked very pale. She did not know what had become of the baby or anything.

"I'll be back in the morning," the doctor said, standing up. "The nurse should be here from St. Ignace by noon and she'll bring everything we need."

He was feeling exalted and talkative as football players are in the dressing room after a game.

"That's one for the medical journal, George," he said. "Doing a Caesarian with a jack-knife and sewing it up with nine-foot, tapered gut leaders."

Uncle George was standing against the wall, looking at his arm.

"Oh, you're a great man, all right," he said.

"Ought to have a look at the proud father. They're usually the worst sufferers in these little affairs," the doctor said. "I must say he took it all pretty quietly."

He pulled back the blanket from the Indian's head. His hand came away wet. He mounted on the edge of the lower bunk with the lamp in one hand and looked in. The Indian lay with his face toward the wall. His throat had been cut from ear to ear. The blood had flowed down into a pool where his body sagged the bunk. His head rested on his left arm. The open razor lay, edge up, in the blankets.

"Take Nick out of the shanty, George," the doctor said.

There was no need of that. Nick, standing in the door of the kitchen, had a good view of the upper bunk when his father, the lamp in one hand, tipped the Indian's head back.

It was just beginning to be daylight when they walked along the logging road back toward the lake.

"I'm terribly sorry I brought you along, Nickie," said his father, all his post-operative exhilaration gone. "It was an awful mess to put you through."

"Do ladies always have such a hard time having babies?" Nick asked.

"No, that was very, very exceptional."

"Why did he kill himself, Daddy?"

"I don't know, Nick. He couldn't stand things, I guess."

"Do many men kill themselves, Daddy?"

"Not very many, Nick."

"Do many women?"

"Hardly ever."

"Don't they ever?"

"Oh, yes. They do sometimes."

"Daddy?"

"Yes."

"Where did Uncle George go?"

"He'll turn up all right."

"Is dying hard, Daddy?"

"No, I think it's pretty easy, Nick. It all depends."

They were seated in the boat, Nick in the stern, his father rowing. The sun was coming up over the hills. A bass jumped, making a circle in the water. Nick trailed his hand in the water. It felt warm in the sharp chill of the morning.

In the early morning on the lake sitting in the stern of the boat with his father rowing, he felt quite sure that he would never die.

JOHN KEATS
After Dark Vapours

————⚮————

JOHN KEATS (1795-1821), the foremost English Romantic poet, was
one of the first to suffuse poetry with sensuous imagery. In "After Dark
Vapours," death is as welcome as the month of May, presaging Keats's
own early death from tuberculosis. It is little known that Keats
completed a course of medical studies. His *Anatomical and
Physiological Note Book* may be of interest to medical students.

After dark vapors have opprese'd our plains
 For a long dreary season, comes a day
 Born of the gentle south, and clears away
From the sick heavens all unseemly stains.
The anxious mouth, relieved from its pains,
 Takes as a long-list right the feel of May,
 The eyelids with the passing coolness play,
Like rose-leaves with the drip of summer rains.
And calmest thoughts come round us—as, of leaves
 Budding,—fruit ripening in stillness,—autumn suns
Smiling at eve upon the quiet sheaves,—
Sweet Sappho's cheek,—a sleeping infant's breath,—
 The gradual sand that through an hour-glass runs,—
A woodland rivulet,—a Poet's death.
 Jan. 1817.

SIR THOMAS MORE
Utopia

———◆∞◆———

THOMAS MORE (1478-1535), English lord chancellor, is known to the modern world as a martyr to Catholic orthodoxy, destroyed by Henry VIII. Paradoxically, in his *Utopia,* More describes an ideal society that proclaims indifference to religious creeds as one of its basic tenets.

The sick, as I said, they see to with great affection, and omit nothing at all in the way of either medicine or good diet whereby they may be restored again to their health. Those that are sick of incurable diseases they comfort with sitting by them, talking with them, and, in brief, with all manner of helps that are at hand. But if the disease is not only incurable, but also full of continual pain and anguish, then the priests and the magistrates exhort the man, seeing he is not able to perform any duty of life, and by outliving his own death is harmful and irksome to others and grievous to himself, that he will determine with himself to cherish no longer that pestilent and painful disease. And seeing his life is to him but a torment, that he be not unwilling to die, but rather take to himself good hope, and either despatch himself out of this painful life, as out of a prison or a rack of torment, or else suffer himself willingly to be rid of it by others. And in so doing they tell him he will do wisely, seeing that by his death he shall lose no comfort, but end his pain. And because in that act he will follow the counsel of the priests, that is to say, of the interpreters of God's will and pleasure, they show him that he will be acting like a godly and virtuous man. They that are thus persuaded, finish their lives willingly, either by hunger, or else die in their sleep without any feeling of death. And they cause none such to die against his will, nor do they use less diligence and attendance about him, believing this to be an honorable death. On the contrary, he that kills himself before the priests and the council have sanctioned the cause of his death, him they cast unburied into some stinking marsh, as unworthy both of the earth and of fire.

GEORGE ORWELL
How the Poor Die

GEORGE ORWELL (1903-1950) is the perennial favorite of undergraduates for his satires of totalitarianism in *Animal Farm* and *1984*. Recurrent hospitalization for tuberculosis gave him the background of social outrage expressed in *How the Poor Die*.

In the year 1929 I spend several weeks in the Hôpital X, in the fifteenth arrondissement of Paris. The clerks put me through the usual third degree at the reception desk, and indeed I was kept answering questions for some twenty minutes before they would let me in. If you have ever had to fill up forms in a Latin country you will know the kind of questions I mean. For some days past I had been unequal to translating Reaumur into Fahrenheit, but I know that my temperature was round about 103, and by the end of the interview I had some difficulty in standing on my feet. At my back a resigned little knot of patients, carrying bundles done up in colored handkerchiefs, waited their turn to be questioned.

After the questioning came the bath—a compulsory routine for all newcomers, apparently, just as in prison or the workhouse. My clothes were taken away from me, and after I had sat shivering for some minutes in five inches of warm water I was given a linen nightshirt and a short blue flannel dressing gown—no slippers, they had none big enough for me, they said—and led out into the open air. This was a night in February and I was suffering from pneumonia. The ward we were going to was two hundred yards away and it seemed that to get to it you had to cross the hospital grounds. Someone stumbled in front of me with a lantern. The gravel path was frosty underfoot, and the wind whipped the nightshirt round my bare calves. When we got into the ward I was aware of a strange feeling of familiarity whose origin I did not succeed in pinning down till later in the night. It was a long, rather low, ill-lit room, full of murmuring voices and with three rows of beds surprisingly close together. There was a foul smell, fecal and yet sweetish. As I lay down I saw on a bed nearly opposite me a small, round-shouldered, sandy-haired man sitting half naked while a doctor and a student performed some strange operation on him. First the doctor produced from his black bag a dozen small glasses like wine glasses, then the student burned a match inside each glass to exhaust the air, then the glass was popped on to the man's back or chest and the vacuum drew up a huge yellow blister. Only after some moments did I realize what they were doing to him. It was something called cupping, a treatment which you can read about in old medical textbooks but which till then I had vaguely thought of as one of those things they do to horses.

The cold air outside had probably lowered my temperature, and I watched this barbarous remedy with detachment and even a certain amount of amusement. The next moment, however, the doctor and the student came across to my bed, hoisted me upright, and without a word began applying the same set of glasses, which had not been sterilized in any way. A few feeble protests that I uttered got no more response than if I had been an animal. I was very much impressed by the impersonal way in which the two men started on me. I had never been in the public ward of a hospital before, and it was my first experience of doctors who handle you without speaking to you or, in a human sense, taking any notice of you. They only put on six glasses in my case, but after doing so they scarified the blisters and applied the glasses again. Each glass now drew out about a dessert-spoonful of dark-colored blood. As I lay down again, humiliated, disgusted, and frightened by the thing that had been done to me, I reflected that now at least they would leave me alone. But no, not a bit of it. There was another treatment coming, the mustard poultice, seemingly a matter of routine like the hot bath. Two slatternly nurses had already got the poultice ready, and they lashed it round my chest as tight as a straitjacket while some men who were wandering about the ward in shirt and trousers began to collect round my bed with half-sympathetic grins. I learned later that watching a patient have a mustard poultice was a favorite pastime in the ward. These things are normally applied for a quarter of an hour and certainly they are funny enough if you don't happen to be the person inside. For the first five minutes the pain is severe, but you believe you can bear it. During the second five minutes this belief evaporates, but the poultice is buckled at the back and you can't get it off. This is the period the onlookers enjoy most. During the last five minutes, I noted, a sort of numbness supervenes. After the poultice had been removed a waterproof pillow packed with ice was thrust beneath my head and I was left alone. I did not sleep, and to the best of my knowledge this was the only night of my life—I mean the only night spent in bed—in which I have not slept at all, not even a minute.

During my first hour in the Hôpital X I had had a whole series of different and contradictory treatments, but this was misleading, for in general you get very little treatment at all, either good or bad, unless you were ill in some interesting and instructive way. At five in the morning the nurses came round, woke the patients, and took their temperatures, but did not wash them. If you were well enough you washed yourself, otherwise you depended on the kindness of some walking patient. It was generally patients, too, who carried the bedbottles and the grim bedpan, nicknamed *la casserole*. At eight breakfast arrived, called army-fashion *la soupe*. It was soup, too, a thin vegetable soup with slimy hunks of bread floating about in it. Later in the day the tall, solemn, black-bearded doctor made his rounds, with an interne and a troop of students following at his heels, but there were about sixty of us in the ward and it was evident that he had other wards to attend to as well. There were many beds past which he walked day after day, sometimes followed by imploring cries. On the other hand if you had some disease with which the students wanted to familiarize themselves you got plenty of attention of a kind. I myself, with an exceptionally fine specimen of a bronchial rattle, sometimes had as many as a dozen students queuing up to listen to my chest. It was a very queer feeling—queer, I mean, because of their intense interest in learning their job, together with a seeming lack of any perception that the patients were human beings. It is strange to relate, but sometimes as some young student stepped forward to take his turn at manipulating you, he would be actually tremulous with excitement, like a boy who has at last got his hands on some expensive piece of machinery. And then ear after ear—ears of young men, of girls, of Negroes—pressed against your back, relays of fingers solemnly but clumsily tapping, and not from any one of them did you get a word of conversation or a look direct in your face. As a non-paying patient, in the uniform nightshirt, you were primarily *a specimen,* a thing I did not resent but could never quite get used to.

After some days I grew well enough to sit up and study the surrounding patients. The stuffy room, with its narrow beds so close together that you could easily touch your neighbor's hand, had every sort of disease in it except, I suppose, acutely infectious cases. My right-hand neighbor was a little red-haired cobbler with one leg shorter than the other, who used to announce the death of any other patient (this happened a number of times, and my neighbor was always the first to hear of it) by whistling to me, exclaiming "Numero 43!" (or whatever it was) and flinging his arms above his head. This man had not much wrong with him, but in most of the other beds within my angle of vision some squalid tragedy or some plain horror was being enacted. In the bed that was foot to foot with mine there lay, until he died (I didn't see him die—they moved him to another bed), a little weazened man who was suffering from I do not know what disease, but something that made his whole body so intensely sensitive that any movement from side to side, sometimes even the weight of the bedclothes, would make him shout out with pain. His worst suffering was when he urinated, which he did with the greatest difficulty. A nurse would bring him the bedbottle and then for a long time stand beside his bed, whistling, as grooms are said to do with horses, until at last with an agonized shriek of *"Je pisse!"* he would get started. In the bed next to him the sandy-haired man whom I had seen being cupped used to cough up blood-streaked mucus at all hours. My left-hand neighbor was a tall, flaccid-looking young man who used periodically to have a tube inserted into his back and astonishing quantities of frothy liquid drawn off from some part of his body. In the bed beyond that a veteran of the war of 1870 was dying, a handsome old man with a white imperial, round whose bed, at all hours when visiting was allowed, four elderly female relatives dressed all in black sat exactly like crows, obviously scheming for some pitiful legacy. In the bed opposite me in the further row was an old bald-headed man with drooping moustaches and greatly swollen face and body, who was suffering from some disease that made him urinate almost incessantly. A huge glass receptacle stood always beside his bed. One day his wife and daughter came to visit him. At sight of them the old man's bloated face lit up with a smile of surprising sweetness, and as his daughter, a pretty girl of about twenty, approached the bed I saw that his hand was slowly working its way from under the bedclothes. I seemed to see in advance the gesture that was coming—the girl kneeling beside the bed, the old man's hand laid on her head in his dying blessing. But no, he merely handed her the bedbottle, which she promptly took from him and emptied into the receptacle.

About a dozen beds away from me was Numero 57—I think that was his number—a cirrhosis of the liver case. Everyone in the ward knew him by sight because he was sometimes the subject of a medical lecture. On two afternoons a week the tall, grave doctor would lecture in the ward to a party of students, and on more than one occasion old Numero 57 was wheeled in on a sort of trolley into the middle of the ward, where the doctor would roll back his nightshirt, dilate with his fingers a huge flabby protuberance on the man's belly—the diseased liver, I suppose—and explain solemnly that this was a disease attributable to alcoholism, commoner in the wine-drinking countries. As usual he neither spoke to his patient nor gave him a smile, a nod or any kind of recognition. While he talked, very grave and upright, he would hold the wasted body beneath his two hands, sometimes giving it a gentle roll to and fro, in just the attitude of a woman handling a rolling-pin. Not that Numero 57 minded this kind of thing. Obviously he was an old hospital inmate, a regular exhibit at lectures, his liver long since marked down for a bottle in some pathological museum. Utterly uninterested in what was said about him, he would lie with his colorless eyes gazing at nothing, while the doctor showed him off like a piece of antique china. He was a man of about sixty, astonishingly shrunken. His face, pale as vellum, had shrunken away till it seemed no bigger than a doll's.

One morning my cobbler neighbor woke me up plucking at my pillow before the nurses arrived. "Numero 57!"—he flung his arms above his head. There was a light in the ward, enough to see by. I could see old Numero 57 lying crumpled up on his side, his face sticking out over the side of the bed, and toward me. He had died some time during the night, nobody knew when. When the nurses came they received the news of his death indifferently and went about their work. After a long time, an hour or more, two other nurses marched in abreast like soldiers, with a great clumping of sabots, and knotted the corpse up in the sheets, but it was not removed till some time later. Meanwhile, in the better light, I had had time for a good look at Numero 57. Indeed I lay on my side to look at him. Curiously enough he was the first dead European I had seen. I had seen dead men before, but always Asiatics and usually people who had died violent deaths. Numero 57's eyes were still open, his mouth also open, his small face contorted into an expression of agony. What most impressed me, however, was the whiteness of his face. It had been pale before, but now it was little darker than the sheets. As I gazed at the tiny, screwed-up face it struck me that this disgusting piece of refuse, waiting to be carted away and dumped on a slab in the dissecting room, was an example of "natural" death, one of the things you pray for in the Litany. There you are, then, I thought, that's what is waiting for you, twenty, thirty, forty years hence: that is how the lucky ones die, the one who lives to be old. One wants to live, of course, indeed one only stays alive by virtue of the fear of death, but I think now, as I thought then, that it's better to die violently and not too old. People talk about the horrors of war, but what weapons has man invented that even approaches in cruelty some of the commoner diseases? "Natural" death, almost by definition, means something slow, smelly, and painful. Even at that, it makes a difference if you can achieve it in your own home and not in a public institution. This poor old wretch who had just flickered out like a candle end was not even important enough to have anyone watching by his deathbed. He was merely a number, then a "subject" for the students' scalpels. And the sordid publicity of dying in such a place! In the Hôpital X the beds were very close together and there were no screens. Fancy, for instance, dying like the little man whose bed was for a while foot to foot with mine, the one who cried out when the bedclothes touched him! I dare say *"Je pisse!"* were his last recorded words. Perhaps the dying don't bother about such things—that at least would be the standard answer: nevertheless dying people are often more or less normal in their minds till within a day or so of the end.

In the public wards of a hospital you see horrors that you don't seem to meet with among people who manage to die in their own homes, as though certain diseases only attacked people at the lower income levels. But it is a fact that you would not in any English hospitals see some of the things I saw in the Hôpital X. This business of people just dying like animals, for instance, with nobody standing by, nobody interested, the death not even noticed till the morning—this happened more than once. You certainly would not see that in England, and still less would you see a corpse left exposed to the view of the other patients. I remember that once in a cottage hospital in England a man died while we were at tea, and though there were only six of us in the ward the nurses managed things so adroitly that the man was dead and his body removed without our even hearing about it till tea was over. A thing we perhaps underrate in England is the advantage we enjoy in having large numbers of well-trained and rigidly disciplined nurses. No doubt English nurses are dumb enough, they may tell fortunes with tea leaves, wear Union Jack badges, and keep photographs of the Queen on their mantelpieces, but at least they don't let you lie unwashed and constipated on an unmade bed, out of sheer laziness. The nurses at the Hôpital X still had a tinge of Mrs. Gamp about them, and later, in the military hospitals of Republican Spain, I was to see nurses almost too ignorant to take a temperature. You wouldn't, either, see in England such dirt as existed in the Hôpital X. Later on, when I was well enough to wash myself in the bathroom, I found that there was kept there a huge packing case into which the scraps of food and dirty dressings from the ward were flung, and the wainscotings were infested by crickets.

When I had got back my clothes and grown strong on my legs I fled from the Hôpital X, before my time was up and without waiting for a medical discharge. It was not the only hospital I have fled from, but its gloom and bareness, its sickly smell and, above all, something in its mental atmosphere stand out in my memory as exceptional. I had been taken there because it was the hospital belonging to my arrondissement, and I did not learn till after I was in it that it bore a bad reputation. A year or two later the celebrated swindler, Madame Hanaud, who was ill while on remand, was taken to the Hôpital X, and after a few days of it she managed to elude her guards, took a taxi, and drove back to the prison, explaining that she was more comfortable there. I have no doubt that the Hôpital X was quite untypical of French hospitals even at that date. But the patients, nearly all of them working men, were surprisingly resigned. Some of them seemed to find the conditions almost comfortable, for at least two were destitute malingerers who found this a good way of getting through the winter. The nurses connived because the malingerers made themselves useful by doing odd jobs. But the attitude of the majority was: of course this is a lousy place, but what else do you expect? It did not seem strange to them that you should be woken at five and then wait three hours before starting the day on watery soup, or that people should die with no one at their bedside, or even that your chance of getting medical attention should depend on catching the doctor's eye as he went past. According to their traditions that was what hospitals were like. If you are seriously ill, and if you are too poor to be treated in your own home, then you must go into hospital, and once there you must put up with harshness and discomfort, just as you would in the army. But on top of this I was interested to find a lingering belief in the old stories that have now almost faded from memory in England—stories, for instance, about doctors cutting you open out of sheer curiosity or thinking it funny to start operating before you were properly "under." There were dark tales about a little operating room said to be situated just beyond the bathroom. Dreadful screams were said to issue from this room. I saw nothing to confirm these stories and no doubt they were all nonsense, though I did see two students kill a sixteen-year-old-boy, or nearly kill him (he appeared to be dying when I left the hospital, but he may have recovered later) by a mischievous experiment which they probably could not have tried on a paying patient. Well within living memory it used to be believed in London that in some of the big hospitals patients were killed off to get dissection subjects. I didn't hear this tale repeated at the Hôpital X, but I should think some of the men there would have found it credible. For it was a hospital in which not the methods, perhaps, but something of the atmosphere of the nineteenth century had managed to survive, and therein lay its peculiar interest.

During the past fifty years or so there has been a great change in the relationship between doctor and patient. If you look at almost any literature before the later part of the nineteenth century, you find that a hospital is popularly regarded as much the same thing as a prison, and an old-fashioned, dungeon-like prison at that. A hospital is a place of filth, torture, and death, a sort of antechamber to the tomb. No one who was not more or less destitute would have thought of going into such a place for treatment. And especially in the early part of the last century, when medical science had grown bolder than before without being any more successful, the whole business of doctoring was looked on with horror and dread by ordinary people. Surgery, in particular, was believed to be no more than a peculiarly gruesome form of sadism, and dissection, possible only with the aid of body-snatchers, was even confused with necromancy. From the nineteenth century you could collect a large horror-literature connected with doctors and hospitals. Think of poor old George III, in his dotage, shrieking for mercy as he sees his surgeons approaching to "bleed him till he faints"! Think of the conversations of Bob Sawyer and Benjamin Allen, which no doubt are hardly parodies, or the field hospitals in *La Débâcle* and *War and Peace,* or that shocking description of an amputation in Melville's *Whitejacket*! Even the names given to doctors in nineteenth-century English fiction, Slasher, Carver, Sawyer, Fillgrave, and so on, and the generic nickname "sawbones," are about as grim as they are comic. The anti-surgery tradition is perhaps best expressed in Tennyson's poem, *The Children's Hospital,* which is essentially a pre-chloroform document though it seems to have been written as late as 1880. Moreover, the outlook which Tennyson records in this poem had a lot to be said for it. When you consider what an operation without anaesthetics must have been like, what it notoriously *was* like, it is difficult not to suspect the motives of people who would undertake such things. For these bloody horrors which the students so eagerly looked forward to ("A magnificent sight if Slasher does it!") were admittedly more or less useless: the patient who did not die of shock usually died of gangrene, a result which was taken for granted. Even now doctors can be found whose motives are questionable. Anyone who has had much illness, or who has listened to medical students talking, will know what I mean. But anaesthetics were a turning point, and disinfectants were another. Nowhere in the world, probably, would you now see the kind of scene described by Axel Munthe in *The Story of San Michele,* when the sinister surgeon in top-hat and frock-coat, his starched shirtfront spattered with blood and pus, carves up patient after patient with the same knife and flings the severed limbs into a pile beside the table. Moreover, national health insurance has partly done away with the idea that a working-class patient is a pauper who deserves little consideration. Well into this century it was usual for "free" patients at the big hospitals to have their teeth extracted with no anaesthetic. They didn't pay, so why should they have an anaesthetic—that was the attitude. That too has changed.

And yet every institution will always bear upon it some lingering memory of its past. A barrack-room is still haunted by the ghost of Kipling, and it is difficult to enter a workhouse without being reminded of *Oliver Twist*.

Hospitals began as a kind of casual ward for lepers and the like to die in, and they continued as places where medical students learned their art on the bodies of the poor. You can still catch a faint suggestion of their history in their characteristically gloomy architecture. I would far from complaining about the treatment I have received in any English hospital, but I do know that it is a sound instinct that warns people to keep out of hospitals if possible, and especially out of the public wards. Whatever the legal position may be, it is unquestionable that you have far less control over your own treatment, far less certainty that frivolous experiments will not be tried on you, when it is a case of "accept the discipline or get out." And it is a great thing to die in your own bed, though it is better still to die in your boots. However great the kindness and the efficiency, in every hospital death there will be some cruel, squalid detail, something perhaps too small to be told but leaving terribly painful memories behind, arising out of the haste, the crowding, the impersonality of a place where every day people are dying among strangers.

The dread of hospitals probably still survives among the very poor, and in all of us it has only recently disappeared. It is a dark patch not far beneath the surface of our minds. I have said earlier that when I entered the ward at the Hôpital X I was conscious of a strange feeling of familiarity. What the scene reminded me of, of course, was the reeking, pain-filled hospitals of the nineteenth century, which I had never seen but of which I had a traditional knowledge. And something, perhaps the black-clad doctor with his frowsy black bag, or perhaps only the sickly smell, played the queer trick of unearthing from my memory that poem of Tennyson's, *The Children's Hospital,* which I had not thought of for twenty years. It happened that as a child I had had it read aloud to me by a sick-nurse whose own working life might have stretched back to the time when Tennyson wrote the poem. The horrors and sufferings of the old-style hospitals were a vivid memory to her. We had shuddered over the poem together, and then seemingly I had forgotten it. Even its name would probably have recalled nothing to me. But the first glimpse of the ill-lit murmurous room, with the beds so close together, suddenly roused the train of thought to which it belonged, and in the night that followed I found myself remembering the whole story and atmosphere of the poem, with many of its lines complete.

WILLIAM SHAKESPEARE
Pericles

ACT III, SCENE II
Enter CERIMON, *a Servant, and some shipwrecked*
Persons.

    Cer. Philemon, ho!

Enter PHILEMON

Philemon. Doth my lord call?
    Cer. Get fire and meat for these poor men:
It has been a turbulent and stormy night.
    Serv. I have been in many; but such a night as this,
Till now, I ne'er endur'd.
    Cer. Your master will be dead ere you return:
There's nothing can be minister'd to nature
That can recover him. Give this to the 'pothecary.
And tell me how it works.   [*To* PHILEMON.
        [*Exeunt* PHILEMON, Servant, *and the rest*.

Enter two Gentlemen.

    1 *Gentleman.*   Good morrow.
    2 *Gent.* Good morrow to your lordship.
    Cer.   Gentlemen,
Why do you stir so early?
    1 *Gent.* Sir.
Our lodings, standing bleak upon the sea,
Shook, as the earth did quake;
The very principals did seem to rend,
And all-to topple. Pure surprise and fear
Made me quit the house.
    2 *Gent.* That is the cause we trouble you so early;
'Tis not our husbandry.
    Cer.   O, you say well.

    1 Gent. But I much marvel that your lordship, having
Rich tire about you, should at these early hours

Shake off the golden slumber of repose.
'Tis most strange,
Nature should be so conversant with pain,
Being thereto not compell'd.
 Cer.   I held it ever,
Virtue and cunning were endowments greater
Than nobleness and riches: careless heirs
May the two latter darken and expend;
But immortality attends the former,
Making a man a god. 'Tis known, I ever
Have studied physic, through which secret art,
By turning o'er authorities, I have
(Together with my practice) made familiar
To me and to my aid, the blest infusions
That dwell in vegetives, in metals, stones;
And can speak of the disturbances that Nature
Works, and of her cures; which doth give me
A more content in course of true delight
Than to be thirsty after tottering honour,
Or tie my treasure in silken bags,
To please the Fool and Death.
 2 Gent. Your honour has through Ephesus pour'd forth
Your charity, and hundreds call themselves
Your creatures, who by you have been restor'd:
And not your knowledge, your personal pain, but even
Your purse, still open, hath built Lord Cerimon
Such strong renown as never shall decay.

Enter two Servants *with a chest.*

 Serv. So; lift there.
 Cer.   What is that?
 Serv.   Sir, even now
Did the sea toss upon our shore this chest:
'Tis of some wreck.
 Cer.   Set it down; let's look upon 't.
 2 Gent. 'Tis like a coffin, sir.
 Cer.   *Whate'er it be,*
'Tis wondrous heavy. Wrench it open straight:
If the sea's stomach be o'ercharg'd with gold,
'Tis a good constraint of fortune it belches upon us.

2 Gent. 'Tis so, my lord.

Cer.   How close 'tis caulk'd and bitum'd.
Did the sea cast it up?

Serv. I never saw so huge a billow, sir,
As toss'd it up on shore.

Cer.   Come, wrench it open.
Soft!—it smells most sweetly in my sense.

2 Gent. A delicate odour.

Cer. —As ever hit my nostril. So, up with it.
O you most potent gods! what's here? a corse?

1 Gent. Most strange!

Cer. Shrouded in cloth of state; balm'd and entreasur'd
With bags full of spices! A passport too:
Apollo, perfect me i' the characters!

                                            [*Unfolds a scroll.*
                                                 [*Reads.*

> *"Here I give to understand,*
> *(If e'er this coffin drive a-land,)*
> *I, King Pericles, have lost*
> *This Queen, worth all our mundane cost.*
> *Who finds her, give her burying;*
> *She was the daughter of a king:*
> *Besides this treasure for a fee,*
> *The gods requite his charity!"*

If thou liv'st, Pericles, thou hast a heart
That even cracks for woe!—This chanc'd to-night.

2 Gent. Most likely, sir.

Cer.   Nay, certainly to-night;
For look, how fresh she looks.—They were too rough
That threw her in the sea. Make fire within:
Fetch hither all the boxes in my closet. [*Exit a Servant.*
Death may usurp on nature many hours,
And yet the fire of life kindle again
The o'erpress'd spirits. I heard of an Egyptian,
That had nine hours lien dead,
Who was by good appliances recover'd.

Enter Servants, *with boxes, napkins, and fire.*

Well said, well said; the fire and the cloths.—
The rough and woful music that we have,
Cause it to sound, beseech you.

The vial once more;—how thou stirr'st, thou block!—
The music there!—I pray you, give her air.
Gentlemen,
This Queen will live: nature awakes: a warmth
Breathes out of her: she hath not been entranc'd
About five hours. See, how she 'gins to blow
Into life's flower again!
   1 *Gent*.   The Heavens,
Through you, increase our wonder, and set up
Your fame for ever.
   Cer.   She is alive! behold,
Her eyelids, cases to those heavenly jewels
Which Pericles hath lost, begin to part
Their fingers of bright gold: the diamonds
Of a most praised water do appear
To make the world twice rich. Live, and make
Us weep to hear your fate, fair creature,
Rare as you seem to be!   [*She moves*.
   Thai.   O dear Diana!
Where am I? Where's my lord? What world is this?
   2 *Gent*. Is not this strange?
   1 *Gent*.   Most rare?
   Cer.   Hush, gentle neighbours!
Lend me your hands; to the next chamber bear her.
Get linen: now this matter must be look'd to,
For her relapse is mortal. Come, come;
And Æsculapius guide us!
                [*Exeunt, carrying out* THAISA.

LEO TOLSTOY
The Death of Ivan Ilych

————◦◦◦————

LEO TOLSTOY (1828-1910) prided himself on his ability to transcend his
aristocratic background in writing about the massive problems of social
justice and the vagaries of human nature, but he was criticized by his
less affluent contemporaries for inconsistencies between his stated
philosophy and his lifestyle. His *War and Peace* is generally regarded
as one of the three or four greatest novels of the Western world. His
particular genius as a writer lay in his gift for throwing a grand loop
around major historical events while dealing with the agonies and
glories of individual human beings. His *The Death of Ivan Ilych*
chronicles the inability of human beings to comprehend the reasons for
their affections and their utter emotional dependence on physicians
who never fully appreciate the importance of their psychological role in
treating patients.

They were all in good health. It could not be called ill health if Ivan Ilych
sometimes said that he had a queer taste in his mouth and felt some
discomfort in his left side.

But this discomfort increased and, though not exactly painful, grew into
a sense of pressure in his side accompanied by ill humour. And his
irritability became worse and worse and began to mar the agreeable, easy,
and correct life that had established itself in the Golovin family. Quarrels
between husband and wife became more and more frequent, and soon the
ease and amenity disappeared and even the decorum was barely maintained. Scenes again became frequent, and very few of those islets
remained on which husband and wife could meet without an explosion.
Praskovya Fëdorovna now had good reason to say that her husband's
temper was trying. With characteristic exaggeration she said he had always
had a dreadful temper, and that it had needed all her good nature to put up
with it for twenty years. It was true that now the quarrels were started by
him. His bursts of temper always came just before dinner, often just as he
began to eat his soup. Sometimes he noticed that a plate or dish was
chipped, or the food was not right, or his son put his elbow on the table, or
his daughter's hair was not done as he liked it, and for all this he blamed
Praskovya Fëdorovna. At first she retorted and said disagreeable things to

399

him, but once or twice he fell into such a rage at the beginning of dinner that she realized it was due to some physical derangement brought on by taking food, and so she restrained herself and did not answer, but only hurried to get the dinner over. She regarded this self-restraint as highly praiseworthy. Having come to the conclusion that her husband had a dreadful temper and made her life miserable, she began to feel sorry for herself, and the more she pitied herself the more she hated her husband. She began to wish he would die; yet she did not want him to die because then his salary would cease. And this irritated her against him still more. She considered herself dreadfully unhappy just because not even his death could save her, and though she concealed her exasperation, that hidden exasperation of hers increased his irritation also.

After one scene in which Ivan Ilych had been particularly unfair and after which he had said in explanation that he certainly was irritable but that it was due to his not being well, she said that if he was ill it should be attended to, and insisted on his going to see a celebrated doctor.

* * *

He said nothing of this, but rose, placed the doctor's fee on the table, and remarked with a sigh: "We sick people probably often put inappropriate questions. But tell me, in general, is this complaint dangerous, or not? . . ."

The doctor looked at him sternly over his spectacles with one eye, as if to say: "Prisoner, if you will not keep to the questions put to you, I shall be obliged to have you removed from the court."

"I have already told you what I consider necessary and proper. The analysis may show something more." And the doctor bowed.

Ivan Ilych went out slowly, seated himself disconsolately in his sledge, and drove home. All the way home he was going over what the doctor had said, trying to translate those complicated, obscure, scientific phrases into plain language and find in them an answer to the question: "Is my condition bad? Is it very bad? Or is there as yet nothing much wrong?" And it seemed to him that the meaning of what the doctor had said was that it was very bad. Everything in the streets seemed depressing. The cabmen, the houses, the passers-by, and the shops, were dismal. His ache, this dull gnawing ache that never ceased for a moment, seemed to have acquired a new and more serious significance from the doctor's dubious remarks. Ivan Ilych now watched it with a new and oppressive feeling.

He reached home and began to tell his wife about it. She listened, but in the middle of his account his daughter came in with her hat on, ready to go out with her mother. She sat down reluctantly to listen to this tedious story, but could not stand it long, and her mother too did not hear him to the end.

"Well, I am very glad," she said. "Mind now to take your medicine regularly. Give me the prescription and I'll send Gerasim to the chemist's." And she went to get ready to go out.

While she was in the room Ivan Ilych had hardly taken time to breathe, but he sighed deeply when she left it.

"Well," he thought, "perhaps it isn't so bad after all."

He began taking his medicine and following the doctor's directions, which had been altered after the examination of the urine. But then it happened that there was a contradiction between the indications drawn from the examination of the urine and the symptoms that showed themselves. It turned out that what was happening differed from what the doctor had told him, and that he had either forgotten, or blundered, or hidden something from him. He could not, however, be blamed for that, and Ivan Ilych still obeyed his orders implicitly and at first derived some comfort from doing so.

From the time of his visit to the doctor, Ivan Ilych's chief occupation was the exact fulfilment of the doctor's instructions regarding hygiene and the taking of medicine, and the observation of his pain and his excretions. His chief interests came to be people's ailments and people's health. When sickness, deaths, or recoveries were mentioned in his presence, especially when the illness resembled his own, he listened with agitation which he tried to hide, asked questions, and applied what he heard to his own case.

The pain did not grow less, but Ivan Ilych made efforts to force himself to think that he was better. And he could do this so long as nothing agitated him. But as soon as he had any unpleasantness with his wife, any lack of success in his official work, or held bad cards at bridge, he was at once acutely sensible of his disease. He had formerly borne such mischances, hoping soon to adjust what was wrong, to master it and attain success, or make a grand slam. But now every mischance upset him and plunged him into despair. He would say to himself: There now, just as I was beginning to get better and the medicine had begun to take effect, comes this accursed misfortune, or unpleasantness. . . ." And he was furious with the mishap, or with the people who were causing the unpleasantness and killing him, for he felt that this fury was killing him but could not restrain it. One would have thought that it should have been clear to him that this exasperation with circumstances and people aggravated his illness, and that he ought therefore to ignore unpleasant occurrences. But he drew the very opposite conclusion: he said that he needed peace, and he watched for everything that might disturb it and became irritable at the slightest infringement of it. His condition was rendered worse by the fact that he read medical books and consulted doctors. The progress of his disease was so gradual that he could deceive himself when comparing one day with another—the difference was so slight. But when he consulted the doctors it seemed to him that he was getting worse, and even very rapidly. Yet despite this he was continually consulting them.

That month he went to see another celebrity, who told him almost the same as the first had done but put his questions rather differently, and the interview with this celebrity only increased Ivan Ilych's doubts and fears. A friend of a friend of his, a very good doctor, diagnosed his illness again quite differently from the others, and though he predicted recovery, his questions and suppositions bewildered Ivan Ilych still more and increased his doubts. A homoeopathist diagnosed the disease in yet another way, and prescribed medicine which Ivan Ilych took secretly for a week. But after a week, not feeling any improvement and having lost confidence both in the former doctor's treatment and in this one's, he became still more despondent. One day a lady acquaintance mentioned a cure effected by a wonder-working icon. Ivan Ilych caught himself listening attentively and beginning to believe that it had occurred. This incident alarmed him. "Has my mind really weakened to such an extent?" he asked himself. "Nonsense! It's all rubbish. I mustn't give way to nervous fears but having chosen a doctor must keep strictly to his treatment. That is what I will do. Now it's all settled. I won't think about it, but will follow the treatment seriously till summer."

*   *   *

He went to see Peter Ivanovich, and together they went to see his friend, the doctor. He was in, and Ivan Ilych had a long talk with him.

Reviewing the anatomical and physiological details of what in the doctor's opinion was going on inside him, he understood it all.

There was something, a small thing, in the vermiform appendix. It might all come right. Only stimulate the energy of one organ and check the activity of another, then absorption would take place and everything would come right. He got home rather late for dinner, ate his dinner, and conversed cheerfully, but could not for a long time bring himself to go back to work in his room. At last, however, he went to his study and did what was necessary, but the consciousness that he had put something aside—an important, intimate matter which he would revert to when his work was done—never left him. When he had finished his work he remembered that this intimate matter was the thought of his vermiform appendix. But he did not give himself up to it, and went to the drawing-room for tea. There were callers there, including the examining magistrate who was a desirable match for his daughter, and they were conversing, playing the piano, and singing. Ivan Ilych, as Praskovya Fëdorovna remarked, spent that evening more cheerfully than usual, but he never for a moment forgot that he had postponed the important matter of the appendix. At eleven o'clock he said good-night and went to his bedroom. Since his illness he had slept alone in a small room next to his study. He undressed and took up a novel by Zola, but instead of reading it he fell into thought, and in his imagination that desired improvement in the vermiform appendix occurred. There was the absorption and evacuation and the re-establishment of normal activity. "Yes, that's it!" he said to himself. "One need only assist nature, that's all." He remembered his medicine, rose, took it, and lay down on his back watching for the beneficent action of the medicine and for it to lessen the pain. "I need only take it regularly and avoid all injurious influences. I am already feeling better, much better." He began touching his side: it was not painful to the touch. "There, I really don't feel it. It's much better already." He put out the light and turned on his side. . . . "The appendix is getting better, absorption is occurring." Suddenly he felt the old, familiar, dull, gnawing pain, stubborn and serious. There was the same familiar loathsome taste in his mouth. His heart sank and he felt dazed. "My God! My God!" he muttered. "Again, again! and it will never cease." And suddenly the matter presented itself in a quite different aspect. "Vermiform appendix! Kidney!" he said to himself. "It's not a question of appendix or kidney, but of life and . . . death. Yes, life was there and now it is going, going and I cannot stop it. Yes. Why deceive myself? Isn't it obvious to everyone but me that I'm dying, and that it's only a question of weeks, days . . . it may happen this moment. There was light and now there is darkness. I was here and now I'm going there! Where?" A chill came over him, his breathing ceased, and he felt only the throbbing of his heart.

"When I am not, what will there be? There will be nothing. Then where shall I be when I am no more? Can this be dying? No, I don't want to!" He jumped up and tried to light the candle, felt for it with trembling hands, dropped candle and candlestick on the floor, and fell back on his pillow.

"What's the use? It makes no difference," he said to himself, staring with wide-open eyes into the darkness. "Death. Yes, death. And none of them know or wish to know it, and they have no pity for me. Now they are playing." (He heard through the door the distant sound of a song and its accompaniment.) "It's all the same to them, but they will die too! Fools! I first, and they later, but it will be the same for them. And now they are merry . . . the beasts!"

Anger choked him and he was agonizingly, unbearably miserable. "It is impossible that all men have been doomed to suffer this awful horror!" He raised himself.

"Something must be wrong. I must calm myself—must think it all over from the beginning." And he again began thinking. "Yes, the beginning of my illness: I knocked my side, but I was still quite well that day and the next. It hurt a little, then rather more. I saw the doctors, then followed despondency and anguish, more doctors, and I drew nearer to the abyss. My strength grew less and I kept coming nearer and nearer, and now I have wasted away and there is no light in my eyes. I think of the appendix—but this is death! I think of mending the appendix, and all the while here is death! Can it really be death?" Again terror seized him and he gasped for breath. He leant down and began feeling for the matches, pressing with his elbow on the stand beside the bed. It was in his way and hurt him, he grew furious with it, pressed on it still harder, and upset it. Breathless and in despair he fell on his back, expecting death to come immediately.

Meanwhile the visitors were leaving. Praskovya Fëdorovna was seeing them off. She heard something fall and came in.

"What has happened?"

"Nothing. I knocked it over accidentally."

She went out and returned with a candle. He lay there panting heavily, like a man who has run a thousand yards, and stared upwards at her with a fixed look.

"What is it, Jean?"

"No . . . o . . . thing. I upset it." ("Why speak of it? She won't understand," he thought.)

And in truth she did not understand. She picked up the stand, lit his candle, and hurried away to see another visitor off. When she came back he still lay on his back, looking upwards.

"What is it? Do you feel worse?"

"Yes."

She shook her head and sat down.

"Do you know, Jean, I think we must ask Leshchetitsky to come and see you here."

This meant calling in the famous specialist, regardless of expense. He smiled malignantly and said ''No.'' She remained a little longer and then went up to him and kissed his forehead.

While she was kissing him he hated her from the bottom of his soul and with difficulty refrained from pushing her away.

''Good-night. Please God you'll sleep.''

''Yes.''

Ivan Ilych saw that he was dying, and he was in continual despair.

In the depth of his heart he knew he was dying, but not only was he not accustomed to the thought, he simply did not and could not grasp it.

The syllogism he had learnt from Kiezewetter's Logic: ''Caius is a man, men are mortal, therefore Caius is mortal,'' had always seemed to him correct as applied to Caius, but certainly not as applied to himself. That Caius—man in the abstract—was mortal, was perfectly correct, but he was not Caius, not an abstract man, but a creature quite, quite separate from all others. He had been little Vanya, with a mamma and a papa, with Mitya and Volodya, with the toys, a coachman and a nurse, afterwards with Katenka and with all the joys, griefs, and delights of childhood, boyhood, and youth. What did Caius know of the smell of that striped leather ball Vanya had been so fond of? Had Caius kissed his mother's hand like that, and did the silk of her dress rustle so for Caius? Had he rioted like that at school when the pastry was bad? Had Caius been in love like that? Could Caius preside at a session as he did? ''Caius really was mortal, and it was right for him to die; but for me, little Vanya, Ivan Ilych, with all my thoughts and emotions, it's altogether a different matter. It cannot be that I ought to die. That would be too terrible.''

Such was his feeling.

''If I had to die like Caius I should have known it was so. An inner voice would have told me so, but there was nothing of the sort in me and I and all my friends felt that our case was quite different from that of Caius. And now here it is!'' he said to himself. ''It can't be. It's impossible! But here it is. How is this? How is one to understand it?''

He could not understand it, and tried to drive this false, incorrect, morbid thought away and to replace it by other proper and healthy thoughts. But that thought, and not the thought only but the reality itself, seemed to come and confront him.

And to replace that thought he called up a succession of others, hoping to find in them some support. He tried to get back into the former current of thoughts that had once screened the thought of death from him. But strange to say, all that had formerly shut off, hidden, and destroyed, his consciousness of death, no longer had that effect. Ivan Ilych now spent most of his time in attempting to re-establish that old current. He would say to himself: "I will take up my duties again—after all I used to live by them." And banishing all doubts he would go to the law courts, enter into conversation with his colleagues, and sit carelessly as was his wont, scanning the crowd with a thoughtful look and leaning both his emaciated arms on the arms of his oak chair; bending over as usual to a colleague and drawing his papers nearer he would interchange whispers with him, and then suddenly raising his eyes and sitting erect would pronounce certain words and open the proceedings. But suddenly in the midst of those proceedings the pain in his side, regardless of the stage the proceedings had reached, would begin its own gnawing work. Ivan Ilych would turn his attention to it and try to drive the thought of it away, but without success. *It* would come and stand before him and look at him, and he would be petrified and the light would die out of his eyes, and he would again begin asking himself whether *It* alone was true. And his colleagues and subordinates would see with surprise and distress that he, the brilliant and subtle judge, was becoming confused and making mistakes. He would shake himself, try to pull himself together, manage somehow to bring the sitting to a close, and return home with the sorrowful consciousness that his judicial labours could not as formerly hide from him what he wanted them to hide, and could not deliver him from *It*.

And what was worst of all was that *It* drew his attention to itself not in order to make him take some action but only that he should look at *It*, look it straight in the face: look at it and without doing anything, suffer inexpressibly.

And to save himself from this condition Ivan Ilych looked for consolations—new screens—and new screens were found and for a while seemed to save him, but then they immediately fell to pieces or rather became transparent, as if *It* penetrated them and nothing could veil *It*.

In these latter days he would go into the drawing-room he had arranged—that drawing-room where he had fallen and for the sake of which (how bitterly ridiculous it seemed) he had sacrificed his life—for he knew that his illness originated with that knock. He would enter and see that something had scratched the polished table. He would look for the cause of this and find that it was the bronze ornamentation of an album, that had got bent. He would take up the expensive album which he had lovingly arranged, and feel vexed with his daughter and her friends for their untidiness—for the album was torn here and there and some of the photographs turned upside down. He would put it carefully in order and bend the ornamentation back into position. Then it would occur to him to place all those things in another corner of the room, near the plants. He could call the footman, but his daughter or wife would come to help him. They would not agree, and his wife would contradict him, and he would dispute and grow angry. But that was all right, for then he did not think about *It*. *It* was invisible.

But then, when he was moving something himself, his wife would say: "Let the servants do it. You will hurt yourself again." And suddenly *It* would flash through the screen and he would see it. It was just a flash, and he hoped it would disappear, but he would involuntarily pay attention to his side. "It sits there as before, gnawing just the same!" And he could no longer forget *It*, but could distinctly see it looking at him from behind the flowers. "What is it all for?"

"It really is so! I lost my life over that curtain as I might have done when storming a fort. Is that possible? How terrible and how stupid. It can't be true! It can't, but it is."

He would go to his study, lie down, and again be alone with *It:* face to face with *It*. And nothing could be done with *It* except to look at it and shudder.

*　　*　　*

How it happened it is impossible to say because it came about step by step, unnoticed, but in the third month of Ivan Ilych's illness, his wife, his daughter, his son, his acquaintances, the doctors, the servants, and above all he himself, were aware that the whole interest he had for other people was whether he would soon vacate his place, and at last release the living from the discomfort caused by his presence and be himself released from his sufferings.

He slept less and less. He was given opium and hypodermic injections of morphine, but this did not relieve him. The dull depression he experienced in a somnolent condition at first gave him a little relief, but only as something new, afterwards it became as distressing as the pain itself or even more so.

Special foods were prepared for him by the doctors' orders, but all those foods became increasingly distasteful and disgusting to him.

For his excretions also special arrangements had to be made, and this was a torment to him every time—a torment from the uncleanliness, the unseemliness, and the smell, and from knowing that another person had to take part in it.

But just through this most unpleasant matter, Ivan Ilych obtained comfort. Gerasim, the butler's young assistant, always came in to carry the things out. Gerasim was a clean, fresh peasant lad, grown stout on town food and always cheerful and bright. At first the sight of him, in his clean Russian peasant costume, engaged in that disgusting task embarrassed Ivan Ilych.

Once when he got up from the commode too weak to draw up his trousers, he dropped into a soft armchair and looked with horror at his bare, enfeebled thighs with the muscles so sharply marked on them.

Gerasim with a firm light tread, his heavy boots emitting a pleasant smell of tar and fresh winter air, came in wearing a clean Hessian apron, the sleeves of his print shirt tucked up over his strong bare young arms; and refraining from looking at his sick master out of consideration for his feelings, and restraining the joy of life that beamed from his face, he went up to the commode.

"Gerasim!" said Ivan Ilych in a weak voice.

Gerasim started, evidently afraid he might have committed some blunder, and with a rapid movement turned his fresh, kind, simple young face which just showed the first downy signs of a beard.

"Yes, sir?"

"That must be very unpleasant for you. You must forgive me. I am helpless."

"Oh, why, sir," said Gerasim's eyes beamed and he showed his glistening white teeth, "what's a little trouble? It's a case of illness with you, sir."

And his deft strong hands did their accustomed task, and he went out of the room stepping lightly. Five minutes later he as lightly returned.

Ivan Ilych was still sitting in the same position in the armchair.

"Gerasim," he said when the latter had replaced the freshly-washed utensil. "Please come here and help me." Gerasim went up to him. "Lift me up. It is hard for me to get up, and I have sent Dmitri away."

Gerasim went up to him, grasped his master with his strong arms deftly but gently, in the same way that he stepped—lifted him, supported him with one hand, and with the other drew up his trousers and would have set him down again, but Ivan Ilych asked to be led to the sofa. Gerasim, without an effort and without apparent pressure, led him, almost lifting him, to the sofa and placed him on it.

"Thank you. How easily and well you do it all!"

Gerasim smiled again and turned to leave the room. But Ivan Ilych felt his presence such a comfort that he did not want to let him go.

"One thing more, please move up that chair. No, the other one—under my feet. It is easier for me when my feet are raised."

Gerasim brought the chair, set it down gently in place, and raised Ivan Ilych's legs on to it. It seemed to Ivan Ilych that he felt better while Gerasim was holding up his legs.

"It's better when my legs are higher," he said. "Place that cushion under them."

Gerasim did so. He again lifted the legs and placed them, and again Ivan Ilych felt better while Gerasim held his legs. When he set them down Ivan Ilych fancied he felt worse.

"Gerasim," he said. "Are you busy now?"

"Not at all, sir," said Gerasim, who had learnt from the townsfolk how to speak to gentlefolk.

"What have you still to do?"

"What have I to do? I've done everything except chopping the logs for tomorrow."

"Then hold my legs a bit higher, can you?"

"Of course I can. Why not?" And Gerasim raised his master's legs higher and Ivan Ilych thought that in that position he did not feel any pain at all.

"And how about the logs?"

"Don't trouble about that, sir. There's plenty of time."

Ivan Ilych told Gerasim to sit down and hold his legs, and began to talk to him. And strange to say it seemed to him that he felt better while Gerasim held his legs up.

After that Ivan Ilych would sometimes call Gerasim and get him to hold his legs on his shoulders, and he liked talking to him. Gerasim did it all easily, willingly, simply, and with a good nature that touched Ivan Ilych. Health, strength, and vitality in other people were offensive to him, but Gerasim's strength and vitality did not mortify but soothed him.

What tormented Ivan Ilych most was the deception, the lie, which for some reason they all accepted, that he was not dying but was simply ill, and that he only need keep quiet and undergo a treatment and then something very good would result. He however knew that do what they would nothing would come of it, only still more agonizing suffering and death. This deception tortured him—their not wishing to admit what they all knew and what he knew, but wanting to lie to him concerning his terrible condition, and wishing and forcing him to participate in that lie. Those lies—lies enacted over him on the eve of his death and destined to degrade this awful, solemn act to the level of their visitings, their curtains, their sturgeon for dinner—were a terrible agony for Ivan Ilych. And strangely enough, many times when they were going through their antics over him he had been within a hairbreadth of calling out to them: "Stop lying! You know and I know that I am dying. Then at least stop lying about it!" But he had never had the spirit to do it. The awful, terrible act of his dying was, he could see, reduced by those about him to the level of a casual, unpleasant, and almost indecorous incident (as if someone entered a drawing-room diffusing an unpleasant odour) and this was done by that very decorum which he had served all his life long. He saw that no one felt for him, because no one even wished to grasp his position. Only Gerasim recognized it and pitied him. And so Ivan Ilych felt at ease only with him. He felt comforted when Gerasim supported his legs (sometimes all night long) and refused to go to bed, saying: "Don't you worry, Ivan Ilych. I'll get sleep enough later on," or when he suddenly became familiar and exclaimed: "If you weren't sick it would be another matter, but as it is, why should I grudge a little trouble?" Gerasim alone did not lie; everything showed that he alone understood the facts of the case and did not consider it necessary to disguise them, but simply felt sorry for his emaciated and enfeebled master. Once when Ivan Ilych was sending him away he even said straight out: "We shall all of us die, so why should I grudge a little trouble?"—expressing the fact that he did not think of his work burdensome, because he was doing it for a dying man and hoped someone would do the same for him when his time came.

Apart from his lying, or because of it, what most tormented Ivan Ilych was that no one pitied him as he wished to be pitied. At certain moments after prolonged suffering he wished most of all (though he would have been ashamed to confess it) for someone to pity him as a sick child is pitied. He longed to be petted and comforted. He knew he was an important functionary, that he had a beard turning grey, and that therefore what he longed for was impossible, but still he longed for it. And in Gerasim's attitude towards him there was something akin to what he wished for, and so that attitude comforted him. Ivan Ilych wanted to weep, wanted to be petted and cried over, and then his colleague Shebek would come, and instead of weeping and being petted, Ivan Ilych would assume a serious, severe, and profound air, and by force of habit would express his opinion on a decision of the Court of Cassation and would stubbornly insist on that view. This falsity around him and within him did more than anything else to poison his last days.

*   *   *

Perhaps it's the doctor? It is. He comes in fresh, hearty, plump, and cheerful, with that look on his face that seems to say: "There now, you're in a panic about something, but we'll arrange it all for you directly!'' The doctor knows this expression is out of place here, but he has put it on once for all and can't take it off—like a man who has put on a frock-coat in the morning to pay a round of calls.

The doctor rubs his hands vigorously and reassuringly.

"Brr! How cold it is! There's such a sharp frost; just let me warm myself!'' he says, as if it were only a matter of waiting till he was warm, and then he would put everything right.

"Well now, how are you?''

Ivan Ilych feels that the doctor would like to say: "Well, how are our affairs?'' but that even he feels that this would not do, and says instead: "What sort of a night have you had?''

Ivan Ilych looks at him as much as to say: "Are you really never ashamed of lying?'' But the doctor does not wish to understand this question, and Ivan Ilych says: "Just as terrible as ever. The pain never leaves me and never subsides. If only something . . .''

"Yes, you sick people are always like that. . . . There, now I think I am warm enough. Even Praskovya Fëdorovna, who is so particular, could find no fault with my temperature. Well, now I can say good-morning,'' and the doctor presses his patient's hand.

Then, dropping his former playfulness, he begins a most serious face to examine the patient, feeling his pulse and taking his temperature, and then begins the sounding and auscultation.

Ivan Ilych knows quite well and definitely that all this is nonsense and pure deception, but when the doctor, getting down on his knee, leans over him, putting his ear first higher then lower, and performs various gymnastic movements over him with a significant expression on his face, Ivan Ilych submits to it all as he used to submit to the speeches of the lawyers, though he knew very well that they were all lying and why they were lying.

The doctor, kneeling on the sofa, is still sounding him when Praskovya Fëdorovna's silk dress rustles at the door and she is heard scolding Peter for not having let her know of the doctor's arrival.

She comes in, kisses her husband, and at once proceeds to prove that she has been up a long time already, and only owing to a misunderstanding failed to be there when the doctor arrived.

Ivan Ilych looks at her, scans her all over, sets against her the whiteness and plumpness and cleanness of her hands and neck, the gloss of her hair, and the sparkle of her vivacious eyes. He hates her with his whole soul. And the thrill of hatred he feels for her makes him suffer from her touch.

Her attitude towards him and his disease is still the same. Just as the doctor had adopted a certain relation to his patient which he could not abandon, so had she formed one towards him—that he was not doing something he ought to do and was himself to blame, and that she reproached him lovingly for this—and she could not now change that attitude.

"You see he doesn't listen to me and doesn't take his medicine at the proper time. And above all he lies in a position that is no doubt bad for him—with his legs up."

She described how he made Gerasim hold his legs up.

The doctor smiled with a contemptuous affability that said :"What's to be done? These sick people do have foolish fancies of that kind, but we must forgive them."

When the examination was over the doctor looked at his watch, and then Praskovya Fëdorovna announced to Ivan Ilych that it was of course as he pleased, but she had sent today for a celebrated specialist who would examine him and have a consultation with Michael Danilovich (their regular doctor).

"Please don't raise any objections. I am doing this for my own sake," she said ironically, letting it be felt that she was doing it all for his sake and only said this to leave him no right to refuse. He remained silent knitting his brows. He felt that he was so surrounded and involved in a mesh of falsity that it was hard to unravel anything.

Everything she did for him was entirely for her own sake, and she told him she was doing for herself what she actually was doing for herself, as if that was so incredible that he must understand the opposite.

At half-past eleven the celebrated specialist arrived. Again the sounding began and the significant conversations in his presence and in another room, about the kidneys and the appendix, and the questions and answers, with such an air of importance that again, instead of the real question of life and death which now alone confronted him, the question arose of the kidney and appendix which were not behaving as they ought to and would now be attacked by Michael Danilovich and the specialist and forced to amend their ways.

The celebrated specialist took leave of him with a serious though not hopeless look, and in reply to the timid question Ivan Ilych, with eyes glistening with fear and hope, put to him as to whether there was a chance of recovery, said that he could not vouch for it but there was a possibility. The look of hope with which Ivan Ilych watched the doctor out was so pathetic that Praskovya Fëdorovna, seeing it, even wept as she left the room to hand the doctor his fee.

MARK TWAIN
Autobiography

———— ◦≫⊱ ————

I had found a place on the *Pennsylvania* for my brother Henry, who was two years my junior. It was not a place of profit, it was only a place of promise. He was "mud" clerk. Mud clerks received no salary, but they were in the line of promotion. They could become, presently, third clerk and second clerk, then chief clerk—that is to say, purser. The dream begins when Henry had been mud clerk about three months. We were lying in port at St. Louis. Pilots and steersmen had nothing to do during the three days that the boat lay in port in St. Louis and New Orleans, but the mud clerk had to begin his labors at dawn and continue them into the night, by the light of pine-knot torches. Henry and I, moneyless and unsalaried, had billeted ourselves upon our brother-in-law, Mr. Moffett, as night lodgers while in port. We took our meals on board the boat. No, I mean *I* lodged at the house, not Henry. He spent the *evenings* at the house, from nine until eleven, then went to the boat to be ready for his early duties. On the night of the dream he started away at eleven, shaking hands with the family, and said good-by according to custom. I may mention that handshaking as a good-by was not merely the custom of that family, but the custom of the region—the custom of Missouri, I may say. In all my life, up to that time, I had never seen one member of the Clemens family kiss another one—except once. When my father lay dying in our home in Hannibal, Missouri—the 24th of March, 1847—he put his arm around my sister's neck and drew her down and kissed her, saying, "Let me die." I remember that, and I remember the death rattle which swiftly followed those words, which were his last. These good-bys were always executed in the family sitting room on the second floor, and Henry went from that room and downstairs without further ceremony. But this time my mother went with him to the head of the stairs and said good-by again. As I remember it, she was moved to this by something in Henry's manner, and she remained at the head of the stairs while he descended. When he reached the door he hesitated, and climbed the stairs and shook hands good-by again. In the morning, when I awoke, I had been dreaming, and the dream was so vivid, so like reality, that it deceived me, and I thought it *was* real. In the dream I had seen Henry a corpse. He lay in a metallic burial case. He was dressed in a suit of my clothing, and on his breast lay a great bouquet of flowers, mainly white roses, with a red rose in the center. The casket stood upon a couple of chairs. I dressed, and moved toward that door, thinking I would go in there and look at it, but I changed my mind. I thought I could not yet bear to meet my mother. I thought I would wait awhile and make some preparation for that ordeal. The house was in Locust Street, a little above Thirteenth, and I walked to Fourteenth and to the middle of the block beyond before it suddenly flashed upon me that there was nothing real about this—it was only a dream. I can still feel something of the grateful upheaval of joy of that moment, and I can also still feel the remnant of doubt, the suspicion that maybe it was real, after all. I returned to the house almost on a run, flew up the stairs two or three steps at a jump, and rushed into that sitting room, and was made glad again, for there was no casket there.

We made the usual eventless trip to New Orleans—no, it was not eventless, for it was on the way down that I had the fight with Mr. Brown[1] which resulted in his requiring that I be left ashore at New Orleans. In New Orleans I always had a job. It was my privilege to watch the freight piles from seven in the evening until seven in the morning, and get three dollars for it. It was a three-night job and occurred every thirty-five days. Henry always joined my watch about nine in the evening, when his own duties were ended, and we often walked my rounds and chatted together until midnight. This time we were to part, and so the night before the boat sailed I gave Henry some advice. I said: "In case of disaster to the boat, don't lose your head—leave that unwisdom to the passengers—they are competent—they'll attend to it. But you rush for the hurricane deck, and astern to the solitary lifeboat lashed aft the wheelhouse on the port side, and obey the mate's orders—thus you will be useful. When the boat is launched, give such help as you can in getting the women and children into it, and be sure you don't try to get into it yourself. It is summer weather, the river is only a mile wide, as a rule, and you can swim ashore without any trouble." Two or three days afterward the boat's boilers exploded at Ship Island, below Memphis, early one morning—and what happened afterward I have already told in *Life on the Mississippi*. As related there, I followed the *Pennsylvania* about a day later, on another boat, and we began to get news of the disaster at every port we touched at, and so by the time we reached Memphis we knew all about it.

I found Henry stretched upon a mattress on the floor of a great building along with thirty or forty other scalded and wounded persons, and was promptly informed, by some indiscreet person, that he had inhaled steam,

[1]See *Life on the Mississippi*.

that his body was badly scalded, and that he would live but a little while; also, I was told that the physicians and nurses were giving their whole attention to persons who had a chance of being saved. They were short-handed in the matter of physicians and nurses, and Henry and such others as were considered to be fatally hurt were receiving only such attention as could be spared, from time to time, from the more urgent cases. But Doctor Peyton, a fine and large-hearted old physician of great reputation in the community, gave me his sympathy and took vigorous hold of the case, and in about a week he had brought Henry around. He never committed himself with prognostications which might not materialize, but at eleven o'clock one night he told me that Henry was out of danger and would get well. Then he said, "At midnight these poor fellows lying here and there and all over this place will begin to mourn and mutter and lament and make outcries, and if this commotion should disturb Henry it will be bad for him; therefore ask the physicians on watch to give him an eighth of a grain of morphine, but this is not to be done unless Henry shall show signs that he is being disturbed."

Oh, well, never mind the rest of it. The physicians on watch were young fellows hardly out of the medical college, and they made a mistake—they had no way of measuring the eighth of a grain of morphine, so they guessed at it and gave him a vast quantity heaped on the end of a knife blade, and the fatal effects were soon apparent. I think he died about dawn, I don't remember as to that. He was carried to the dead-room and I went away for a while to a citizen's house and slept off some of my accumulated fatigue— and meantime something was happening. The coffins provided for the dead were of unpainted white pine, but in this instance some of the ladies of Memphis had made up a fund of sixty dollars and bought a metallic case, and when I came back and entered the dead-room Henry lay in that open case, and he was dressed in a suit of my clothing. I recognized instantly that my dream of several weeks before was here exactly reproduced, so far as these details went—and I think I missed one detail, but that one was immediately supplied, for just then an elderly lady entered the place with a large bouquet consisting mainly of white roses, and in the center of it was a red rose, and she laid it on his breast.

I told the dream there in the club that night just as I have told it here, I suppose.

VIRGINIA WOOLF
Mrs. Dalloway

———❧———

Holmes was coming upstairs. Holmes would burst open the door. Holmes would say "In a funk, eh?" Holmes would get him. But no; not Holmes; not Bradshaw. Getting up rather unsteadily, hopping indeed from foot to foot, he considered Mrs. Filmer's nice clean bread knife with "Bread" carved on the handle. Ah, but one mustn't spoil that. The gas fire? But it was too late now. Holmes was coming. Razors he might have got, but Rezia, who alway did that sort of thing, had packed them. There remained only the window, the large Bloomsbury-lodging house window, the tiresome, the troublesome, and rather melodramatic business of opening the window and throwing himself out. It was their idea of tragedy, not his or Rezia's (for she was with him). Holmes and Bradshaw like that sort of thing. (He sat on the sill.) But he would wait till the very last moment. He did not want to die. Life was good. The sun hot. Only human beings—what did *they* want? Coming down the staircase opposite an old man stopped and stared at him. Holmes was at the door. "I'll give it you!" he cried, and flung himself vigorously, violently down on to Mrs. Filmer's area railings.

"The coward!" cried Dr. Holmes, bursting the door open. Rezia ran to the window, she saw; she understood. Dr. Holmes and Mrs. Filmer collided with each other. Mrs. Filmer flapped her apron and made her hide her eyes in the bedroom. There was a great deal of running up and down stairs. Dr. Holmes came in—white as a sheet, shaking all over, with a glass in his hand. She must be brave and drink something, he said (What was it? Something sweet), for her husband was horribly mangled, would not recover consciousness, she must not see him, must be spared as much as possible, would have the inquest to go through, poor young woman. Who could have foretold it? A sudden impulse, no one was in the least to blame (he told Mrs. Filmer). And why the devil he did it, Dr. Holmes could not conceive.

It seemed to her as she drank the sweet stuff that she was opening long windows, stepping out into some garden. But where? The clock was striking—one, two, three: how sensible the sound was; compared with all this thumping and whispering; like Septimus himself. She was falling asleep. But the clock went on striking, four, five, six and Mrs. Filmer waving her apron (they wouldn't bring the body in here, would they?)

seemed part of that garden; or a flag. She had once seen a flag slowly rippling out from a mast when she stayed with her aunt at Venice. Men killed in battle were thus saluted, and Septimus had been through the War. Of her memories, most were happy.

She put on her hat, and ran through cornfields—where could it have been?—on to some hill, somewhere near the sea, for there were ships, gulls, butterflies; they sat on a cliff. In London too, there they sat, and, half dreaming, came to her through the bedroom door, rain falling, whisperings, stirrings among dry corn, the caress of the sea, as it seemed to her, hollowing them in its arched shell and murmuring to her laid on shore, strewn she felt, like flying flowers over some tomb.

"He is dead," she said, smiling at the poor old woman who guarded her with her honest light-blue eyes fixed on the door. (They wouldn't bring him in here, would they?) But Mrs. Filmer pooh-poohed. Oh no, oh no! They were carrying him away now. Ought she not to be told? Married people ought to be together, Mrs. Filmer thought. But they must do as the doctor said.

"Let her sleep," said Dr. Holmes, feeling her pulse. She saw the large outline of his body standing dark against the window. So that was Dr. Holmes.

*   *   *

Sinking her voice, drawing Mrs. Dalloway into the shelter of common femininity, a common pride in the illustrious qualities of husbands and their sad tendency to overwork, Lady Bradshaw (poor goose—one didn't dislike her) murmured how, "just as we were starting, my husband was called up on the telephone, a very sad case. A young man (that is what Sir William is telling Mr. Dalloway) had killed himself. He had been in the army." Oh! thought Clarissa, in the middle of my party, here's death, she thought.

She went on, into the little room where the Prime Minister had gone with Lady Bruton. Perhaps there was somebody there. But there was nobody. The chairs still kept the impress of the Prime Minister and Lady Bruton, she turned deferentially, he sitting four-square, authoritatively. They had been talking about India. There was nobody. The party's splendour fell to the floor, so strange it was to come in alone in her finery.

What business had the Bradshaws to talk of death at her party? A young man had killed himself. And they talked of it at her party—the Bradshaws, talked of death. He had killed himself—but how? Always her body went through it first, when she was told, suddenly, of an accident; her dress flamed, her body burnt. He had thrown himself from a window. Up had flashed the ground; through him, blundering, bruising, went the rusty spikes. There he lay with a thud, thud, thud in his brain, and then a suffocation of blackness. So she saw it. But why had he done it? And the Bradshaws talked of it at her party!

She had once thrown a shilling into the Serpentine, never anything more. But he had flung it away. They went on living (she would have to go back; the rooms were still crowded; people kept on coming). They (all day she had been thinking of Bourton, of Peter, of Sally), they would grow old. A thing there was that mattered; a thing, wreathed about with chatter, defaced, obscured in her own life, let drop every day in corruption, lies, chatter. This he had preserved. Death was defiance. Death was an attempt to communicate; people feeling the impossibility of reaching the centre which, mystically, evaded them; closeness drew apart; rapture faded, one was alone. There was an embrace in death.

But this young man who had killed himself—had he plunged holding his treasure? "If it were now to die, 'twere now to be most happy," she had said to herself once, coming down in white.

Or there were the poets and thinkers. Suppose he had had that passion, and had gone to Sir William Bradshaw, a great doctor yet to her obscurely evil, without sex or lust, extremely polite to women, but capable of some indescribable outrage—forcing your soul, that was it—if this young man had gone to him, and Sir William had impressed him, like that, with his power, might he not then have said (indeed she felt it now), Life is made intolerable; they make life intolerable, men like that?

Then (she had felt it only this morning) there was the terror; the overwhelming incapacity, one's parents giving it into one's hands, this life, to be lived to the end, to be walked with serenely; there was in the depths of her heart an awful fear. Even now, quite often if Richard had not been there reading the *Times*, so that she could crouch like a bird and gradually revive, send roaring up that immeasurable delight, rubbing stick to stick, one thing with another, she must have perished. But that young man had killed himself.

Somehow it was her disaster—her disgrace. It was her punishment to see sink and disappear here a man, there a woman, in this profound darkness, and she forced to stand here in her evening dress. She had schemed; she had pilfered. She was never wholly admirable. She had wanted success. Lady Bexborough and the rest of it. And once she had walked on the terrace at Bourton.

It was due to Richard; she had never been so happy. Nothing could be slow enough; nothing last too long. No pleasure could equal, she thought, straightening the chairs, pushing in one book on the shelf, this having done with the triumphs of youth, lost herself in the process of living, to find it, with a shock of delight, as the sun rose, as the day sank. Many a time had she gone, at Bourton when they were all talking, to look at the sky; or seen it between people's shoulders at dinner; seen it in London when she could not sleep. She walked to the window.

It held, foolish as the idea was, something of her own in it, this country sky, this sky above Westminster. She parted the curtains; she looked. Oh, but how surprising!—in the room opposite the old lady stared straight at her! She was going to bed. And the sky. It will be a solemn sky, she had thought, it will be a dusky sky, turning away its cheek in beauty. But there it was—ashen pale, raced over quickly by tapering vast clouds. It was new to her. The wind must have risen. She was going to bed, in the room opposite. It was fascinating to watch her, moving about, that old lady, crossing the room, coming to the window. Could she see her? It was fascinating, with people still laughing and shouting in the drawing-room, to watch that old woman, quite quietly, going to bed. She pulled the blind now. The clock began striking. The young man had killed himself; but she did not pity him; with the clock striking the hour, one, two, three, she did not pity him, with all this going on. There! the old lady had put out her light! the whole house was dark now with this going on, she repeated, and the words came to her, Fear no more the heat of the sun. She must go back to them. But what an extraordinary night! She felt somehow very like him—the young man who had killed himself. She felt glad that he had done it; thrown it away. The clock was striking. The leaden circles dissolved in the air. He made her feel the beauty; made her feel the fun. But she must go back. She must assemble. She must find Sally and Peter. And she came in from the little room.

HANS ZINSSER
As I Remember Him

---—❦—---

As his disease caught up with him, R. S. felt increasingly grateful for the fact that death was coming to him with due warning, and gradually. So many times in his active life he had been near sudden death by accident, violence, or acute disease; and always he had thought that rapid and unexpected extinction would be most merciful. But now he was thankful that he had time to compose his spirit, and to spend a last year in affectionate and actually merry association with those dear to him. He set down his feelings in his last sonnet:—

> Now is death merciful. He calls me hence
> Gently, with friendly soothing of my fears
> Of ugly age and feeble impotence
> And cruel disintegration of slow years.
> Nor does he leap upon me unaware
> Like some wild beast that hungers for its prey,
> But gives me kindly warning to prepare:
> Before I go, to kiss your tears away.
>
> How sweet the summer! And the autumn shone
> Late warmth within our hearts as in the sky,
> Ripening rich harvests that our love had sown.
> How good that 'ere the winter comes, I die!
> The, ageless, in your heart I'll come to rest
> Serene and proud, as when you loved me best.[1]

EMILE ZOLA
Dr. Pascal

———————✦———————

ÉMILE ZOLA (1840-1902) portrayed contemporary society in what came to be called naturalism. His technique of candid disclosure went even beyond Flaubert. He immersed himself in the principal causes of his time, and will probably be forever identified in the popular mind with the famous Dreyfus case. *Dr. Pascal* is but one example of Zola's zeal for social reforms.

The instant he pushed open the door of the kitchen on the left of the hall, a horrible odor escaped from it; an odor of burned flesh and bones. When he entered the room he could hardly breathe, so filled was it by a thick vapor, a stagnant and nauseous cloud, which choked and blinded him. The sunbeams that filtered through the cracks made only a dim light. He hurried to the fireplace, thinking that perhaps there had been a fire, but the fireplace was empty, and the articles of furniture around appeared to be uninjured. Bewildered, and feeling himself growing faint in the poisoned atmosphere, he ran to the window and threw the shutters wide open. A flood of light entered.

Then the place presented to the doctor's view filled him with amazement. Everything was in its place, the glass and the empty bottle of spirits were on the table; only the chair in which Uncle Macquart must have been sitting bore traces of fire, the front legs were blackened and the straw was partially consumed. What had become of Macquart? Where could he have disappeared? In front of the chair, on the brick floor, which was saturated with grease, there was a little heap of ashes, beside which lay the pipe—a black pipe which had not even broken in falling. All of Uncle Macquart was there, in this handful of fine ashes; and he was in the red cloud, also, which floated through the open window; in the layer of soot which carpeted the entire kitchen; the horrible grease of burnt flesh, enveloping everything, sticky and foul to the touch.

It was the finest case of spontaneous combustion the physician had ever seen. The doctor had, indeed, read in medical papers of surprising cases, among others that of a shoemaker's wife, a drunken woman who had fallen asleep over her foot warmer, and of whom they had found only a hand and foot. He had, until now, put little faith in these cases, unwilling to admit, like the ancients, that a body impregnated with alcohol could disengage an unknown gas, capable of taking fire spontaneously and consuming the flesh and the bones. But he denied the truth of them no longer; besides, everything became clear to him as he reconstructed the scene—the coma of drunkenness producing absolute insensibility; the pipe falling on the clothes, which had taken fire; the flesh, saturated with liquor, burning and cracking; the fat melting, part of it running over the ground and part of it aiding the combustion, and all, at last—muscles, organs, and bones—consumed in a general blaze. Uncle Macquart was all there, with his blue cloth suit, and his fur cap, which he wore from one year's end to the other. Doubtless, as soon as he had begun to burn like a bonfire he had fallen forward, which would account for the chair being only blackened; and nothing of him was left, not a bone, not a tooth, not a nail, nothing but this little heap of gray dust which the draught of air from the door threatened at every moment to sweep away.

THE PATIENT

The gravitational center of medicine is not the physician's office or the medical school but the patient himself. Medical scientists may emerge from their laboratories with spectacular answers to disease; technology may produce new marvels; hospitals may find new ways of caring for the seriously ill. But it is the response of the patient to all the science and the caring that represents the final verdict. And, in an Age of Consumerism, the physician discovers that his communications skills may be hardly less important than the nature and quality of the information being communicated.

W. H. AUDEN
Surgical Ward

They are and suffer; that is all they do;
A bandage hides the place where each is living,
His knowledge of the world restricted to
The treatment that the instruments are giving.

And lie apart like epochs from each other
—Truth in their sense is how much they can bear;
It is not talk like ours, but groans they smother—
And are remote as plants; we stand elsewhere.

For who when healthy can become a foot?
Even a scratch we can't recall when cured,
But are boist'rous in a moment and believe

In the common world of the uninjured, and cannot
Imagine isolation. Only happiness is shared,
And anger, and the idea of love.

JEAN COCTEAU
Opium: The Diary of a Cure

————⤫————

JEAN COCTEAU (1891-1973) was an avant-garde artist, a poet, novelist, dramatist, and film-maker. He was part of nearly every experimental art movement of the early twentieth century. Cocteau detailed his own experiences in *Opium: The Diary of a Cure*. He rhapsodizes over the world of artificial euphoria and excoriates doctors who waste their time purging patients of it instead of finding ways to render it harmless.

To begin with, I could not have been thoroughly cured the first time. Many courageous drug addicts do not know the pitfalls of being cured, they are content merely to give up and emerge ravaged by a useless ordeal, their cells weakened and further prevented from regaining their vitality through alcohol and sport.

Incredible phenomena are attached to the cure; medicine is powerless against them, beyond making the padded cell look like a hotel-room and demanding of the doctor or nurse patience, attendance and sensitivity. I shall explain later that the phenomena should be not those of an organism in a state of decomposition but on the contrary the uncommunicated symptoms of a baby at the breast and of vegetables in spring.

A tree must suffer from the rising of its sap and not feel the falling of its leaves.

"Le Sacre Du Printemps" orchestrates a cure with a scrupulous precision of which Stravinsky is not even aware.

I therefore became an opium addict again because the doctors who cure—one should really say, quite simply, who purge—do not seek to cure the troubles which first cause the addiction; I had found again my unbalanced state of mind; and I preferred an artificial equilibrium to no equilibrium at all. This moral disguise is more misleading than a disordered appearance: it is human, almost feminine, to have recourse to it.

I became addicted with caution and under medical supervision. There *are* doctors capable of pity. I never exceeded ten pipes. I smoked them at the rate of three in the morning (at nine o'clock), four in the afternoon (at five o'clock), three in the evening (at eleven o'clock). I believed that, in this way, I was reducing the chances of addiction. With opium I suckled new cells, which were restored to the world after five months of abstinence, and

I suckled them with countless unknown alkaloids, whereas a morphine addict, whose habits frighten me, fills his veins with a single known poison and surrenders himself far less to the unknown.

*   *   *

There is still no such thing as a scientific cure. No sooner are the alkaloids in the blood, than they fix upon certain tissues. Morphine becomes a phantom, a shadow, a fairy. One can imagine how the known and unknown opium alkaloids work, their Chinese invasion. To overcome them, one must have recourse to the methods of Molière. One drains the patient, cleans him out, stirs up his bile and, whether one likes it or not, goes back to those tales according to which evil spirits were supposed to be chased out by herbs, charms, purges and emetics.

*   *   *

Do not expect me to be a traitor. Of course opium remains unique and the euphoria it induces superior to that of health. I owe it my perfect hours. It is a pity that instead of perfecting curative techniques, medicine does not try to render opium harmless.

But here we come back to the problem of progress. Is suffering a regulation or a lyrical interlude?

It seems to me that on an earth so old, so wrinkled, so painted, where so many compromises and laughable conventions are rife, opium (if its harmful effects could be eliminated) would soften people's manners and would cause more good than the fever of activity causes harm.

My nurse says to me: "You are the first patient whom I have seen writing on the eighth day."

I full realise that I am planting a spoon in the soft tapioca of my young cells, that I am delaying matters, but I am burning myself up and will always do so. In two weeks, despite these notes, I shall no longer believe in what I am experiencing now. One must leave behind a trace of this journey which memory forgets. One must, when this is impossible, write or draw without responding to the romantic solicitations of pain, without enjoying suffering like music, tieing a pen to one's foot if need be, helping the doctors who can learn nothing from laziness.

During an attack of neuritis one night, I asked B.: "You, who do not practise and are up to your eyes in work at the Salpêtrière and are preparing your thesis, why do you attend me at my home day and night? I know doctors. You like me very much but you like medicine more." He replied that he had at last found a patient who talked, that he learnt more from me, because I was capable of describing my symptoms, than at the Salpêtrière where the question: "Where does it hurt?" invariably brought the same reply: "Don't know, doctor."

*   *   *

We are no longer, alas, a race of farmers and shepherds. The fact that we need another system of therapy to defend our over-worked nervous system cannot be questioned. For that reason it is imperative to discover some means of rendering harmless those beneficial substances which the body eliminates so unsatisfactorily, or of shielding the nerve cells.

*   *   *

Tell this obvious truth to a doctor and he will shrug his shoulders. He talks of literature, Utopia, and the obsessions of the drug addict.

Nevertheless, I contend that one day we shall use those soothing substances without danger, that we shall avoid habit-making, that we shall laugh at the bugaboo of the drug and that opium, once tamed, will assuage the evil of towns where trees die on their feet.

*   *   *

While I am drawing, E . . ., who is a replacement, is writing to her brother: "I'm taking advantage of the fact that my patient has found a pastime for the moment in writing to you." She pronounces the word *Quiès* (ear-plugs called Quiès) *Cuisses* (thighs). Mlle d'A . . . would never have been able to go to sleep without putting her Cuisses in her ears.

Do not forget that no visitors are allowed, that a nervous case, a semi-lunatic who ought to be entertained, is shut up alone with his nurse for months on end. The chief medical officer comes in for a minute. If the patient is all right, he stays longer. If the patient is not well, he beats a retreat. The psychiatrist attached to the establishment is young, agreeable and lively. He cannot help but be liked. If he is liked, a long visit vexes the chief medical officer, who is disliked. He stays ten minutes.

Any nurse is allotted to any patient. Yet the choice of a nurse is of paramount importance for nervous cases. Smiles: "Ah! If we also had to worry about details like that . . ." And the nervous patient is treated like an old dodderer. The composition of the medicines is kept hidden from him. Human contacts are avoided. The doctor must be inhuman. The doctor who talks and makes contact with the patient is never taken seriously. "Yes, he's a good talker, but if I were very ill I should send for someone else." Psychology is the enemy of medicine. Rather than tackle the question of opium with the patient who is obsessed by it, they avoid it. A real doctor does not stay long in the room, he conceals his tricks for lack of tricks. This method has corrupted the patients. They suspect the doctor who listens to them, the human doctor. Dr. M. has killed all my family and treated my brother's broken nose for erysipelas. His frock coat and bald pate were reassuring.

*   *   *

I wanted to take notes during my stay in the clinic and above all to contradict myself in order to follow the stages of the treatment. It was a question of talking about opium without embarrassment, without literature and without any medical knowledge.[1]

The specialists seem to be unaware of the world which separates the opium addict from the other victims of poisons, 'the drug,' and drugs.

I am not trying to defend the drug; I am trying to see clearly in the dark, to make blunders and to come face to face with the problems which are always approached from the side.

I imagine that young doctors are beginning to shake off the yoke, to revolt against the ridiculous prejudices and follow new developments.

A strange thing. Our physical safety accepts doctors who correspond to the artists whom our moral safety rejects. Imagine being cared for by someone like Ziem, Henner or Jean Aicard.

Will the young doctors discover either an active type of cure (the present method remains passive), or a regime which would enable us to withstand the blessings of the poppy?

The medical faculty detests intuition or risks; it wants practitioners, forgetting that they only arise thanks to discoveries which in the first place come up against scepticism, one of the worst forms of comfort.

There will be objections—art and science follow different paths. This is not true.

*   *   *

[1] Consult *Le Livre de la Feuemés* by Louis Laloy, the only good modern work on opium.

After the cure. The worst moment, the worst danger. Health with this void and an immense sadness. The doctors honestly hand you over to suicide.

*   *   *

I was therefore eliminating through ink, and even after the official elimination there was an unofficial elimination with a flow which became solid through my desire to write and draw. I allowed these drawings or notes only the value of frankness, and they seemed to me to be a derivative, a discipline for the nerves, but they became the faithful graph of the last stage. Sweat and bile precede some phantom substance which would have dissolved, leaving no other trace behind except a deep depression, if a fountain pen had not given it a direction, relief and shape.

Waiting for a period of calm to write these notes was trying to relive a state which is inconceivable as soon as the organism is no longer in it. Since I have never granted the slightest importance to the setting and since I was using opium as a remedy, I was not unhappy at seeing my state disappear. Whatever one renounces is a dead letter for those who imagine that the setting plays a part . . . I hope that this reportage finds a place among doctors' pamphlets and the literature of opium; may it serve as a guide to the novices who do not recognise, beneath the slowness of opium, one of the most dangerous faces of speed.

JAMES DICKEY
Diabetes

————◦∞◦————

JAMES DICKEY (1923-   ) is in the top rank of American poets. His fascination with power, his nostalgia, and his terse, energetic style are uniquely American. His strength lies in his simplicity, as in his agonized account of the patient in "Diabetes."

I

Sugar

One night I thirsted like a prince
Then like a king
Then like an empire   like a world
On fire. I rose and flowed away and fell
Once more to sleep. In an hour I was back
In the kingdom   staggering, my belly going round with self-
Made night-water, wondering what
The hell. Months of having a tongue
Of flame convinced me: I had better not go
On this way. The doctor was young

And nice. He said, I must tell you,
My friend, that it is needless moderation
And exercise. You don't want to look forward
To gangrene and kidney

Failure   boils blindness infection akin trouble falling
Teeth coma and death.
O.K.
In sleep my mouth went dry
With my answer   and in it burned the sands
Of time with new fury. Sleep could give me no water
But my own. Gangrene in white
Was in my wife's hand at breakfast
Heaped like a mountain. Moderation, moderation,

431

My friend, and exercise. Each time the barbell
  Rose each time a foot fell
   Jogging, it counted itself
  One death two death three death and resurrection
For a little while. Not bad! I always knew it would have to be
            somewhere around
    The house: the real
   Symbol of Time I could eat
  And live with, coming true when I opened my mouth:
   True in the coffee and the child's birthday
   Cake helping sickness be fire-
   tongued, sleepless and water-
   logged but not bad, sweet sand
   Of time, my friend, an everyday—
    A livable death at last.

II

Under Buzzards

[for Robert Penn Warren]

Heavy summer. Heavy. Companion, if we climb our mortal bodies
  High with great effort, we shall find ourselves
    Flying with the life
   Of the birds of death. We have come up
    Under buzzards they face us

 Slowly slowly circling and as we watch them they turn us
    Around, and you and I spin
    Slowly, slowly rounding
    Out the hill. We are level
  Exactly on this moment: exactly on the same bird-

plane with those deaths. They are the salvation of our sense
 Of glorious movement. Brother, it is right for us to face
 Them every which way, and come to ourselves and come
    From every direction
   There is. Whirl and stand fast!
   Whence cometh death, O Lord?
   On the downwind, riding fire,

Of Hogback Ridge.
But listen: what is dead here?
They are not falling but waiting   but waiting
Riding, and they may know
The rotten, nervous sweetness of my blood.
Somewhere riding the updraft
Of a far forest fire, they sensed the city sugar
The doctors found in time.
My eyes are green as lettuce with my diet,
My weight is down,

One pocket nailed with needles and injections, the other dragging
With sugar cubes to balance me in life
And hold my blood
Level, level. Tell me, black riders, does this do any good?
Tell me what I need to know about my time
In the world. O out of the fiery

Furnace of pine-woods, in the sap-smoke and crownfire of needles,
Say when I'll die. When will the sugar rise boiling
Against me, and my brain be sweetened
to death?
In heavy summer, like this day.
All right! Physicians, witness! I will shoot my veins
Full of insulin. Let the needle burn
In. From your terrible heads
The flight-blood drains   and you are falling back
Back to the body-raising

Fire.
Heavy summer. Heavy. My blood is clear
For a time. Is it too clear? Heat waves are rising
Without birds. But something is gone from me,
Friend. This is too sensible. Really it is better
To know when to die   better for my blood
To stream with the death-wish of birds.
You know, I had just as soon crush
This doomed syringe
Between two mountain rocks, and bury this needle in needles

Of trees. Companion, open that beer.
How the body works   how hard it works
For its medical books is not
Everything: everything is how
Much glory is in it: heavy summer is right

For a long drink of beer. Red sugar of my eyeballs
Feels them turn blindly
In the fire   rising   turning   turning
Back to Hogback Ridge, and it is all
Delicious, brother: my body is turning   is flashing unbalanced
Sweetness everywhere, and I am calling my birds.

WILLIAM ERNEST HENLEY
In Hospital

CLINICAL

Hist? . . .
Through the corridor's echoes
Louder and nearer
Comes a great shuffling of feet.
Quick, every one of you,
Straight your quilts, and be decent!
Here's the Professor.

In he comes first
With the bright look we know,
From the broad, white brows the kind eyes
Soothing yet nerving you. Here at his elbow,
White-capped, white-aproned, the Nurse,
Towel on arm and her inkstand
Fretful with quills.
Here in the ruck, anyhow.

Surging along,
Louts, duffers, exquisites, students, and prigs—
Whiskers and foreheads, scarf-pins and spectacles—
Hustles the Class! And they ring themselves
Round the first bed, where the Chief
(His dressers and clerks at attention),
Bends in inspection already.

So shows the ring
Seen from behind round a conjurer
Doing his pitch in the street.

BEN JONSON
To Dr. Empirick

———❧———

When men a dangerous disease did 'scape
Of old, they gave a cock to Aesculape.
Let me give two, that doubly am got free
From my disease's danger, and from thee.

THOMAS MANN
The Magic Mountain

———◆◆◆———

THOMAS MANN (1875-1955) won the Nobel Prize for his first novel, *Buddenbrooks,* a mirror of bourgeois life in pre-war Germany. In this selection from *The Magic Mountain* he draws upon his experiences in visiting his tubercular wife in a Swiss sanitarium. Disease becomes a metaphor for the spiritual malaise of Western civilization. Mann won wide acclaim in the United States for the philosophical content of his novels and for his descriptive powers.

And what was Dr. Krokowski saying? What was his line of thought? Hans Castorp summoned his wits to discover, not immediately succeeding, however, since he had not heard the beginning and lost still more while musing on Frau Chauchat's flabby back. It was about a power, the power which—in short, it was about the power of love. Yes, of course; the subject was already given out in the general title of the whole course, and, moreover, this was Dr. Krokowski's special field; of what else should he be talking? It was a bit odd, to be sure, listening to a lecture on such a theme, when previously Hans Castorp's courses had dealt only with such matters as geared transmission in shipbuilding. No, really, how did one go about to discuss a subject of this delicate and private nature, in broad daylight, before a mixed audience? Dr. Krokowski did it by adopting a mingled terminology, partly poetic and partly erudite; ruthlessly scientific, yet with a vibrating, singsong delivery, which impressed young Hans Castorp as being unsuitable, but may have been the reason why the ladies looked flushed and the gentlemen flicked their ears to make them hear better. In particular the speaker employed the word love in a somewhat ambiguous sense, so that you were never quite sure where you were with it, or whether he had reference to its sacred or its passionate and fleshy aspect—and this doubt gave one a slightly seasick feeling. Never in all his life had Hans Castorp heard the word uttered so many times on end as he was hearing it now. When he reflected, it seemed to him he had never taken it in his own mouth, nor ever heard it from a stranger's. That might not be the case, but whether it were or no, the word did not seem to him to repay such frequent repetition. The slippery monosyllable, with its lingual and labial, and the bleating vowel between—it came to sound positively offensive; it suggested watered milk, or anything else that was pale and insipid; the more so considering the meat for strong men Dr. Krokowski was in fact serving up. For it was plain that when one set about it like that, one could go pretty far without shocking anybody. He was not content to allude, with exquisite tact, to certain matters which are known to everybody, but which most people are content to pass over in silence. He demolished illusions, he was ruthlessly enlightened, he relentlessly destroyed all faith in the dignity of silver hairs and the innocence of the sucking babe. And he wore, with the frock-coat his négligé collar, sandals, and grey woollen socks, and, thus attired, made an impression profoundly otherworldly, though at the same time not a little startling to young Hans Castorp. He supported his statements with a wealth of illustration and anecdote from the books and loose notes on the table before him; several times he even quoted poetry. And he discussed certain startling manifestations of the power of love, certain extraordinary, painful, uncanny variations, which the majestic phenomenon at times displayed. It was, he said, the most unstable, the most unreliable of man's instincts, the most prone of its very essence to error and fatal perversion. In the which there was nothing that should cause surprise. For this mighty force did not consist of a single impulse, it was of its nature complex; it was built up out of components which, however legitimate they might be in composition, were, taken each by itself, sheer perversity. But—continued Dr. Krokowski—since we refuse, and rightly, to deduce the perversity of the whole from the perversity of its parts, we are driven to claim, for the component perversities, some part at least, though perhaps not all, of the justification which attaches to their united product. We were driven by sheer force of logic to this conclusion; Dr. Krokowski implored his hearers, having arrived at it, to hold it fast. Now there were physical correctives, forces working in the other direction, instincts tending to conformability and regularity—he would almost have liked to characterize them as bourgeois; and these influences had the effect of merging the perverse components into a valid and irreproachable whole: a frequent and gratifying result, which, Dr. Krokowski almost contemptuously added, was, as such, of no further concern to the thinker and the physician. But on the other hand, there were cases where this result was not obtained, could not and should not be obtained; and who, Dr. Krokowski asked, would dare to say that these cases did not, physically considered, form a higher, more exclusive type? For in these cases the two opposing groups of instincts—the compulsive force of love, and the sum of the impulses urging in the other direction, among which he would particularly mention shame and disgust—both exhibited an extraordinary and abnormal height and intensity when measured by the ordinary bourgeois standards; and the conflict between them which took place in the abysses of the soul prevented the erring instinct from attaining to that safe, sheltered, and civilized state which alone could resolve its difficulties in the prescribed harmonies of the love-life as experienced by the average human being. This conflict between the powers of love and chastity—for that was what it really amounted to—what was its issue? It ended, apparently, in the triumph of chastity. Love was suppressed, held in darkness and chains, by fear, conventionality, aversion, or a tremulous yearning to be pure. Her confused and tumultuous claims were never allowed to rise to consciousness or to come to proof in anything like their entire strength or multiformity. But this triumph of chastity was only an apparent, a pyrrhic victory; for the claims of love could not be crippled or enforced by any such means. The love thus suppressed was not dead; it lived, it laboured after fulfilment in the darkest and secretest depths of the being. It would break through the ban of chastity, it would emerge—if in a form so altered as to be unrecognizable. But what then was this form, this mask, in which suppressed, unchartered love would reappear? Dr. Krokowski asked the question, and looked along the listening rows as though in all seriousness expecting an answer. But he had to say it himself, who had said so much else already. No one knew save him, but it was plain that he did. Indeed, with his ardent eyes, his black beard setting off the waxen pallor of his face, his monkish sandals and grey woollen socks, he seemed to symbolize in his own person that conflict between passion and chastity which was his theme. At least so thought Hans Castorp, as with the others he waited in the greatest suspense to hear in what form love driven below the surface would reappear. The ladies barely breathed. Lawyer Paravant rattled his ear anew, that the critical moment might find it open and receptive. And Dr. Krokowski answered his own question, and said: "In the form of illness. Symptoms of disease are nothing but a disguised manifestation of the power of love; and all disease is only love transformed."

JEAN STAFFORD
The Interior Castle

------◆◇◆------

J EAN S TAFFORD (1915-1979) wrote sensitive, well-crafted stories of
American life. Her cool tone belies the vulnerability of her pro-
tagonists, as in "The Interior Castle," in which she describes excruciating medical treatment from the vantage point of the captive
patient.

Dr. Nicholas came at nine o'clock to prepare her for the operation. With
him came an entourage of white-frocked acolytes, and one of them wheeled
in a wagon on which lay knives and scissors and pincers, cans of swabs and
gauze. In the midst of these was a bowl of liquid whose rich purple color
made it seem strange like the brew of an alchemist.

"All set?" the surgeon asked her, smiling. "A little nervous, what? I
don't blame you. I've often said I'd rather break a leg than have a
submucous resection." Pansy thought for a moment he was going to touch
his nose. His approach to her was roundabout. He moved through the
yellow light shed by the globe in the ceiling which gave his forehead a liquid
gloss; he paused by the bureau and touched a blossom of the cyclamen; he
looked out the window and said, to no one and to all, "I couldn't start my
car this morning. Came in a cab." Then he came forward. As he came, he
removed a speculum from the pocket of his short-sleeved coat and like a
cat, inquiring of the nature of a surface with its paws, he put out his hand
toward her and drew it back, gently murmuring, "You must not be afraid,
my dear. There is no danger, you know. Do you think for a minute I would
operate if there were?"

Dr. Nicholas, young, brilliant, and handsome, was an aristocrat, a
husband, a father, a clubman, a Christian, a kind counselor, and a trustee of
his preparatory school. Like many of the medical profession, even those
whose specialty was centered on the organ of the basest sense, he
interested himself in the psychology of his patients: in several instances, for
example, he had found that severe attacks of sinusitis were coincident with
emotional crises. Miss Vanneman more than ordinarily captured his fancy
since her skull had been fractured and her behavior throughout had been so
extraordinary that he felt he was observing at first hand some of the results
of shock, that incommensurable element, which frequently were too subtle

440

to see. There was, for example, the matter of her complete passivity during a lumbar puncture, reports of which were written down in her history and were enlarged upon for him by Dr. Rivers' interne who had been in charge. Except for a tremor in her throat and a deepening of pallor, there were no signs at all that she was aware of what was happening to her. She made no sound, did not close her eyes nor clench her fists. She had had several punctures; her only reaction had been to the very first one, the morning after she had been brought in. When the interne explained to her that he was going to drain off cerebrospinal fluid which was pressing against her brain, she exclaimed, "My God!" but it was not an exclamation of fear. The young man had been unable to name what it was he had heard in her voice; he could only say that it had not been fear as he had observed it in other patients.

Dr. Nicholas wondered about her. There was no way of guessing whether she had always had a nature of so tolerant and undemanding a complexion. It gave him a melancholy pleasure to think that before her accident she had been high-spirited and loquacious; he was moved to think that perhaps she had been a beauty and that when she had first seen her face in the looking glass she had lost all joy in herself. It was very difficult to tell what the face had been, for it was so bruised and swollen, so hacked-up and lopsided. The black stitches the length of the nose, across the saddle, across the cheekbone, showed that there would be unsightly scars. He had ventured once to give her the name of a plastic surgeon but she had only replied with a vague, refusing smile. He had hoisted a manly shoulder and said, "You're the doctor."

Much as he pondered, coming to no conclusions, about what went on inside that pitiable skull, he was, of course, far more interested in the nose, deranged so badly that it would require his topmost skill to restore its functions to it. He would be obliged not only to make a submucous resection, a simple run-of-the-mill operation, but to remove the vomer, always a delicate task but further complicated in this case by the proximity of the bone to the frontal fracture line which conceivably was not entirely closed. If it were not and he operated too soon and if a cold germ then found its way into the opening, his patient would be carried off by meningitis in the twinkling of an eye. He wondered if she knew in what potential danger she lay; he desired to assure her that he had brought his craft to its nearest perfection and that she had nothing to fear of him, but feeling that she was perhaps both ignorant and unimaginative and that such consolation would create a fear rather than dispel one, he held his tongue and came nearer to the bed.

Watching him, Pansy could already feel the prongs of his pliers opening her nostrils for the insertion of his fine probers. The pain he caused her with his instruments was of a different kind from that she felt unaided: it was a naked, clean, and vivid pain that made her faint and ill and made her wish to die. Once she had fainted as he ruthlessly explored and after she was brought around, he continued until he had finished his investigation. The memory of this outrage had afterward several times made her cry.

This morning she looked at him and listened to him with hatred. Fixing her eyes upon the middle of his high, protuberant brow, she imagined the clutter behind it and she despised its obtuse imperfection. In his bland unawareness, this nobody, this nose-bigot, was about to play with fire and she wished him ill.

He said, "I can't blame you. No, I expect you're not looking forward to our little party. But you'll be glad to be able to breathe again."

He stationed his lieutenants. The interne stood opposite him on the left side of the bed. The surgical nurse wheeled the wagon within easy reach of his hands and stood beside it. Another nurse stood at the foot of the bed. A third drew the shades at the windows and attached a blinding light that shone down on the patient hotly, and then she left the room, softly closing the door. Pansy stared at the silver ribbon tied in a great bow round the green crepe paper of one of the flowerpots. It made her realize for the first time that one of the days she had lain here had been Christmas, but she had no time to consider this strange and thrilling fact, for Dr. Nicholas was genially explaining his anesthetic. He would soak packs of gauze in the purple fluid, a cocaine solution, and he would place them then in her nostrils, leaving them there for an hour. He warned her that the packing would be disagreeable (he did not say "painful") but that it would be well worth a few minutes of discomfort not to be in the least sick after the operation. He asked her if she were ready and when she nodded her head, he adjusted the mirror on his forehead and began.

At the first touch of his speculum, Pansy's fingers mechanically bent to the palms of her hands and she stiffened. He said, "A pack, Miss Kennedy," and Pansy closed her eyes. There was a rush of plunging pain as he drove the sodden gobbet of gauze high up into her nose and something bitter burned in her throat so that she retched. The doctor paused a moment and the surgical nurse wiped Pansy's mouth. He returned to her with another pack, pushing it with his bodkin doggedly until it lodged against the first. Stop! Stop! cried all her nerves, wailing along the surface of her skin. The coats that covered them were torn off and they shuddered like naked people screaming, Stop! Stop! But Dr. Nicholas did not hear. Time and again he came back with a fresh pack and did not pause at all until one nostril was finished. She opened her eyes and saw him wipe the sweat off his forehead and saw the dark interne bending over her, fascinated. Miss Kennedy bathed her temples in ice water and Dr. Nicholas said, "There. It won't be much longer. I'll tell them to send you some coffee, though I'm afraid you won't be able to use it. Ever drink coffee with chicory in it? I have no use for it."

She snatched at his irrelevancy and, though she had never tasted chicory, she said severely, "I love it."

Dr. Nicholas chuckled. "De gustibus. Ready? A pack, Miss Kennedy."

The second nostril was harder to pack since the other side was now distended and this passage was anyhow much narrower, as narrow, he had once remarked, as that in the nose of an infant. In such pain as passed all language and even the farthest fetched analogies, she turned her eyes inward, thinking that under the obscuring cloak of the surgeon's pain she could see her brain without the knowledge of its keeper. But Dr. Nicholas and his aides would give her no peace. They surrounded her with their murmuring and their foot-shuffling and the rustling of their starched uniforms, and her eyelids continually flew back in embarrassment and mistrust. She was claimed entirely by this present, meaningless pain and suddenly and sharply she forgot what she had meant to do. She was aware of nothing but her ascent to the summit of something; what it was she did not know, whether it was a tower or a peak or Jacob's ladder. Now she was an abstract word, now she was a theorem of geometry, now she was a kite flying, a top spinning, a prism flashing, a kaleidoscope turning.

But none of the others in the room could see inside and when the surgeon was finished, the nurse at the foot of the bed said, "Now you must take a look in the mirror. It's simply too comical." And they all laughed intimately like old, fast friends. She smiled politely and looked at her reflection: over the gruesomely fastened snout, her scarlet eyes stared in fixed reproach upon her upturned lips, gray with bruises. But even in its smile of betrayal, the mouth itself was puzzled: it reminded her that something had been left behind, but she could not recall what it was. She was hollowed out and was as dry as a white bone.

*   *   *

They strapped her ankles to the operating table and put leather nooses round her wrists. Over her head was a mirror with a thousand facets in which she saw a thousand travesties of her face. At her right side was the table, shrouded in white, where lay the glittering blades of the many knives, thrusting out fitful rays of light. All the cloth was frosty; everything was white or silver and as cold as snow. Dr. Nicholas, a tall snowman with silver eyes and silver fingernails, came into the room soundlessly, for he walked on layers and layers of snow that deadened his footsteps; behind him came the interne, a smaller snowman, less impressively proportioned. At the foot of the table, a snow figure put her frozen hands upon Pansy's helpless feet. The doctor plucked the packs from the cold, numb nose. His laugh was like a cry on a bitter, still night: "I will show you now," he called across the expanse of snow, "that you can feel nothing." The pincers bit at nothing, snapped at the air and cracked a nerveless icicle. Pansy called back and heard her own voice echo: "I feel nothing."

Here the walls were gray, not tan. Suddenly the face of the nurse at the foot of the table broke apart and Pansy first thought it was in grief. But it was a smile and she said, "Did you enjoy your coffee?" Down the gray corridors of the maze, the words rippled, ran like mice, birds, broken beads: Did you enjoy your coffee? your coffee? your coffee? Similarly once in another room that also had gray walls, the same voice had said, "Shall I give her some whisky?" She was overcome with gratitude that this young woman (how pretty she was with her white hair and her white face and her china-blue eyes!) had been with her that first night and was with her now.

In the great stillness of the winter, the operation began. The knives carved snow. Pansy was happy.

WILLIAM CARLOS WILLIAMS
The Injury

From this hospital bed
I can hear an engine
breathing—somewhere
    in the night:

—Soft coal, soft coal,
    soft coal!

And I know it is men
    breathing
shoveling, resting—

—Go about it
the slow way, if you can
find any way—
        Christ!
who's a bastard?
      —quit
and quit shoveling.

A man breathing
    and it quiets and
the puff of steady
work begins
      slowly: Chug.
Chug. Chug. Chug. . . .
    fading off.
Enough coal at least
    for this small job

    Soft! Soft!
—enough for one small
engine, enough for that.

A man shoveling
working and not lying here
        in this
hospital bed—powerless
—with the white-throat
        calling in the
poplars before dawn, his
faint flute-call,
triple tongued, piercing
the shingled curtain
of the new leaves;
        drowned out by
        car wheels
singing now on the rails,
taking the curve,
        slowly,
            a long wail,
high pitched:
        rounding
            the curve—
—the slow way because
(if you can find any way) that is
the only way left now
                    for you.

AN ENDURING TRADITION

The chronological distance from Bacon to Williams loses it vastness when the philosophical connections come into view. The authors and thinkers in history who have preoccupied themselves with the human condition may be addressing themselves to an evolving species under circumstances of constant change, but they all recognize an enduring aspect in the way human beings reach out for and accept help. People need more than "treatment." They need to be understood. They need to know that there is a dimension not just of competence but of caring in the kind of help they seek. Every person, as Robert Burton wrote in *Anatomy of Melancholy,* needs help. If that were not so, he added, we might fulfill the prediction of Paracelsus and live 400 years.

If the mind, that rules the body, ever so far forgets itself as to trample on its slave, the slave is never generous enough to forgive the injury, but will rise and smite the oppressor.

Longfellow.

Dyspepsia is the remorse of a guilty stomach.

A. Kerr.

Anguish of mind has driven thousands to suicide; anguish of body, none. This proves that the health of the mind is of far more consequence to our happiness than the health of the body, although both are deserving of much more attention than either receives.

Colton.

SIR FRANCIS BACON
Advancement of Learning

———⸺◦∞◦⸺———

Another article of this knowledge is the inquiry touching the affections; for as in medicining of the body it is in order first to know the divers complexions and constitutions, secondly the diseases, and lastly the cures; so in medicining of the mind, after knowledge of the divers characters of men's natures, it followeth in order to know the diseases and infirmities of the mind, which are no other than, the perturbations and distempers of the affections. For as the ancient politiques in popular estates were wont to compare the people to the sea and the orators to the winds, because as the sea would of itself be calm and quiet if the winds did not move and trouble it, so the people would be peaceable and tractable if the seditious orators did not set them in working and agitation; so it may be fitly said, that the mind in the nature thereof would be temperate and stayed, if the affections, as winds, did not put it into tumult and perturbation. And here again I find strange, as before, that Aristotle should have written divers volumes of Ethics, and never handled the affections, which is the principal subject thereof; and yet in his Rhetorics, where they are considered but collaterally and in a second degree (*as they may be moved by speech*), he findeth place for them, and handleth them well for the quantity; but where their true place is, he pretermitteth them. For it is not his disputations about pleasure and pain that can satisfy this inquiry, no more than he that should generally handle the nature of light can be said to handle the nature of colours; for pleasure and pain are to the particular affections as light is to particular colours. Better travails I suppose had the Stoics taken in this argument, as far as I can gather by that which we have at second hand: but yet it is like it was after their manner, rather in subtilty of definitions (which in a subject of this nature are but curiosities) than in active and ample descriptions and observations. So likewise I find some particular writings of an elegant nature touching some of the affections; as of *anger,* of *comfort upon adverse accidents,* of *tenderness of countenance,* and other. But the poets and writers of histories are the best doctors of this knowledge.

ROBERT BURTON
Anatomy of Melancholy

---◇---

SUBSECTION 3—
Terrors and Affrights, Causes of Melancholy

Tully (in the 4th of his Tusculans) distinguisheth these terrors which arise from the apprehension of some terrible object heard or seen from other fears, and so doth Patritius. Of all fears they are most pernicious and violent, and so suddenly alter the whole temperature of the body, move the soul & spirits, strike such a deep impression, that the parties can never be recovered, causing more grievous and fiercer Melancholy, (as Felix Plater speaks out of his experience,) than any inward cause whatsoever: *and imprints itself so forcibly in the spirits, brain, humours, that, if all the mass of blood were let out of the body, it could hardly be extracted. This horrible kind of Melancholy* (for so he terms it) *had been often brought before him, and troubles and affrights commonly men and women, young and old, of all sorts.* Hercules de Saxonia calls this kind of Melancholy by a peculiar name, it comes from the agitation, motion, contraction, dilatation of spirits, not from any distemperature of humours, and produceth strong effects. This terror is most usually caused, as Plutarch will have, *from some imminent danger, when a terrible object is at hand,* heard, seen, or conceived, *truly appearing, or in a dream:* and many times the more sudden the accident, it is the more violent.

> *Their soul's affright, their heart amazed quakes,*
> *The trembling liver pants i' th' veins, and aches.* (SENECA)

Artemidorus the Grammarian lost his wits by the unexpected sight of a Crocodile. The Massacre at Lyons, 1572, in the reign of Charles the 9th, was so terrible and fearful, that many ran mad, some died, great-bellied women were brought to bed before their time, generally all affrighted and aghast. Many lose their wits *by the sudden sight of some spectrum or devil, a thing very common in all ages,* saith Lavater, as Orestes did at the sight of the Furies, which appeared to him in black (as Pausanias records). The Greeks call them mormoluches,* which so terrify their souls. Or if they be

---

* In the text, in Greek letters, mormolykeia, but "mormoluche" appears elsewhere in Burton as a translation of the word. "Mormo" was a Greek she-monster of hideous aspect; "lykeia" refers to Mt. Lykaion, of which gruesome tales were told. There was a Lykaian Zeus, in whose festival the central rite was a human sacrifice, and he who tasted of the entrails of this sacrifice was turned into a wolf. But the word for wolf is "lykos." Perhaps, therefore, "werewolf" best suggests the meaning of the "mormoluche." The word is also seen in English, as in H. G. Wells' "Time Machine," as "Morlock."

but affrighted by some counterfeit devils in jest, as children in the dark conceive hobgoblins, and are sore afraid, they are the worse for it all their lives; some by sudden fires, earthquakes, inundations, or any such dismal objects. Themison the Physician fell into an *Hydrophobia* by seeing one sick of that disease, or by the sight of a monster, a carcase, they are disquieted many months following, & cannot endure the room where a corse had been, for a world would not be alone with a dead man, or lie in that bed many years after in which a man hath died. At Basil a many little children in the spring time went to gather flowers in a meadow at the town's end, where a malefactor hung in gibbets; all gazing at it, one by chance flung a stone, and made it stir, by which accident the children affrighted ran away; one, slower than the rest, looking back, and seeing the stirred carcase wag towards her, cried out it came after, & was so terribly affrighted, that for many days she could not rest, eat, sleep, she could not be pacified, but melancholy died. In the same town another child, beyond the Rhine, saw a grave opened, & upon the sight of the carcase was so troubled in mind, that she could not be comforted, but a little after departed, and was buried by it. A Gentlewoman of the same city saw a fat hog cut up; when the entails were opened, and a noisome savour offended her nose, she much misliked, and would not longer abide: a Physician in presence told her, as that hog, so was she, full of filthy excrements, and aggravated the matter by some other loathsome instances, in so much this nice Gentlewoman apprehended it so deeply, that she fell forthwith a vomiting, was so mightily distempered in mind and body, that, with all his art and persuasions, for some months after, he could not restore her to herself again, she could not forget it, or remove the object out of her sight. (F. Plater). Many cannot endure to see a wound opened, but they are offended, a man executed, or labour of any fearful disease, as possession, apoplexies, one bewitched, or if they read by chance of some terrible thing, the symptoms alone of such a disease, or that which they dislike, they are instantly troubled in mind, aghast, ready to apply it to themselves, they are as much disquieted as if they had seen it, or were so affected themselves. They dream and continually think of it. As lamentable effects are caused by such terrible objects heard, read, or seen; as Plutarch holds, no sense makes greater alteration of body & mind: sudden speech sometimes, unexpected news, be they good or bad, will move as much, as a Philosopher observes, will take away our sleep, and appetite, disturb and quite overturn us. Let them bear witness that have heard those tragical alarums, out-cries, hideous noises, which are many times suddenly heard in the dead of the night by irruption of enemies & accidental fires, &c., those panick fears, which often drive men out of their wits, bereave them of sense, under-standing and all, some for a time, some for their whole lives, they never recover it. The Midianites were so affrighted by Gideon's soldiers, they breaking but every one a pitcher; and Hannibal's army by such a panick fear was discomfited at the walls of Rome. Augusta Livia, hearing a few tragical verses recited out of Virgil, fell down dead in a swoon. Edinus, King of Denmark, by a sudden sound which he heard, *was turned into fury, with all his men*. Amatus Lusitanus had a patient, that by reason of bad tidings became *epileptic*. Cardan saw one that lost his wits by mistaking of an *echo*. If one sense alone can cause such violent commotions of the mind, what may we think when hearing, sight & those other senses, are all troubled at once, as by some earth-quakes, thunder, lightning, tempests, &c.? At Bologna in Italy, in the year 1504, there was such a fearful earth-quake about eleven a clock in the night (as Beroaldus, in his book On the Motion of the Earth, hath commended to posterity) that all the city trembled, the people thought the world was at an end; such a fearful noise it made, such a detestable smell, the inhabitants were infinitely affrighted, and some ran mad. Hear a strange story, and worthy to be chronicled (mine author adds), I had a servant at the same time called Fulco Argelanus, a bold proper man, so grievously terrified with it, that he was first melancholy, after doted, at last mad, & made away himself. At Fuscinum in Japan *there was such an earth-quake and darkness on a sudden, that many men were offended with headache, many overwhelmed with sorrow and melancholy*. At Meacum *whole streets & goodly palaces were overturned at the same time, & there was such an hideous noise withal, like thunder, and filthy small, that their hair stared for fear, and their hearts quaked; men and beasts were incredibly terrified*. In Sacal, another city, *the same earthquake was so terrible unto them, that many were bereft of their senses; and others by that horrible spectacle so much amazed, that they knew not what they did*. Blasius, a Christian, the reporter of the news, was so affrighted for his part that, though it were two months after, he was scarce his own man, neither could he drive the remembrance of it out of his mind. Many times some years following they will tremble afresh at the remembrance or conceit of such a terrible object, even all their lives long, if mention be made of it. Cornelius Agrippa relates out of Gulielmus Parisiensis a story of one, that, after a distasteful purge which a Physician had prescribed unto him, was so much moved, *that at the very sight of physick he would be distempered;* though he never so much as smelled to it, the box of physick long after would give him a purge; nay, the very remembrance of it did effect it; *like travellers and sea-men,* saith Plutarch, *that when they have been stranded, or dashed on a rock, for ever after fear not that mischance only, but all such dangers whatsoever*.

D. H. LAWRENCE
Psychoanalysis and the Unconscious

————— ◦◦◦ —————

D. H. LAWRENCE (1885-1930) sent shock waves through English letters with his direct way of dealing with contemporary psychology and sexuality. He was the inspiration for a literary cult. His "Psychology and the Unconscious," from which this chapter is drawn, is an indictment of Freud for thwarting the "blood consciousness," as he called it, in which both intellectual and physical passions should be allowed free rein.

PSYCHOANALYSIS *vs*. MORALITY

Psychoanalysis has sprung many surprises on us, performed more than one *volte-face* before our indignant eyes. No sooner had we got used to the psychiatric quack who vehemently demonstrated the serpent of sex coiled round the root of all our actions, no sooner had we begun to feel honestly uneasy about our lurking complexes, than lo and behold the psychoanalytic gentleman reappeared on the stage with a theory of pure psychology. The medical faculty, which was on hot bricks over the therapeutic innovations, heaved a sigh of relief as it watched the ground warming under the feet of the professional psychologists.

This, however, was not the end. The ears of the ethnologist began to tingle, the philosopher felt his gorge rise, and at last the moralist knew he must rush in. By this time psychoanalysis had become a public danger. The mob was on the alert. The Œdipus complex was a household word, the incest motive a commonplace of tea-table chat. Amateur analyses became the vogue. "Wait till you've been analysed," said one man to another, with varying intonation. A sinister look came into the eyes of the initiates—the famous, or infamous, Freud look. You could recognize it everywhere, wherever you went.

Psychoanalysts know what the end will be. They have crept in among us as healers and physicians; growing bolder, they have asserted their authority as scientists; two more minutes and they will appear as apostles. Have we not seen and heard the *ex cathedrâ* Jung? And does it need a prophet to discern that Freud is on the brink of a Weltanschauung—or at least a Menschenschauung, which is a much more risky affair? What detains him? Two things. First and foremost, the moral issue. And next, but more vital, he can't get down to the rock on which he must build his church.

Let us look to ourselves. This new doctrine—it will be called no less—has been subtly and insidiously suggested to us, gradually inoculated into us. It is true that doctors are the priests, nay worse, the medicine-men of our decadent society. Psychoanalysis has made the most of the opportunity.

First and foremost the issue is a moral issue. It is not here a matter of reform, new moral values. It is the life or death of all morality. The leaders among the psychoanalysts know what they have in hand. Probably most of their followers are ignorant, and therefore pseudo-innocent. But it all amounts to the same thing. Psychoanalysis is out, under a therapeutic disguise, to do away entirely with the moral faculty in man. Let us fling the challenge, and then we can take sides in all fairness.

The psychoanalytic leaders know what they are about, and shrewdly keep quiet, going gently. Yet, however gently they go, they set the moral stones rolling. At every step the most innocent and unsuspecting analyst starts a little landslide. The old world is yielding under us. Without any direct attack, it comes loose under the march of the psychoanalyst, and we hear the dull rumble of the incipient avalanche. We are in for a *débâcle*.

But at least let us know what we are in for. If we are to rear a serpent against ourselves, let us at least refuse to nurse it in our temples or to call it the cock of Æsculapius. It is time the white garb of the therapeutic cant was stripped off the psychoanalyst. And now that we feel the strange crackling and convulsion in our moral foundations, let us at least look at the house which we are bringing down over our heads so blithely.

Long ago we watched in frightened anticipation when Freud set out on his adventure into the hinterland of human consciousness. He was seeking for the unknown sources of the mysterious stream of consciousness. Immortal phrase of the immortal James! Oh stream of hell which undermined my adolescence! The stream of consciousness! I felt it streaming through my brain, in at one ear and out at the other. And again I was sure it went round in my cranium, like Homer's Ocean, encircling my established mind. And sometimes I felt it must bubble up in the cerebellum and wind its way through all the convolutions of the true brain. Horrid stream! Whence did it come, and whither was it bound? The stream of consciousness!

And so, who could remain unmoved when Freud seemed suddenly to plunge towards the origins? Suddenly he stepped out of the conscious into the unconscious, out of the everywhere into the nowhere, like some supreme explorer. He walks straight through the wall of sleep, and we hear him rumbling in the cavern of dreams. The impenetrable is not impenetrable, unconsciousness is not nothingness. It is sleep, that wall of darkness which limits our day. Walk bang into the wall, and behold the wall isn't there. It is the vast darkness of a cavern's mouth, the cavern of anterior darkness whence issues the stream of consciousness.

With dilated hearts we watched Freud disappearing into the cavern of darkness, which is sleep and unconsciousness to us, darkness which issues in the foam of all our day's consciousness. He was making for the origins. We watched his ideal candle flutter and go small. Then we waited, as men do wait, always expecting the wonder of wonders. He came back with dreams to sell.

But sweet heaven, what merchandise! What dreams, dear heart! What was there in the cave? Alas that we ever looked! Nothing but a huge slimy serpent of sex, and heaps of excrement, and a myriad repulsive little horrors spawned between sex and excrement.

Is it true? Does the great unknown of sleep contain nothing else? No lovely spirits in the anterior regions of our being? None! Imagine the unspeakable horror of the *repressions* Freud brought home to us. Gagged, bound, maniacal repressions, sexual complexes, fæcal inhibitions, dream-monsters. We tried to repudiate them. But no, they were there, demonstrable. These were the horrid things that ate our souls and caused our helpless neuroses.

We had felt that perhaps we were wrong inside, but we had never imagined it so bad. However, in the name of healing and medicine we prepared to accept it all. If it was all just a result of illness, we were prepared to go through with it. The analyst promised us that the tangle of complexes would be unravelled, the obsessions would evaporate, the monstrosities would dissolve, sublimate, when brought into the light of day. Once all the dream-horrors were translated into full consciousness, they would sublimate into—well, we don't quite know what. But anyhow, they would sublimate. Such is the charm of a new phrase that we accepted this sublimation process without further question. If our complexes were going to sublimate once they were surgically exposed to full mental consciousness, why, best perform the operation.

Thus analysis set off gaily on its therapeutic course. But like Hippolytus, we ran too near the sea's edge. After all, if complexes exist only as abnormalities which can be removed, psychoanalysis has not far to go. Our own horses ran away with us. We began to realize that complexes were not just abnormalities. They were part of the stock-in-trade of the normal unconscious. The only abnormality, so far, lies in bringing them into consciousness.

This creates a new issue. Psychoanalysis, the moment it begins to demonstrate the nature of the unconscious, is assuming the rôle of psychology. Thus the new science of psychology proceeds to inform us that our complexes are not just mere interlockings in the mechanism of the psyche, as was taught by one of the first and most brilliant of the analysts, a man now forgotten. He fully realized that even the psyche itself depends on a certain organic, mechanistic activity, even as life depends on the mechanistic organism of the body. The mechanism of the psyche could have its hitches, certain parts could stop working, even as the parts of the body can stop their functioning. This arrest in some part of the functioning psyche gave rise to a complex, even as the stopping of one little cog-wheel in a machine will arrest a whole section of that machine. This was the origin of the complex-theory, purely mechanistic. Now the analyst found that a complex did not necessarily vanish when brought into consciousness. Why should it? Hence he decided that it did not arise from the stoppage of any little wheel. For it refused to disappear, no matter how many psychic wheels were started. Finally, then, a complex could not be regarded as the result of an inhibition.

Here is the new problem. If a complex is not caused by the inhibition of some so-called normal sex-impulse, what on earth is it caused by? It obviously refuses to sublimate—or to come undone when exposed and prodded. It refuses to answer to the promptings of normal sex-impulse. You can remove all possible inhibitions of the normal sex desire, and still you cannot remove the complex. All you have done is to make conscious a desire which previously was unconscious.

This is the moral dilemma of psychoanalysis. The analyst set out to cure neurotic humanity by removing the cause of the neurosis. He finds that the cause of neurosis lies in some unadmitted sex desire. After all he has said about inhibition of normal sex, he is brought at last to realize that at the root of almost every neurosis lies some incest-craving, and that this incest-craving is *not the result of inhibition of normal sex-craving*. Now we see the dilemma—it is a fearful one. If the incest-craving is not the outcome of any inhibition of normal desire, if it actually exists and refuses to give way before any criticism, what then? What remains but to accept it as part of the normal sex-manifestation?

Here is an issue which analysis is perfectly willing to face. Among themselves the analysts are bound to accept the incest-craving as part of the normal sexuality of man, normal, but suppressed, because of moral and perhaps biological fear. Once, however, you accept the incest-craving as part of the normal sexuality of man, you must remove all repression of incest itself. In fact, you must admit incest as you now admit sexual marriage, as a duty even. Since at last it works out that neurosis is not the result of inhibition of so-called *normal* sex, but of inhibition of incest-craving. Any inhibition must be wrong, since inevitably in the end it causes neurosis and insanity. Therefore the inhibition of incest-craving is wrong, and this wrong is the cause of practically all modern neurosis and insanity.

Psychoanalysis will never openly state this conclusion. But it is to this conclusion that every analyst must, willy-nilly, consciously or unconsciously, bring his patient.

Trigant Burrow says that Freud's *unconscious* does but represent our conception of conscious sexual life as this latter exists in a state of repression. Thus Freud's unconscious amounts practically to no more than our repressed incest impulses. Again, Burrow says that it is knowledge of sex that constitutes sin, and not sex itself. It is when the mind turns to consider and *know* the great affective-passional functions and emotions that sin enters. Adam and Eve fell, not because they had sex, or even because they committed the sexual act, but because they became aware of their sex and of the possibility of the act. When sex became to them a mental object—that is, when they discovered that they could deliberately enter upon and enjoy and even provoke sexual activity in themselves, then they were cursed and cast out of Eden. Then man became self-responsible; he entered on his own career.

Both these assertions by Burrow seem to us brilliantly true. But must we inevitably draw the conclusion psychoanalysis draws? Because we discover in the unconscious the repressed body of our incest-craving, and because the recognition of *desire,* the making a mental objective of a certain desire causes the introduction of the sin motive, the desire in itself being beyond criticism or moral judgment, must we therefore accept the incest-craving as part of our natural desire and proceed to put it into practice, as being at any rate a lesser evil than neurosis and insanity?

It is a question. One thing, however, psychoanalysis all along the line fails to determine, and that is the nature of the pristine unconscious in man. The incest-craving is or is not inherent in the pristine psyche. When Adam and Eve became aware of sex in themselves, they became aware of that which was pristine in them, and which preceded all knowing. But when the analyst discovers the incest motive in the unconscious, surely he is only discovering a term of humanity's repressed *idea* of sex. It is not even *suppressed* sex-consciousness, but *repressed.* That is, it is nothing pristine and anterior to mentality. It is in itself the mind's ulterior motive. That is, the incest-craving is propagated in the pristine unconscious by the mind itself, even though unconsciously. The mind acts as incubus and procreator of its own horrors, *deliberately unconsciously*. And the incest motive is in its origin not a pristine impulse, but a logical extension of the existent idea of sex and love. The mind, that is, transfers the idea of incest into the affective-passional psyche, and keeps it there as a repressed motive.

This is as yet a mere assertion. It cannot be made good until we determine the nature of the true, pristine unconscious, in which all our genuine impulse arises—a very different affair from that sack of horrors which psychoanalysts would have us believe is source of motivity. The Freudian unconscious is the cellar in which the mind keeps its own bastard spawn. The true unconscious is the wellhead, the fountain of real motivity. The sex of which Adam and Eve became conscious derived from the very God who bade them be not conscious of it—it was not spawn produced by secondary propagation from the mental consciousness itself.

GEORGE MEREDITH
Melampus

———⟨∞⟩———

George Meredith (1828-1909) is only rarely found these days on college booklists. His work is almost non-existent in paperback editions, though he was the most esteemed author in England in his day. As a novelist, he liked to deal with moral issues. He was far ahead of his time in his evocative imagery and unconcern for the niceties of narration. When Meredith wrote about physicians, he did so against the background of his chronic back trouble, which confined him to a wheel chair late in life. In Greek mythology, Melampus, the hero of Meredith's tale, was the first mortal to practice the art of healing.

I

With love exceeding a simple love of the things
    That glide in grasses and rubble of woody wreck;
Or change their perch on a beat of quivering wings
    From branch to branch, only restful to pipe and peck;
Or, bristled, curl at a touch their snouts in a ball;
    Or cast their web between bramble and thorny hook;
The good physician Melampus, loving them all,
    Among them walked, as a scholar who reads a book.

II

For him the woods were a home and gave him the key
    Of knowledge, thirst for their treasures in herbs and flowers.
The secrets held by the creatures nearer than we
    To earth he sought, and the link of their life with ours:
And where alike we are, unlike where, and the veined
    Division, veined parallel, of a blood that flows
In them, in us, from the source by man unattained
    Save marks he well what the mystical woods disclose.

III

And this he deemed might be boon of love to a breast
   Embracing tenderly each little motive shape,
The prone, the flitting, who seek their food whither best
   Their wits direct, whither best from their foes escape:
For closer drawn to our mother's natural milk,
   As babes they learn where her motherly help is great:
They know the juice for the honey, juice for the silk,
   And need they medical antidotes find them straight.

IV

Of earth and sun they are wise, they nourish their broods,
   Weave, build, hive, burrow and battle, take joy and pain
Like swimmers varying billows: never in woods
   Runs white insanity fleeing itself: all sane
The woods revolve: as the tree its shadowing limns
   To some resemblance in motion, the rooted life
Restrains disorder: you hear the primitive hymns
   Of earth in woods issue wild of the web of strife.

V

Now sleeping once on a day of marvellous fire,
   A brood of snakes he had cherished in grave regret
That death his people had dealt their dam and their sire,
   Through savage dread of them, crept to his neck, and set
Their tongues to lick him: the swift affectionate tongue
   Of each ran licking the slumberer: then his ears
A forked red tongue tickled shrewdly: sudden upsprung,
   He heard a voice piping: Ay, for he has no fears!

VI

A bird said that, in the notes of birds, and the speech
   Of men, it seemed: and another renewed: He moves
To learn and not to pursue, he gathers to teach;
   He feeds his young as do we, and as we love loves.

No fears have I of a man who goes with his head
   To earth, chance looking aloft at us, kind of hand:
I feel to him as to earth of whom we are fed;
   I pipe him much for his good could be understand.

VII

Melampus touched at his ears, laid finger on wrist:
   He was not dreaming, he sensibly felt and heard.
Above, through leaves, where the tree-twigs thick intertwist,
   He spied the birds and the bill of the speaking bird.
His cushion mosses in shades of various green,
   The lumped, the antlered, he pressed, while the sunny snake
Slipped under: draughts he had drunk of clear Hippocrene,
   It seemed, and sat with a gift of the Gods awake.

VIII

Divinely thrilled was the man, exultingly full,
   As quick well-waters that come of the heart of earth,
Ere yet they dart in a brook are one bubble-pool
   To light and sound, wedding both at the leap of birth.
The soul of light vivid shone, a stream within stream;
   The soul of sound from a musical shell outflew;
Where others hear but a hum and see but a beam,
   The tongue and eye of the fountain of life he knew.

IX

He knew the Hours: they were round him, laden with seed
   Of hours bestrewn upon vapour, and one by one
They winged as ripened in fruit the burden decreed
   For each to scatter; they flushed like the buds in sun,
Bequeathing seed to successive similar rings,
   Their sisters, bearers to men of what men have earned:
He knew them, talked with the yet unreddened; the stings,
   The sweets, they warmed at their bosoms divined, discerned.

X

Not unsolicited, sought by diligent feet,
   By riddling fingers expanded, oft watched in growth
With brooding deep as the noon-ray's quickening wheat,
   Ere touch'd, the pendulous flower of the plants of sloth,
The plants of rigidness, answered question and squeeze,
   Revealing wherefore it bloomed uninviting, bent,
Yet making harmony breathe of life and disease,
   The deeper chord of a wonderful instrument.

XI

So passed he luminous-eyed for earth and the fates
   We arm to bruise or caress us: his ears were charged
With tones of love in a whirl of voluble hates,
   With music wrought of distraction his heart enlarged.
Celestial-shining, though mortal, singer, though mute,
   He drew the Master of harmonies, voiced or stilled,
To seek him; heard at the silent medicine-root
   A song, beheld in fulfilment the unfulfilled.

XII

Him Phoebus, lending to darkness colour and form
   Of light's excess, many lessons and counsels gave;
Showed Wisdom lord of the human intricate swarm,
   And whence prophetic it looks on the hives that rave,
And how acquired, of the zeal of love to acquire,
   And where it stands, in the centre of life a sphere;
And Measure, mood of the lyre, the rapturous lyre,
   He said was Wisdom, and struck him the notes to hear.

XIII

Sweet, sweet: 't was glory of vision, honey, the breeze
   In heat, the run of the river on root and stone,
All senses joined, as the sister Pierides
   Are one, uplifting their chorus, the Nine, his own.
In stately order, evolved of sound into sight,

From sight to sound intershifting, the man descried
The growths of earth, his adored, like day out of night,
   Ascend in song, seeing nature and song allied.

XIV

And there vitality, there, there solely in song,
   Resides, where earth and her uses to men, their needs,
Their forceful cravings, the theme are: there is it strong,
   The Master said: and the studious eye that reads,
(Yea, even as earth to the crown of Gods on the mount),
   In links divine with the lyrical tongue is bound.
Pursue thy craft: it is music drawn of a fount
   To spring perennial; well-spring is common ground.

XV

Melampus dwelt among men: physician and sage,
   He served them, loving them, healing them; sick or maimed
Or them that frenzied in some delirious rage
   Outran the measure, his juice of the woods reclaimed.
He played on men, as his master, Phoebus, on strings
   Melodious: as the God did he drive and check,
Through love exceeding a simple love of the things
   That glide in grasses and rubble of woody wreck.

PLATO
Symposium

⎯⎯⎯❧⎯⎯⎯

PLATO (427 B.C.—348 B.C.) spent a lifetime writing and teaching a philosophy of ideas in the hope that philosophers might become kings and kings philosophers.

Then, said The Physician Eryximachus, the weak heads like myself. Aristodemus, Phaedrus, and others who never can drink are fortunate in finding that the stronger ones are not in a drinking mood. (I do not include Socrates, who is able neither to drink or to abstain, and will not mind, whichever we do.) Well, as none of the company seem disposed to drink much, I may be forgiven for saying, as a physician, that drinking deep is a bad practice, which I never follow, if I can help, and certainly do not recommend to another, least of all to any one who still feels the effects of yesterday's carouse.

I always do what you advise, and especially what you prescribe as a physician, rejoined Phaedrus the Myrrhinusian, and the rest of the company, if they are wise, will do the same.

It was agreed that drinking was not to be the order of the day, but that they were all to drink only so much as they pleased.

Then, said Eryximachus, as you are all agreed that drinking is to be voluntary, and that there is to be no compulsion, I move, in the next place, that the flute-girl, who has just made her appearance, be told to go away and play to herself, or, if she likes, to the women who are within. To-day let us have conversation instead; and, if you will allow me, I will tell you what sort of conversation. This proposal having been accepted, Eryximachus proceeded as follows:—

I will begin, he said, after the manner of Melanippe in Euripides,

"Not mine the word"

which I am about to speak, but that of Phaedrus. For often he says to me in an indignant tone:—"What a strange thing it is, Eryximachus, that, whereas other gods have poems and hymns made in their honour, the great

464

and glorious god, Love, has no encomiast among all the poets who are so many. There are the worthy Sophists too—the excellent Prodicus, for example—who have descanted in prose on the virtues of Heracles and other heroes;

*   *   *

Eryximachus the physician, who was reclining on the couch below him. Eryximachus, he said, you ought either to stop my hiccough, or to speak in my turn until I have left off.

I will do both, said Eryximachus: I will speak in your turn, and do you speak in mine; and while I am speaking let me recommend you to hold your breath, and if after you have done so for some time the hiccough is no better, then gargle with a little water; and if it still continues, tickle your nose with something and sneeze; and if you sneeze once or twice, even the most violent hiccough is sure to go. I will do as you prescribe, said Aristophanes, and now get on.

Eryximachus spoke as follows: Seeing that Pausanias made a fair beginning, and but a lame ending, I must endeavour to supply his deficiency. I think that he has rightly distinguished two kinds of love. But my art further informs me that the double love is not merely an affection of the soul of man towards the fair, or towards anything, but is to be found in the bodies of all animals and in productions of the earth, and I may say in all that is; such is the conclusion which I seem to have gathered from my own art of medicine, whence I learn how great and wonderful and universal is the deity of love, whose empire extends over all things, divine as well as human. And from medicine I will begin that I may do honour to my art. There are in the human body these two kinds of love, which are confessedly different and unlike, and being unlike, they have loves and desires which are unlike; and the desire of the healthy is one, and the desire of the diseased is another; and as Pausanias was just now saying that to indulge good men is honourable, and bad men dishonourable:—so too in the body the good and healthy elements are to be indulged, and the bad elements and the elements of disease are not to be indulged, but discouraged. And this is what the physician has to do, and in this the art of medicine consists: for medicine may be regarded generally as the knowledge of the loves and desires of the body, and how to satisfy them or not; and the best physician is he who is able to separate fair love from foul, or to convert one into the other; and he who knows how to eradicate and how to implant love, whichever is required, and can reconcile the most hostile elements in the constitution and make them loving friends, is a skillful practitioner. Now the most hostile are the most opposite, such as hot and cold, bitter and sweet, moist and dry, and the like. And my ancestor, Asclepius, knowing how to implant friendship and accord in these elements, was the creator of our art, as our friends the poets here tell us, and I believe them; and not only medicine in every branch, but the arts of gymnastic and husbandry are under his dominion. Any one who pays the least attention to the subject will also perceive that in music there is the same reconciliation of opposites; and I suppose that this must have been the meaning of Heracleitus, although his words are not accurate; for he says that The One is united by disunion, like the harmony of the bow and the lyre. Now there is an absurdity in saying that harmony is discord or is composed of elements which are still in a state of discord. But what he probably meant was, that harmony is composed of differing notes of higher or lower pitch which disagreed once, but are now reconciled by the art of music; for if the higher and lower notes still disagreed, there could be no harmony,—clearly not. For harmony is a symphony, and symphony is an agreement; but an agreement of disagreements while they disagree there cannot be; you cannot harmonize that which disagrees. In like manner rhythm is compounded of elements short and long once differing and now in accord; which accordance, as in the former instance, medicine, so in all these other cases, music implants, making love and unison to grow up among them; and thus music, too, is concerned with the principles of love in their application to harmony and rhythm. Again, in the essential nature of harmony and rhythm there is no difficulty in discerning love which has not yet become double. But when you want to use them in actual life, either in the composition of songs or in the correct performance of airs or metres composed already, which latter is called education, then the difficulty begins, and the good artist is needed. Then the old tale has to be repeated of fair and heavenly love—the love of Urania the fair and heavenly muse, and of the duty of accepting the temperate, and those who are as yet intemperate only that they may become temperate, and of preserving their love; and again, of the vulgar Polyhymnia, who must be used with circumspection that the pleasure be enjoyed, but may not generate licentiousness; just as in my own art it is a great matter so to regulate the desires of the epicure that he may gratify his tastes without the attendant evil of disease. Whence I infer that in music, in medicine, in all other things human as well as divine, both loves ought to be noted as far as may be, for they are both present.

The course of the seasons is also full of both these principles; and when, as I was saying, the elements of hot and cold, moist and dry, attain the harmonious love of one another and blend in temperance and harmony, they bring to men, animals, and plants health and plenty, and do them no harm; whereas the wanton love, getting the upper hand and affecting the seasons of the year, is very destructive and injurious, being the source of pestilence, and bringing many other kinds of diseases on animals and plants; for hoarfrost and hail and blight spring from the excesses and disorders of these elements of love, which to know in relation to the revolutions of the heavenly bodies and the seasons of the year is termed astronomy. Furthermore, all sacrifices and the whole province of divination, which is the art of communion between gods and men—these, I say, are concerned only with the preservation of the good and the cure of the evil love. For all manner of impiety is likely to ensue if, instead of accepting and honouring and reverencing the harmonious love in all his actions, a man honours the other love, whether in his feelings towards gods or parents, towards the living or the dead. Wherefore the business of divination is to see these loves and to heal them, and divination is the peacemaker of gods and men, working by a knowledge of the religious or irreligious tendencies which exist in human loves. Such is the great and mighty, or rather omnipotent force of love in general. And the love, more especially, which is concerned with the good, and which is perfected in company with temperance and justice, whether among gods or men, has the greatest power, and is the source of all our happiness and harmony, and makes us friends with the gods who are above us, and with one another. I dare say that I too have omitted several things which might be said in praise of Love, but this was not intentional, and you, Aristophanes, may now supply the omission or take some other line of commendation; for I perceive that you are rid of the hiccough.

Yes, said Aristophanes, who followed, the hiccough is gone; not, however, until I applied the sneezing; and I wonder whether the harmony of the body has a love of such noises and ticklings, for I no sooner applied the sneezing than I was cured.

Eryximachus said: Beware, friend Aristophanes, although you are going to speak, you are making fun of me; and I shall have to watch and see whether I cannot have a laugh at your expense, when you might speak in peace.

ARTHUR SCHNITZLER
My Youth in Vienna

———— ◦❈◦ ————

Yet it was no longer quite the same daily grind. Signs pointed to the fact that I was gradually, very gradually, progressing, sometimes in one direction, then again in another. I had begun to practice hypnotism, an interest which had been aroused in me above all by the research of Charcot and Bernheim, and had succeeded in treating successfully several cases of aphonia, that is to day, the loss of voice without any organic change in the vocal cords, by hypnotizing the patient, or simply by the power of suggestion, and had published some case histories in the *Internationale Klinische Rundschau*. Since I had found several excellent mediums, I did not limit myself to this form of therapy in the field of laryngology only, but in emulation of the famous hypnotists, tried all sorts of psychological experiments, which although not uninteresting, did not result in any new information. I jotted them down but never worked them out scientifically. Certainly my happiest achievement from a medical viewpoint was when I was able to induce a partial anesthesia without putting the medium to sleep, simply by power of suggestion, so that it was possible to perform painlessly a minor operation on the larynx, and in one case even a tooth extraction. More stimulating but of little importance medically was when I had my medium experience under hypnosis all sorts of situations and sensations, whatever I felt inclined to invent; or when from one day to the next I arranged for a murder attempt against myself, which I was able to parry successfully because I was prepared for it, and the patient chose to use a dull letter-opener instead of a dagger. Not only my colleagues in the department, but various doctors from the Polyclinic and other hospitals sometimes came to watch my experiments. Those who came most frequently spread the word, spitefully, that I was putting on shows at the Polyclinic, which led to my stopping outsiders from watching what I was doing, although for a while I continued to let my closer associates be present as observers. But here again I failed to proceed and draw the consequences of the way I had chosen, and when I began to notice that my most interesting mediums seemed to suffer a loss of will and a certain damage to their health by the repeated experiments, I desisted from any further experimentation of a purely psychological nature, and used hypnosis only in certain cases and for strictly defined healing purposes.

WILLIAM SHAKESPEARE
Sonnet CXLVII.

My love is as a fever, longing still
For that which longer nurseth the disease,
Feeding on that which doth preserve the ill,
The uncertain sickly appetite to please.
My reason, the physician to my love,
Angry that his prescriptions are not kept,
Hath left me, and I desperate now approve
Desire is death, which physic did except.
Past cure I am, now reason is past care,
And frantic-mad with evermore unrest;
My thoughts and my discourse as madmen's are,
At random from the truth vainly express'd;
   For I have sworn thee fair and thought thee bright
   Who art as black as hell, as dark as night.

GEORGE BERNARD SHAW
Back to Methuselah

CREATIVE EVOLUTION

But this dismal creed does not discourage those who believe that the impulse that produces evolution is creative. They have observed the simple fact that the will to do anything can and does, at a certain pitch of intensity set up by conviction of its necessity, create and organize new tissue to do it with. To them therefore mankind is by no means played out yet. If the weight lifter, under the trivial stimulus of an athletic competition, can 'put up a muscle,' it seems reasonable to believe that an equally earnest and convinced philosopher could 'put up a brain.' Both are directions of vitality to a certain end. Evolution shows us this direction of vitality doing all sorts of things: providing the centipede with a hundred legs, and ridding the fish of any legs at all; building lungs and arms for the land and gills and fins for the sea; enabling the mammal to gestate its young inside its body, and the fowl to incubate hers outside it; offering us, we may say, our choice of any sort of bodily contrivance to maintain our activity and increase our resources.

MARK TWAIN
Autobiography

———◦∞◦———

Down the forest slopes to the left were the swings. They were made of bark stripped from hickory saplings. When they became dry they were dangerous. They usually broke when a child was forty feet in the air, and this was why so many bones had to be mended every year. I had no ill luck myself, but none of my cousins escaped. There were eight of them, and at one time and another they broke fourteen arms among them. But it cost next to nothing, for the doctor worked by the year—twenty-five dollars for the whole family. I remember two of the Florida doctors, Chowning and Meredith. They not only tended an entire family for twenty-five dollars a year, but furnished the medicines themselves. Good measure, too. Only the largest persons could hold a whole dose. Castor oil was the principal beverage. The dose was half a dipperful, with half a dipperful of New Orleans molasses added to help it down and make it taste good, which it never did. The next standby was calomel; the next, rhubarb; and the next, jalap. Then they bled the patient, and put mustard plasters on him. It was a dreadful system, and yet the death rate was not heavy. The calomel was nearly sure to salivate the patient and cost him some of his teeth. There were no dentists. When teeth became touched with decay or were otherwise ailing, the doctor knew of but one thing to do—he fetched his tongs and dragged them out. If the jaw remained, it was not his fault. Doctors were not called in cases of ordinary illness; the family grandmother attended to those. Every old woman was a doctor, and gathered her own medicines in the woods, and knew how to compound doses that would stir the vitals of a cast-iron dog. And then there was the "Indian doctor"; a grave savage, remnant of his tribe, deeply read in the mysteries of nature and the secret properties of herbs; and most backwoodsmen had high faith in his powers and could tell of wonderful cures achieved by him. In Mauritius, away off yonder in the solitudes of the Indian Ocean, there is a person who answers to our Indian doctor of the old times. He is a negro, and has had no teaching as a doctor, yet there is one disease which he is master of and can cure and the doctors can't. They send for him when they have a case. It is a child's disease of a strange and deadly sort, and the negro cures it with a herb medicine which he makes, himself, from a prescription which has come down to him from his father and grandfather. He will not let anyone see it. He keeps the secret of its components to himself, and it is feared that he will die without divulging it; then there will be consternation in Mauritius. I was told these things by the people there, in 1896.

We had the "faith doctor," too, in those early days—a woman. Her specialty was toothache. She was a farmer's old wife and lived five miles from Hannibal. She would lay her hand on the patient's jaw and say, "Believe!" and the cure was prompt. Mrs. Utterback. I remember her very well. Twice I rode out there behind my mother, horseback, and saw the cure performed. My mother was the patient.

Doctor Meredith removed to Hannibal, by and by, and was our family physician there, and saved my life several times. Still, he was a good man and meant well. Let it go.

I was always told that I was a sickly and precarious and tiresome and uncertain child, and lived mainly on allopathic medicines during the first seven years of my life. I asked my mother about this, in her old age—she was in her eighty-eighth year—and said:

"I suppose that during all that time you were uneasy about me?"

"Yes, the whole time."

"Afraid I wouldn't live?"

After a reflective pause—ostensibly to think out the facts—"No—afraid you would."

WILLIAM CARLOS WILLIAMS
Autobiography

—◆◆◆—

OF MEDICINE AND POETRY

When they ask me, as of late they frequently do, how I have for so many years continued an equal interest in medicine and the poem, I reply that they amount for me to nearly the same thing. Any worth-his-salt physician knows that no one is "cured." We recover from some somatic, some bodily "fever" where as observers we have seen various engagements between our battalions of cells playing at this or that lethal maneuver with other natural elements. It has been interesting. Various sewers or feed-mains have given way here or there under pressure: various new patterns have been thrown up for us upon the screen of our knowledge. But a cure is absurd, as absurd as calling these deployments "diseases." Sometimes the home team wins, sometimes the visitors. Great excitement. It is noteworthy that the sulfonamides, penicillin, came in about simultaneously with Ted Williams, Ralph Kiner and the rubber ball. We want home runs, antibiotics to "cure" man with a single shot in the buttocks.

But after you've knocked the ball into the center-field bleachers and won the game, you still have to go home to supper. So what? The ball park lies empty-eyed until the next game, the next season, the next bomb. Peanuts.

Medicine, as an art, never had much attraction for me, though it fascinated me, especially the physiology of the nervous system. That's something. Surgery always seemed to me particularly unsatisfying. What is there to cut off or out that will "cure" us? And to stand there for a lifetime sawing away! You'd better be a chef, if not a butcher. There is a joy in it, I realize, to know that you've really cut the cancer out and that the guy will come in to score, but I never wanted to be a surgeon. Marvelous men—I take off my hat to them. I knew one once who whenever he'd get into a malignant growth would take a hunk of it and rub it into his armpit afterward. Never knew why. It never hurt him, and he lived to a great old age. He had imagination, curiosity and a sense of humor, I suppose.

The cured man, I want to say, is no different from any other. It is a trivial business unless you add the zest, whatever that is, to the picture. That's how I came to find writing such a necessity, to relieve me from such a dilemma. I found by practice, by trial and error, that to treat a man as something to which surgery, drugs and hoodoo applied was an indifferent matter; to treat him as material for a work of art made him somehow come alive to me.

What I wanted to do with him (or her, or it) fascinated me. And it didn't make any difference, apparently, that he was in himself distinguished or otherwise. It wasn't that I wanted to save him because he was a good and useful member of society. Death had no respect for him and for that reason, neither does the artist, neither did I. As far as I can tell that kind of "use" doesn't enter into it; I am myself curious as to what I do find. The attraction is bizarre.

Thus I have said "the mind." And the mind? I can't say that I have ever been interested in a completely mindless person. But I have known one or two that are close to mindless, certainly useless, even fatal to their families, or what remains of their families, whom yet I find far more interesting than plenty of others whom I serve.

These are the matters which obsess me so that I cannot stop writing. I can recall many from the past, boys and girls, bad pupils, renegades, dirty-minded and -fisted, that I miss keenly. When some old woman tells me of her daughter now happily married to a handicapper at the Garden City track, that she has two fine sons, I want to sing and dance. I am happy. I am stimulated. She is still alive. Why should I feel that way? She almost caused me to flunk out of grammar school. I almost ruined my young days over her.

But I didn't. I love her, ignorant, fulsome bit of flesh that she was, and some other really vicious bits of childhood who ruined the record of the whole class—dead of their excesses, most of them. They flatter my memory. The thing, the thing, of which I am in chase. The thing I cannot quite name was there then. My writing, the necessity for a continued assertion, the need for me to go on will not let me stop. To this day I am in pursuit of it, actually—not there, in the academies, nor even in the pursuit of a remote and difficult knowledge or skill.

They had no knowledge and no skill at all. They flunked out, got jailed, got "Mamie" with child, and fell away, if they survived, from their perfections.

There again, a word: their perfections. They were perfect, they seem to have been born perfect, to need nothing else. They were there, living before me, and I lived beside them, associated with them. Their very presence denied the need of "study," that is study by degrees to elucidate them. They were, living, the theme that all my life I have labored to elucidate, and when I could not elucidate them I have tried to put them down, to lay them upon the paper to record them: for to do that is, after all, a sort of elucidation.

It isn't because they fascinated me by their evildoings that they were "bad" boys or girls. Not at all. It was because they were there full of a perfection of the longest leap, the most unmitigated daring, the longest chances.

This immediacy, the thing, as I went on writing, living as I could, thinking a secret life I wanted to tell openly—if only I could—how it lives, secretly about us as much now as ever. It is the history, the anatomy of this, not subject to surgery, plumbing or cures, that I wanted to tell. I don't know why. Why tell that which no one wants to hear? But I saw that when I was successful in portraying something, by accident, of that secret world of perfection, that they did want to listen. Definitely. And my "medicine" was the thing which gained me entrance to these secret gardens of the self. It lay there, another world, in the self. I was permitted by my medical badge to follow the poor, defeated body into those gulfs and grottos. And the astonishing thing is that as such times and such places—foul as they may be with the stinking ischio-rectal abscesses of our comings and goings—just there, the thing, in all its greatest beauty, may for a moment be freed to fly for a moment guiltily about the room. In illness, in the permission I as a physician have had to be present at deaths and births, at the tormented battles between daughter and diabolic mother, shattered by a gone brain —just there—for a split second—from one side or the other, it has fluttered before me for a moment, a phrase which I quickly write down on anything at hand, any piece of paper I can grab.

It is an identifiable thing, and its characteristic, its chief character is that it is sure, all of a piece and, as I have said, instant and perfect: it comes, it is there, and it vanishes. But I have seen it, clearly. I have seen it. I know it because there it is. I have been possessed by it just as I was in the fifth grade—when she leaned over the back of the seat before me and greeted me with some obscene remarks—which I cannot repeat even if made by a child forty years ago, because no one would or could understand what I am saying that then, there, it had appeared.

The great world never much interested me (except at the back of my head) since its effects, from what I observed, were so disastrously trivial—other than in their bulk; smelled the same as most public places. As Bob McAlmon said after the well-dressed Spanish woman passed us in Juarez (I had said, Wow! there's perfume for you!):

"You mean that?" he said. "That's not perfume, I just call that whores."

HANS ZINSSER
As I Remember Him

————◆◆◆————

Speaking of Dr. T. reminds me of a case in which I was credited with saving a life under peculiar circumstances. While still House Physician at the hospital, during Dr. T.'s visiting period, we had a poor fellow on the male ward who appeared to suffer from advanced nephritis. Dr. T., as I have remarked, was a virtuoso at compounding drugs. During his short annual reign of three months, the order sheets of every patient were covered with the red ink in which medication orders were entered. They got something or other "t.i.d." (three times a day), other things with meals, something else on waking up, another before the lights went out, and a few odd pills or injections "p.r.n." (*pro re nata*). Many of them had to be waked out of sound sleep to get one of his "black draughts" or "blue pills" or "brown decoctions"—all of them proudly originated by the Chief himself, and most of them quite complicated, with strong medicaments. The particular old boy of whom I write was getting a formidable sequence of daily doses and was slipping out of our hands—taking it patiently, with good humor and courage. We all liked him, and during his month on the ward he became a favorite. One night, when he was pretty low, I was making my midnight rounds with the ward nurse. We stopped at his bed and held a whispered conversation. He was in bad condition, the nurse said, and she didn't think he'd last long. She hated to force all that medicine down his throat. It bothered him and didn't seem to be doing him any good.

"All right," I said. "He's going to die soon anyway, and we'll stop all medication. Just leave the orders on the chart, and we'll steer the old boy around him as well as we can. Give him anything he wants to eat, within reason, and a shot of my Scotch when you come on at night. I'll bring you a bottle. He might as well die happy."

From that moment, our friend began to improve. Pretty soon, by respectful and adroit suggestion, I arranged to have official sanction for the omission of one pill and "draught" after another. In two weeks our patient began to sit up in bed for extraordinarily hearty meals. In three weeks he was up—his old self, he said. In four, he was out and I forgot about him.

The sequel came one Sunday afternoon during the following winter, when I was sitting in my office. The doorbell rang, and in walked a short, fat, ruddy man of about sixty, behind him a shorter, fatter, and ruddier boy of twenty or so. Neither of them did I recognize. Yet the older man stuck out his ham of a hand and said: "God bless you, doctor, how are you?" Then I suddenly remembered him. "I hope you're not sick again," I said.

"Oh, no, doctor! I'm fine. I just brought in my son" (who, apparently in the horse business, was embarrassedly rolling a flat-topped derby in one hand while he kept adjusting a white piqué tie with a horseshoe pin) "to show him the man who saved my life. You remember, doctor, that night in the hospital when I was nigh dead? You came around about midnight with the nurse. I was feelin' awful low, an' everybody thought I was goin' to die. I was thinkin' so my own self. You thought I was sleepin', but I wasn't. I was just pretendin'. You had a long talk with the nurse in front of my bed an' then you give her some orders. From that minute, I begun to mend.

"This is the man, my boy, as pulled your Pa out of the claws of the Reaper," he said poetically.